THE CELLULAR
wellness
SOLUTION

Tap Into Your Full Health Potential
with the **Science-Backed Power of Herbs**

BILL RAWLS, MD

FirstDoNoHarm
PUBLISHING

Printed in the United States of America

First Printing, 2022

ISBN: 978-0-9823225-6-7

FirstDoNoHarm Publishing
2409 Crabtree Blvd.
Suite 107
Raleigh, NC 27604

CellularWellness.com

Note to the reader:

Dr. Bill Rawls is the co-founder and Medical Director of Vital Plan, Inc., a holistic health and wellness company that offers herbal supplements, education, and support.

As the author of *The Cellular Wellness Solution*, Dr. Bill Rawls does not provide this material in his capacity as a licensed medical doctor. The information in this book should not be considered medical advice, diagnosis, treatment, or a substitute for the professional judgment of a qualified health care professional. All information provided in this book is solely for informational and educational purposes only. Your reliance upon any information provided in this book, including the use of any herbs, other botanicals, or other treatments, is solely at your own risk. Please consult a physician or other health care professional for advice regarding any medical condition or treatment thereof.

This book is dedicated to the many scientific researchers worldwide who have advanced our knowledge of the complex chemistry of herbs. Without their efforts, this book would not have been possible.

Contents

Part One
Unlocking Wellness

Part Two
Embracing Herbs

Part Three
Staying Well & Living Well

Part Four
Problem Solving

Foreword

By Joe & Terry Graedon

We have long been fascinated by natural approaches to healing. After all, Joe's grandfather was a pharmacist who practiced at the turn of the 20th century. Many of the medicines he dispensed were herbal products he had compounded. By the time we attended graduate school, however, botanical remedies had fallen out of favor in mainstream medicine. Instead, doctors embraced drugs developed by the pharmaceutical industry and marketed as the primary way to address disease or illness. Unfortunately, they don't always work as well as patients expect. Perhaps we need a new paradigm for enjoying optimal health.

Over the last 40 years, we have had the honor of interviewing hundreds of health experts on our nationally syndicated public radio program, *The People's Pharmacy*. Scientists who study diet and nutrition, infectious disease experts, exercise physiologists, microbiologists, ecologists, and those knowledgeable in herbal medicine have all offered us insights. We have learned a great deal about the microbiome and its relationship to health and disease. Hopefully, so have our listeners. The insights we have gleaned on chronic health conditions from Dr. Bill Rawls and other experts have been valuable.

Now, Dr. Rawls has integrated all of these fields into an accessible guide to using herbal medicines to achieve optimal health. He has pulled together all of the critical factors that lead to chronic illness with a focus we have not encountered elsewhere. Better yet, he tells readers how to prevent, avoid or treat those causes.

The discussion of intracellular infections you will read about helps explain how infectious agents cause so much confusion, controversy, and challenge. Dr. Rawls helps us understand how the interactions between our immune systems and the microbes we live with can contribute to chronic conditions. But he also describes how we can support cellular wellness with herbal medicines.

A lot of writers pay lip service to the idea of identifying the underlying causes of illness, but relatively few offer a path to achieving and maintaining wellness. Dr. Rawls' own experience as a patient as well as a healer informs his approach to overcoming chronic conditions such as those associated with Borrelia, Chlamydia, or Bartonella microbes. He knows well about the challenges and possibilities. Millions of people now suffering from long COVID pose a mystery to the medical profession, which has very little to offer them to aid recovery. Many of the principles that Dr. Rawls lays out in this book may have value for long haulers, although those studies are yet to be done.

The Cellular Wellness Solution is well-researched, supported by scientific evidence, and written clearly without jargon. While it will satisfy those who demand scientific underpinnings for recommendations, readers who have not studied chemistry, biology, or pharmacology will not find it too challenging. Each chapter concludes with a helpful summary of the points covered. Dr. Rawls' guidelines are straightforward, and he provides readers with the criteria to judge which everyday herbs or antimicrobial herbs might be most beneficial for their use. His argument for utilizing herbs "to cultivate wellness at the cellular level" is clear and his descriptions of the specific herbs he recommends are extremely helpful. We are confident that you will find *The Cellular Wellness Solution* to be a most valuable addition to your health library so that you, too, can chart a path to cellular wellness.

Joe & Terry Graedon
Hosts of the nationally syndicated public radio program,
The People's Pharmacy

Introduction

"The first wealth is health."
-Ralph Waldo Emerson
American philosopher, 1860

This well-known quote from Ralph Waldo Emerson is so powerful and true. Whether you are rich or poor, sick or in perfect health, the importance of wellness unifies us all. It is the foundation on which we build our lives and pursue our passions.

Good health is precious, perhaps more important than anything else in life. We all want to feel smarter about our health and empowered to make healthy decisions. Yet, wellness is surprisingly fragile and easily lost.

Reflexively, most people turn to the healthcare system to keep them well, but as a physician for over thirty years, I've come to appreciate that it's asking the system for more than it was designed for. Our healthcare system evolved to treat illness and injury, not to maintain wellness.

An Insider's Look at Health Care

I grew up in a medical family. Relatives in three generations before me devoted their lives to compassionately treating the sick. Both my maternal grandfather and my father were physicians, so no matter if I was at home or visiting my grandparents, conversation flowed about patients and diseases. As a child, I heard and reheard family lore of both triumphs and tragedies.

One oft-told story was about my great-grandfather, a horse-and-buggy doctor in the early 1900s. He raced out one night and saved a little girl's life by performing an emergency appendectomy on the family's kitchen table. He came home and died that same night of a heart condition assumed to be related to rheumatic heart disease (a heart condition that can occur after untreated strep throat or scarlet fever). Sadly, those were infections for which the medical system of that time had nothing to offer.

A generation later, my grandfather served as a general practitioner in a small North Carolina town. When I became old enough, I sometimes got to tag along with Granddad when he went on house calls. Tucked into his black bag were surgical tools to alleviate a range of acute maladies, such as boils, lacerations, and broken limbs. When childbirth was stalled, he had forceps to assist the delivery. His black bag also held pills and injectable drugs to ease the pain of injury and childbirth. Among those vials, he carried a new weapon against illness that my great-grandfather didn't have: penicillin. That gave my grandfather the ability to treat strep throat, which could have prevented the rheumatic heart disease that had likely taken his father's life.

For chronic illnesses, however, Granddad didn't have much to offer. On those home visits, I remember meeting some people who were "sickly" with some unidentified chronic illness, but there wasn't much in the black bag for them. Of course, my grandfather would offer compassion and any medications he had to ease the symptoms, but nothing that was curative.

My father entered the medical profession in the late 1960s. It was a time that many consider to be the heyday of modern medicine. Synthetic antibiotics and new vaccines had dramatically lessened the risk of the life-threatening infectious diseases that had plagued humankind for centuries (at least in developed countries that could afford these new cures). An ongoing explosion of new drug therapies and surgical technologies offered novel options for ailments once considered untreatable, such as epilepsy and mental illnesses. But it also came with a false sense of security that the medical system could cure all diseases.

By the time I was in medical training in the 1980s, the world was changing. Despite all the medical advances of the twentieth century, the incidences of chronic illnesses, such as heart disease, diabetes, autoimmune disease, and cancer, were rising steadily. Chronic illness remained an enigma for which medical science didn't have good answers (and still doesn't). People who become chronically ill typically never get well and require medical therapy for the remainder of their lives; yet, each year they become sicker and more dependent on the medical system.

It was one of the factors that led me to specialize in obstetrics and gynecology (Ob-Gyn). Of all the medical specialties, Ob-Gyn had the least involvement with long-term management of chronic illness. Most of the patients were young and healthy. When patients did become ill, the treatments were straightforward, and the patients typically got well. Besides that, nothing quite matched the feeling of bringing a baby into the world!

A long career practicing Ob-Gyn wasn't to be, however. Fate had other ideas for me. Right at the peak of my career, my life was completely disrupted by what I feared most: a personal encounter with chronic illness.

Realizing Limitations of the Healthcare System

I wasn't alone in that experience. In 2005, around the time of my struggle, the Centers for Disease Control and Prevention (CDC) stated that 44% of the American population was stricken with some type of incurable chronic illness requiring ongoing medical management. As of 2020, that figure had risen beyond the 50% mark.

Of course, no one intends to become ill. You may be fifty and feeling just fine, but statistics say that as you age—and we all want to live longer—you're likely to tack on a diagnosis or two. In fact, by age 65, well over 80% of the population takes at least one prescription drug, and half of those people take more than four prescriptions. In the modern world, getting older has become synonymous with taking medications and becoming dependent on the medical system.

Management of chronic illness is quite costly. Ninety percent of our health care budget goes to treat the chronically ill. Shockingly, the U.S. spends more on health care than any country on earth, yet we rank poorly compared to other developed countries in terms of wellness and life expectancy.

Even more alarming is the fact that drugs appear to be part of the problem. In an article published in 2013 by Harvard's Center for Ethics, Donald W. Light, Ph.D. related that properly prescribed drugs account for about 1.9 million hospitalizations per year and 128,000 deaths per year.[1] That makes drug therapy the fourth leading cause of death in the United States.

---

1   Light DW. New Prescription Drugs: A Major Health Risk With Few Offsetting Advantages. June 27, 2014. https://ethics.harvard.edu/blog/new-prescription-drugs-major-health-risk-few-offsetting-advantages. Accessed February 25, 2022.
Light DW, Lexchin J, Darrow JJ. Institutional corruption of pharmaceuticals and the myth of safe and effective drugs. *J Law Med Ethics*. 2013;14(3):590-610.

Losing my own health put me in an odd position. Being an insider, I knew how the medical system worked. If I chose to stay loyal to my medical roots, I could foresee living in a compromised state and becoming dependent on the medical system for the rest of my life. My medical expenses would go up every year, yet my health was sure to worsen.

Charting a Pathway to Wellness

Instead, I chose to search for a different pathway. It wasn't easy; it required rethinking everything I had learned and opening up to possibilities beyond conventional medical therapies. Ultimately, that allowed me to do something that few people struggling with chronic illness are ever able to do: *I regained wellness.*

My search led me to explore wellness down to the cellular level. The human body is a complex collection of living cells. If you feel well, it's because your cells are healthy and fully functional. However, the opposite is true if you're chronically ill. As such, the key to staying well at any age is keeping your cells healthy.

In that regard, the most surprising discovery of my journey was herbal therapy. Whereas drugs had held my illness in place, herbs were a key factor in boosting my health beyond chronic illness and back to wellness. After such a remarkable experience, I became intrigued: How could herbs have made such a difference? Searching for and ultimately finding the answers changed my life and career forever.

Recovering my health enabled me to start a new chapter in my career as a physician. Applying the same principles that I used in my recovery, I've been able to help thousands of people recapture wellness. Importantly, it always centers around empowering people to be proactive about their own health.

The experience of helping others served as the foundation for writing this book. The pathway detailed in these pages provides everything you need to unlock your full potential for wellness. Whether you're struggling with chronic symptoms or just wanting to live free of symptoms as you age, you can benefit. The information applies to any age and any level of health.

I consider herbs to be a critical part of the health equation. No matter what you've thought about herbs before, I invite you to consider them with an open mind. Though humans have been using herbs for thousands of years, it's only been within the past few decades that scientists have started unraveling how they actually work. What they've found provides an important key to achieving wellness at the cellular level. It is this new way of thinking about herbs that I want to share with you.

In regards to our society's approach to health and healthcare, we're due for a paradigm shift. The healthcare system offers a lot of good that shouldn't be ignored. Routine screening for diseases at an early stage, such as colon cancer, has saved millions of lives. In early stages of illness, medical therapies can be very important for reducing symptoms and stabilizing progression of illness. And we would all be at a loss without modern anesthesia and innovative surgical technologies. **Medical therapies, however, have little capacity to prevent illness from happening or restore wellness once it's lost.**

That part is up to us. We each have a responsibility to take care of our own health. When people become proactive about their health, reliance on the healthcare system typically lessens. If we do this as a society, the system is allowed to function as it was originally intended—to be there for things we can't control or predict. All it takes is enough people making simple changes to have an impact. My goal with this book is to provide a pathway that makes it possible.

Getting the Best Use of This Book

This book will provide the information you need to take charge of your health. This isn't the kind of information you'll typically find in a doctor's office. It's about cultivating wellness as opposed to treating illness.

The book is divided into four primary parts, for easy use:

PART ONE: Unlocking Wellness

In the first three chapters, you'll learn an elegantly simple model for understanding why chronic illnesses (including cancers) occur and what you can do to avoid those outcomes as you age. At the core of this explanation is an understanding of wellness at the cellular level and the surprising role that microbes play in accelerating illness and aging. We will then explore the crucial role that plant chemicals play in protecting health at the cellular level and why our modern lifestyles are missing this key protection.

PART TWO: Embracing Herbs

This section provides everything you need to know to make herbs part of your life. I'll teach you the science behind herbal therapy and what matters regarding safety and efficacy. This section will serve as your complete guide to understanding herbs and getting started.

PART THREE: Staying Well & Living Well

This section of this book presents the lifestyle model that I follow myself and have used with patients for many years. In these chapters, I detail health habits that set the foundation for vibrant health. My goal with this section of the book is to present simple lifestyle practices that you can immediately begin incorporating into your life. The plan presented in this section is customizable and is not an 'all or nothing' approach. I encourage you to take what works for you. Even small changes can make a big difference, and often that's the approach that sticks long term.

PART FOUR: Problem Solving

This last section of the book offers targeted guidance for specific health areas, such as cardiovascular health or joint support. It includes recommendations for additional supplement and lifestyle support that can be layered on top of the foundational plan recommended in Parts 2 and 3. I invite you to skip around this section to find the topics that are most pertinent to you.

Change starts with you. No matter your current health status, you can always reach for and gain a higher level of health. This book is designed to empower you to make the simple changes necessary to ensure lasting wellness throughout your life.

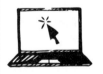

For additional tools, charts, and other resources to print, share, and reference the health approaches covered in this book, visit **CellularWellness.com/Extras**

Part One

Unlocking Wellness

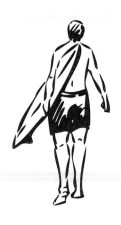

In the first part of this four-part book, we'll explore the concepts that define cellular wellness. You'll get an idea of where you are along the wellness-illness continuum and how the choices you make as you go through life impact your risk of developing disease. You'll also learn the powerful, science-based ways that plants and, specifically, herbs can offer protection for our health. But unlike me, you don't have to wait until a health crisis happens to reap the benefits. These concepts are the foundation for staying well throughout your life.

Here's what you'll learn in Part One:

- The spectrum between wellness and illness

- What your symptoms say about the health of your cells

- Five stress factors that set the stage for chronic illness and cancer

- The role that microbes play in illness

- Aging and its impact on wellness

- How herbs are your pathway to wellness

- The powerhouse properties of plant phytochemicals

- How phytochemicals have gone missing from food plants

1

From Health Crisis to Life-Changing Discovery

L *ying on the beach with my chest heaving and struggling to catch my breath, I wondered if my life was about to end. I was only forty-seven.*

It had been a classic summer day on the North Carolina coast with perfect waves for surfing. I'd been struggling with health issues and knew my body wasn't up to it, but I just had to get out there. Vigorous exercise, preferably out on the water, had always been how I dealt with stress. After riding only a couple waves, however, my heart was beating so erratically and my body ached so intensely, that I had to make my way back to the beach. After reaching the shore, I flopped down on the sand to recover.

Looking back on how I came to that moment of crisis, I can see that it had been building for years.

When I was in my thirties, I could get away with not sleeping, eating on the run, and working under stress. Juggling a busy job, raising a family, and making the most out of every hour I wasn't working, I thought I could do it all. I prided myself in my ability to bounce back after being up all night delivering babies. But being an obstetrician-gynecologist (Ob-Gyn) came with a tremendous amount of stress and a rigorous night-call schedule that left me sleep deprived much of the time.

As I moved beyond my thirties, my ability to bounce back began to fade.

Symptoms had started creeping in—reflux, weight gain, mild joint discomfort, loss of stamina—but life was too busy to do anything about it. As long as over-the-counter medications eased the discomfort, I kept right on pushing through.

I think most people can relate to this scenario. We all experience symptoms. But, as long as they don't interfere with normal life, we tend to be complacent about them. After all, dealing with symptoms is sometimes more inconvenient and more uncomfortable than putting up with them. So, I put up with them—but the symptoms kept accumulating.

When routine checkups at my doctor's office showed that my blood pressure was going up, along with my cholesterol and blood sugar, I couldn't ignore that my health was changing. My doctor prescribed medications to control these issues. However, there was no discussion about what might be causing these abnormalities or if they could be reversed. In our society, accumulating chronic symptoms is accepted as a normal part of aging.

Had I known then what I know now, I might have made simple adjustments that would have saved me a lot of misery. However, I hadn't been trained to think that way. Medical school specifically prepared me to diagnose and treat established illness. There was little emphasis on prevention of illness and even less on restoring wellness.

As I entered my mid-forties, my health kept slipping. I started having days where I woke up feeling like I had the flu. Life became dominated by working around chronic body aches, fatigue, brain fog, heart palpitations, and intestinal dysfunction. My stamina was at rock bottom. My knees and hips sometimes hurt so badly that it was uncomfortable to walk. Worst of all, I had lost the ability to sleep normally. Gradually, my condition deteriorated to the point that I couldn't take night call. It became hard to plan for the future because I wasn't sure what my health would be like.

Visits to doctor's offices became like a revolving door. My internist ran the appropriate tests and diagnostic protocols, but they were all negative. The only exception was that my thyroid function was slightly off, but taking thyroid hormone replacement did nothing to improve my symptoms. Referrals to various specialists also failed to turn up a reason for my malaise. All they had to offer were more tests, followed by more prescriptions.

That day on the beach, everything came to a head. Once I caught my breath, I composed myself enough to drive to the emergency room. There, an EKG showed mild ischemia, a condition in which the heart muscle was being deprived of oxygen. But, it was chronic, not acute. In other words, I wasn't having a heart attack. My doctor arranged a consultation with a cardiologist, who scheduled a cardiac catheterization. That procedure showed that my coronary vessels were clear. The doctor had no explanation for why my heart was beating so erratically or why I was having chest pain. All he had to offer was a prescription for a medication to block the abnormal heartbeats—another prescription to add to my growing list.

For several years after that, I remained trapped—dependent on the medical system, but not being helped by it either.

Being an insider in the medical profession, I knew my experience wasn't unique. A large portion of people who are chronically ill remain undiagnosed. In other words, they don't check all the boxes for any specific diagnosis. It's because symptoms of different chronic illnesses tend to overlap, and lab tests aren't always reliable or specific. This leaves patients in a situation of endlessly searching for the "right" diagnosis. It's a real handicap in the healthcare system—without a firm diagnosis, patients remain untreated.

Even when a definitive diagnosis is made, the capacity of the medical system to restore someone struggling with chronic illness back to normal health is often limited. For most chronic illnesses, medical therapies have the capacity to artificially inhibit dysfunctional processes associated with the illness, but little more. While this can reduce symptoms and slow progression of the illness, the chances of the patient being restored to a normal state of wellness are small. The most a patient can hope for is a never-ending state of chronic illness managed with drug therapy. As the body continues to break down with advancing age, an ever-deepening state of dependence on medical therapies is inevitable

A unique exception where cures for chronic illnesses routinely happen is with cancer therapy. Due to modern innovations in cancer therapy, the death rate for all cancers has dropped significantly in the past several decades. The problem is that little has been done to prevent cancer, and more people are getting cancer than ever before. And despite being given the "all clear," anyone who has had cancer knows that the risk of recurrence or new cancers popping up is always there.

Searching for Answers

Being trapped in a state of managed illness wasn't how I wanted to spend the rest of my life. Somehow, I knew there must be a solution, and I was determined to find it. My goal was regaining wellness. Yet, to move forward, I had to define exactly what that meant.

For most of us, wellness is about being able to interact with other people, work, travel, have relationships, pursue passions, and remain productive. The definition also includes enjoying mental clarity and sharpness, not being limited by pain or physical restrictions, maintaining general contentment and happiness, and being able to care for yourself, especially with advancing age.

From a medical standpoint, wellness is mostly about minimizing symptoms. However, as I found out, that's more about treating illness than restoring wellness. The two aren't necessarily one and the same.

Wellness and illness are mirror opposites of one another. The area between the two, however, isn't distinct. It's more like a continuum. At one end of the spectrum, you might find a twenty-year-old athlete in top condition. At the other end might be a person in a desperate struggle with an autoimmune illness or cancer. Most of us fall somewhere in between and gradually move through life from the wellness end of the spectrum to the illness end.

I've been at both ends of the spectrum, both personally and professionally. The first half of my career was focused on treating illness, primarily with drugs and surgery. Although I was able to help a lot of people and I'm proud of my work during that phase, retrospectively, there was very little emphasis on preventing illness from happening. Problems weren't addressed until they occurred. Ironically, the demands of my career promoted a lifestyle that was anything but healthful. Thus, while I was dutifully "stamping out illness," I became ill myself. I joined the millions of Americans whose lives are compromised by chronic illness.

That phase of my career ended when my condition deteriorated to the point of not being able to take night call. That left me with no choice but to give up my position in the Ob-Gyn practice group I was in. Phase two of my career started when I opened a solo practice in gynecology and primary care. Not having the burden of obstetrics call gave me the freedom I needed to work on improving my health. Little did I know how much my life and career would change in the years that followed.

The Wellness Spectrum

I knew there must be a way to break free from being ill and regain wellness, but I wasn't getting there with anything my conventional training had to offer. It was time to go back to the drawing board—literally. I took out a sheet of 8 ½ x 11 paper and turned it sideways. On the left side of the paper, I wrote the word, WELLNESS. On the right side, I wrote the word, ILLNESS. I drew two straight lines in parallel across the middle of the page, one with an arrow at the end pointing toward wellness and the other with an arrow pointing toward illness. At the top of the page, I wrote: Factors that Promote Wellness. At the bottom I wrote: Factors that Promote Illness.

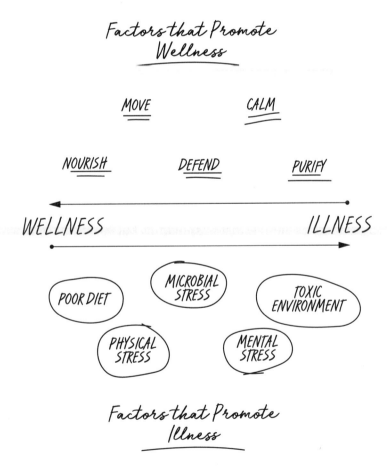

Over subsequent months and years of intense research and study, I filled that paper full of information. It became my roadmap to wellness. It also gave me hope because it provided an alternative to simply suppressing symptoms with drugs.

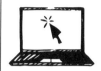 **Create your own roadmap to wellness:** for a printable, blank version of the Wellness Spectrum chart that you fill in yourself, visit **CellularWellness.com/Extras**

Recognizing the Factors that Promote Illness

Everything in the universe results from cause and effect, including all types of illness. Even cancer results from causes that are finite and quantifiable. If you can identify the underlying causes of an event, then you can either prevent it from ever happening or help it to resolve if it has already occurred.

In all, it sifts down to five categories of stress factors that have been recognized by science as having the capacity to promote chronic illness and cancer. These factors come together to create the physical manifestations we experience as symptoms. The five categories are (1) poor diet, (2) toxic environment, (3) mental stress, (4) physical stress, and (5) microbial stress. I listed the categories across the bottom of my Wellness—Illness worksheet and took personal stock of how each might have contributed to my situation.

Poor Diet

Some of my health stressors were obvious. Poor food choices had not only contributed to my expanding midsection, but also elevated blood sugar and cholesterol. The fact that one-third of the American population is defined as obese is directly tied to poor dietary choices. Poor food choices are a primary contributor to high rates of diabetes and heart disease, but also set the stage for many other illnesses.

My meal plan needed some immediate changes. I started by cutting out products made with flour and sugar. I shifted to eating whole foods and made a pledge to eat more vegetables than anything else—every day, no exceptions. These simple changes allowed me to drop thirty pounds over a couple years and get back down to a healthy weight.

Toxic Environment

I was also aware that we're all affected by low-grade exposure to toxic substances. Air pollution, both outside and indoors, and toxic substances present in food and water have all been identified as contributors to chronic respiratory conditions, cardiovascular illnesses, autoimmune diseases, and a range of other chronic conditions. Although I didn't smoke and had all but given up alcohol, I wanted to reduce my exposure to toxic substances as much as possible. I installed a water filter at home, stopped drinking water from plastic bottles, purchased organic food whenever it was practical, and placed air filters in my office and house.

Mental Stress

Chronic mental stress is a well-recognized contributor to all major illnesses. It was the biggest contributor to my chronic condition. There weren't many hours in a day when I wasn't mentally overstimulated, and I spent too many hours awake. Chronic stress also disrupts sleep. But, in my case, I hadn't allowed time for adequate sleep. Wellness just isn't possible without seven to eight hours of sleep every night.

Twenty years of sleep deprivation had left me with brittle sleep. I had to train my body to sleep again. Not being burdened with night call was a step in the right direction. I learned to control my sleep environment (along with my caffeine intake), forced myself to turn off lighted screens by 9 p.m., and made a habit of being in bed by 10:30 every night. These changes were something I had never done before. Gradually, sleep improved, but it took constant effort.

Physical Stress

Physical factors, such as trauma or excessive physical strain, have an obvious detrimental effect on the body, but being sedentary is destructive in a different way. The body is designed to move and when regular movement doesn't occur, everything in the body stagnates.

I not only enjoyed being physically active, but it was also my primary way to relieve stress. Losing the capacity to do high-intensity exercise, such as windsurfing and surfing, was a real blow. I had to be satisfied with walking. I became a regular at a state park trail. At first, I could only walk half a mile before hitting a wall of fatigue. Some days were better than others. Over time, I worked my way up to greater distances. I also started attending yoga classes a couple times a week. It would take several years to get back up to normal capacity for my age.

Microbial Stress

Regarding the last category, I understood that infections with bacteria, viruses, and other microbes have always played a major role in human suffering. At the time, however, I hadn't defined an infection as contributing to my declining health. Even though I experienced "flu-like" symptoms every day, my tests for mononucleosis and Lyme disease had been negative. And doctors assured me that my illness wasn't from an infection. The fact that my symptoms didn't go away seemed to support this. I always assumed that infections are transient. Given time, the body would naturally recover from it.

Changing my health habits was beneficial, but it was hard to be consistent and keep up with regular life. The stress of running a busy solo medical practice could sometimes be unrelenting. Though my sleep habits had improved, my ability to sleep still wasn't perfect. Even so, my efforts were enough to allow me to make it through the workday and enjoy low-intensity physical activity such as kayaking and hiking again. By the middle of the afternoon, however, my energy would run dry. And I was still struggling with irregular heartbeats, joint and muscle aches, and more.

Something was holding my symptoms in place, but I just couldn't quite put my finger on what it was.

New Clues

Life went on like this for several years until a retest suggested that I was carrying the bacteria that caused Lyme disease. For a short while, I thought I'd found the reason for my misery—finally, a treatable diagnosis! But after multiple rounds of antibiotics made me worse instead of better, the possibility of Lyme disease generated more questions than answers.

The fact that my symptoms didn't respond to antibiotics made me question the Lyme disease diagnosis altogether. When Lyme disease becomes chronic, both false positive and false negative tests for the bacteria are not uncommon. Which had mine been? Not only that, the conventional medical community doesn't even recognize chronic Lyme disease as a diagnosis. Infectious disease experts maintain that the recommended two-week course of antibiotics always eradicates the bacteria from the body, and any symptoms that persist aren't associated with Lyme disease.

Ultimately, I would uncover evidence that proved this assumption to be false. Numerous case reports and clinical studies published in scientific journals have confirmed that Borrelia, the bacteria associated with Lyme disease, can persist in the body despite prolonged antibiotic therapy, along with chronic symptoms. Not only that, I found that Borrelia was one of many possibilities. Most people identifying with the chronic form of Lyme disease are found to be harboring a variety of different bacteria along with Borrelia. What's more, any of those bacteria can cause all the symptoms I was having without Borrelia even being present.

Fast-forward a decade, and I've uncovered quite a number of different microbes—including viruses, bacteria, and protozoa—that can cause chronic symptoms similar to the ones I was having. These microbes have also been linked to a wide variety of chronic illnesses. At that particular point in time, however, all I cared about was getting my life and health back. Like most people who identify with chronic Lyme disease, I didn't know which microbe might be causing my illness or have absolute proof that it was a microbe at all. But one thing was for sure: I was tired of feeling miserable and needed to do something about it—ASAP.

Discovering Herbs

While still sorting my situation out and wondering whether I did or didn't have Lyme disease, I happened upon an herbal protocol created by an herbalist named Stephen Buhner. Other people had successfully used his treatment protocol to overcome the chronic manifestations of Lyme disease. By then, I had exhausted all options and was willing to try almost anything.

The protocol consisted of multiple herbs. But, instead of the average supplements or teas that you might find at a grocery store, the recommendations were for high-grade standardized extracts of specific herbs with documented antimicrobial properties.

I pieced together the regimen from niche retailers. Many of the herbs felt exotic to me at the time, given my limited exposure to herbs. The primary Lyme treatment herbs had names like Japanese knotweed, andrographis, cat's claw, garlic extract, Chinese skullcap, cordyceps, and reishi mushrooms.

My decision wasn't a leap of faith. I was encouraged by the science presented by Buhner and the fact that thousands of people had reported significant benefit from the protocol. However, I did my own research verifying the safety and efficacy of the different herbs.

Even so, I'll have to admit that I didn't have high expectations. My medical training had left me with the biased opinion that herbs were just weak versions of drugs that offered little in the way of therapeutic value. But I didn't see any better options, so I gave the herbs a chance.

Little did I know how much this simple decision would forever change my life and my career pathway as a physician.

I remember the day the herbs arrived. There were almost a dozen bottles from a pieced-together collection of brands. Over a week or two, I worked up to taking several capsules from each bottle—a handful of capsules collectively—twice a day. (My wife thought I had lost my mind.) Being very sensitive to drugs, I expected side effects, but none ever occurred. This included the absence of any gastrointestinal side effects, which had always been a problem when I took antibiotics. In fact, the longer I took the herbs, the more my gut function improved!

Change was slow and subtle. It took several weeks before I noticed any benefit at all. By the time three months had passed, however, I was at least fifty percent improved. The achiness in my joints had subsided. Remarkably, I was able to sleep normally again. My brain fog had cleared. And, best of all, I still had energy at the end of the day. The herbs were working!

Once I started feeling better, I would occasionally forget to order more herbs, and they would eventually run out. I would be fine for a while, but with the first bit of stress, the symptoms would flare up again. Then, I would go back on the herbs, and, like before, the symptoms would subside. It went back and forth like this for several years until I decided just to continue taking the herbs indefinitely. I wasn't having any side effects. And I sure felt better whenever I was taking them.

That's when I noticed something truly extraordinary. For every year that I was on the herbs, my health got steadily better. Eventually, I got back everything I had lost—and then some.

Stamina improved. Gut function returned to normal. Joint discomfort resolved, along with that annoying crunch in my knees. Even some of my more stubborn symptoms—the burning in my feet and irregular heartbeats—gradually resolved. As my mental functions sharpened, my mood became brighter and more positive. By the time I reached my mid-fifties, my health was finally back to what I considered normal.

The benefits provided by the herbs exceeded all my expectations. It was obvious they were doing much more than just eliminating microbes. Beyond clearing the symptoms that I had associated with Lyme disease, I was dumbfounded to witness my blood pressure, cholesterol, and blood sugar levels normalizing, too. My skin even felt better. The benefits provided by the herbs were truly remarkable.

A New Life and a New Passion

More than fifteen years have elapsed since that day on the beach. Despite the fact that I've aged, I've been able to achieve and retain good health. Gratefully, my life is no longer restricted by symptoms. In fact, I have fewer symptoms now than I did in my thirties and forties. What's more, I have plenty of energy to pursue passions and maintain purpose in life.

I give herbs credit for that. Although I don't take the quantities of herbs that I did during my recovery, I still take a basic regimen every day. It's enough to prevent me from sliding back to where I was. To give them the attention they deserve, I wrote the word, HERBS, at a central place in my wellness diagram.

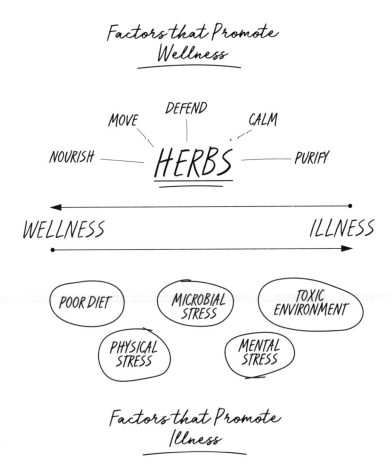

Beyond providing my personal pathway to wellness, the diagram became my guide for practicing medicine. As my recovery progressed, my practice gradually shifted from primary care and gynecology to helping people overcome chronic health conditions that don't respond to conventional medical therapies. Instead of using drugs to treat symptoms, I show people how to rebuild wellness into their lives. The healing power of herbs is central to that pathway. With time, I found that these same principles could be applied to any health condition—including maintaining wellness as you age.

Chapter Highlights

- Life is a continuum between wellness and illness.

- Medical therapies are valuable for reducing symptoms and slowing disease progression, but for chronic illness they have low capacity to actually restore wellness.

- Aging is a reality but it need not be accompanied by chronic disease.

- The key to maintaining or restoring wellness entails addressing the underlying causes of illness.

- Herbs work differently than drugs and do things that drugs can't do.

2

Understanding Symptoms at the Cellular Level

My current job involves doing consultations to help people overcome various kinds of health challenges. It's a real bright spot in my life. Because of my unique health experiences, I can often see what other health care providers can't. I talk to people all over the country and sometimes from around the world. Often they've had extensive evaluations at major medical centers, only to come away without a firm diagnosis or a clear pathway to wellness. Many of them have been searching for years.

I sift through the person's health history looking for clues to their health issues. My approach is very different from what you might find in a conventional doctor's office. Instead of trying to issue a diagnosis, I focus my efforts on determining how the person's health issues evolved. Once the underlying causes are sorted out, I can often put that person on a clear pathway to wellness. The healing power of herbs is central to that pathway.

I see people with a wide range of health conditions. That includes everything from people struggling with chronic illnesses to people who don't consider themselves ill at all. I've worked with professional athletes who wanted to up their game or stay active longer as they age. People who are healthy and want to stay that way as they age routinely seek my advice. The earlier I can catch someone before they start having significant symptoms, the easier it is to keep them well (reader, take notice).

Anne, a fifty-seven-year-old woman who I worked with recently, had developed a series of seemingly unrelated symptoms. She had always considered herself a healthy person, but as of late, she had become easily stressed and often didn't sleep well at night. Her energy level wasn't what it once was, and she wasn't able to think as clearly as she once did. That sometimes made doing her job as an accountant challenging.

A significant part of her story was that her father had died of Parkinson's disease with associated dementia about five years prior. Up until his death, Anne had been his primary caregiver. Caring for her father while maintaining a full-time job as a CPA, had come with an extreme amount of mental and emotional stress. Her one outlet was running, and she ran a few miles every day. About a year before her father died, she slipped on an ice patch after a late spring freeze and broke her arm. She needed surgery to put in a temporary pin to hold the bone in place. The wound became infected, and she was put on antibiotics for six weeks.

For years, it had been one unanticipated stress on top of another. And though her stress had leveled off, she hadn't been able to get back on her feet. Despite the fact that her arm had healed completely, she started having pain in her joints, especially her knees. That made running difficult. Also, her gut was never quite the same after the antibiotics. Symptoms of gas and bloating and occasional constipation had become chronic. Although she tried to eat a healthy diet and was taking a probiotic, the symptoms were persistent.

Her primary care provider had reassured her that these were normal signs of aging, and perhaps lingering symptoms of menopause that she had gone through several years prior. Tests were run, but other than a mildly elevated cholesterol level (it had always been normal before), nothing came up of concern. Her only other significant finding was mildly elevated blood pressure, but that was attributed to stress. She was referred to a neurologist, but that doctor found no evidence of Parkinson's disease or dementia (much to her relief). Each of the doctors issued prescriptions to ease her various symptoms, but that was the limit of what they had to offer.

Although nobody wants to have symptoms, most people intuitively know that just suppressing symptoms with drug therapy isn't necessarily addressing the underlying problem. Drugs simply mask the symptoms along with the illness lurking within. In fact, drug therapy often interrupts the healing process that would allow the symptoms to resolve naturally. Instead of getting well, the patient lives with illness masked by medications.

Anne was looking for more. She wanted to be well again.

Defining Symptoms

While symptoms are often thought of as unpleasant sensations that need to be eliminated or suppressed, they are actually *telling you something*.

Symptoms define where you are along The Wellness Spectrum. The greater the symptoms, the closer you are to the illness end of the spectrum. In contrast, you know your health is improving when symptoms are resolving. Spontaneous resolution of symptoms is the most definitive sign of healing.

On a deeper level, what symptoms are telling you is that cells in your body are stressed or injured.

Although we tend to think of the body as a whole, it's actually a complex, interconnected collection of cells. Depending on your age, your body contains anywhere from 20 to 40 trillion cells.[2] All of your tissues and organs are made of cells. Absolutely everything that happens inside your body results from the actions of cells. Whether it's your heart beating or brain impulses firing, it's done by individual cells working in synchrony with other cells. In total, there are over 200 different cell types required to keep your body humming along.

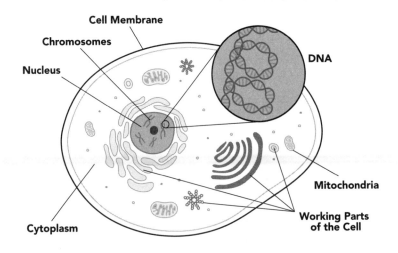

If all the cells in your body are healthy and functioning in synchrony, then your energy will be good, you'll feel calm and focused, and symptoms will not be present. Symptoms *only* occur when cells in

2   Bianconi E, Piovesan A, Facchin F, et al. An estimation of the number of cells in the human body. *Ann Hum Biol.* 2013;40(6):463-471.

the body are stressed or injured. Because there are many types of cells in the body, and cells can be stressed in different ways, a wide variety of symptoms are possible.

Taking symptoms down to the cellular level was the ah-ha moment that changed my perspective forever. It provides an elegantly simple model for understanding illness—and how to avoid it. Symptoms point to the cells in the body that are stressed or injured and indicate the degree of injury. It's often a more sensitive indicator of an internal problem than labs or diagnostic tests. You just have to pay attention to what the body is saying.

When cells become injured or stressed, two things happen:

- Injured cells release chemical substances that activate nerves and send an "SOS" signal to your brain. If enough cells are stressed or damaged, your brain registers it as a nagging or unpleasant sensation that you feel as a symptom. In other words, your cells are trying to get your brain's attention. The intensity of a symptom is a reflection of the number of cells being affected—the greater the number of cells that are stressed or injured, the more intense the discomfort.

- More significantly, when cells are stressed or injured, they can't do their jobs—those functions are lost or become dysfunctional. Because all the cells in the body are networked together and depend on each other, loss of function in one group of cells can affect other cells, sending a ripple effect throughout the entire body.

To illustrate, if you misstep and twist your ankle, cells in the ankle joint and supporting ligaments have been injured. You know about it immediately: when those injured cells activate nerves, you feel it as pain at the injury site. Because that function has been compromised, the pain forces you to favor that ankle every time you try to put weight on it. The degree of cellular injury defines the level of disability.

Of course, some cells in the body are more essential than others. A twisted ankle might put you on crutches for a while, but the injury doesn't directly affect other cells in the body. A similar degree of injury to heart muscle cells, however, can be catastrophic because all the cells in the body depend on the heart pumping blood.

Healing at the Cellular Level

If you pamper a sprained ankle for a while, it will heal, and you'll be able to walk on it normally again. "Healing" is another one of those things that we know conceptually, but have a hard time defining. Again, thinking at the cellular level gives you the answer. Specifically, healing is the ability of cells to recover from stress or injury.

One of the most remarkable features of our cells is the ability to continually repair internal damage caused by wear and tear. Even when stress or injury causes excessive wear and tear, as long as the stress isn't ongoing or the injury isn't catastrophic, a cell can recover and return to its normal functional capacity. In the case of cells being mortally wounded, other cells can regenerate into new cells to replace those that went missing.

The collective ability of cells in the body to repair and regenerate defines the remarkable healing capacity of the human body.

Of course, some cells in the body have greater regenerative capacity than others. Skin and intestinal cells are constantly being shed and have a high capacity to regenerate. Liver cells have a medium capacity for regeneration. Muscle cells have a low capacity to regenerate. An injury to muscles or ligaments can take months to heal completely. Heart muscle is especially slow to heal because the heart never stops beating. The only downtime that heart cells get is between beats. Nerve cells have the lowest capacity to regenerate of any cell in the body. A major brain or spinal cord injury exceeds the capacity of nerve tissue to regenerate. This is why protecting your head with a well-designed helmet is really important if you enjoy activities such as skiing, biking, or playing contact sports.

The healing capacity of the human body is affected by aging. Aging is marked by the gradual loss of functional cells over time. Because healing is a cellular process, fewer functional cells lowers the body's capacity for healing. It is why recovery from injury or illness is much slower in older adults.

The Inflammatory Response vs. Chronic Inflammation

The immune system plays a key role in the healing process. When you twist an ankle, cells that are mortally injured die and break apart. This creates debris that congests the spaces around living cells, which inhibits the flow of the water, oxygen, and nutrients that surviving cells need to survive. As long as congestion is present, cellular healing is compromised.

To clean up the mess, the immune system sends in specialized white blood cells called *macrophages*. Macrophages are the garbage collectors of the immune system. They scoop up the debris from dead and dying cells, break it down with potent acid and free radicals, and haul it away. Macrophages and other immune cells also kill any microbes that may have invaded the area. This essential part of the healing process is called the *inflammatory response*.

When illness becomes chronic, cells throughout the body are stressed. Stressed cells die off faster. This creates debris that accumulates faster than macrophages can clear it. Tissues become a toxic stew of dead cells and debris, a state called *chronic inflammation*. You feel it as joint discomfort, stiffness, general achiness, fatigue, low stamina, brain fog, slow mental activity, depressed mood, and intolerance to any type of stress. Simply put, you feel "inflamed".

Many drugs used for chronic illness, including steroids and newer targeted immune-blocking drugs (such as Humira) target chronic inflammation by blocking the ability of the immune system to mount an inflammatory response. While this can reduce the destructive effects of inflammation, it also compromises the body's ability to heal itself. Quite simply, the inflammatory response is an essential part of healing. Although short-term use of anti-inflammatory drugs can be highly beneficial, chronic use of inflammation-blocking drugs inhibits healing.

When Symptoms Become Chronic

Cells can only recover from being stressed if the stress is lifted. If the stress never lets up, then cells don't have an opportunity to recover, and symptoms become persistent. For instance, if you push through the pain and keep walking on a twisted ankle, the injured cells never have an opportunity to heal. With time, the injury will worsen as cells continue to break down until the symptoms of ankle pain and weakness become chronic. If enough cells are damaged beyond recovery, the joint becomes permanently compromised.

Any type of injury or illness can become chronic. Illness is defined as chronic when it doesn't resolve spontaneously and requires ongoing therapy. Some of the most common examples are cardiovascular diseases, diabetes, arthritis, and gastrointestinal illnesses. In the past century, autoimmune illnesses, cancer, and diseases commonly associated with aging, such as Parkinson's disease, Alzheimer's disease and other forms of dementia, and osteoporosis have also become quite prevalent. There are chronic illnesses for every system and tissue in the body.

In other words, there are a lot of ways not to be well.

Unlike a twisted ankle, however, most chronic illnesses are considered *multifactorial*. This simply means that it's not just one stress factor but multiple factors affecting different types of cells throughout the body. Not surprisingly, different chronic illnesses frequently share common symptoms because of the overlap of the cells being stressed. Also, it's not uncommon for a person to have multiple diagnoses. In other words, it's not one thing falling apart, but everything all at once. Because the underlying stress factors are subtle and add up over time, it's often challenging (but not impossible) to define what's driving the symptoms.

It's easy to see why a doctor might be more enthusiastic about treating someone with a twisted ankle, where the cause is obvious and the solution is straightforward, than a patient like Anne, who has multiple chronic symptoms with less well-defined causes. With a sprained ankle, all the doctor has to do is put a brace on it and give the patient a pair of crutches along with a prescription for an anti-inflammatory agent. Within a few weeks, that ankle will be healed, and the patient will be walking normally again.

No matter what the situation, however, the same principles can be applied. If you can identify the underlying stress factors that might be contributing to a person's symptoms and ease those stressors in some way, the stressed cells can recover, and the symptoms will resolve. Identifying the underlying stressors isn't as difficult as it might seem.

This isn't standard procedure in the conventional medical system, however. Medical therapies used to treat chronic illnesses are designed to artificially block the manifestations (symptoms and processes) of chronic illness, not address underlying causes of cellular stress. While there is value in alleviating symptoms and slowing the progression of illness, restoration of wellness is unlikely without addressing the underlying causes of an illness. For Anne, I had more to offer than just prescriptions.

Chronic Illness is a State of Low Energy

Chronic illness is really about energy—or the lack thereof. All cells require energy to function. When cells are stressed, energy demands go up. When cells are chronically stressed and don't get an opportunity to recover, cellular capacity to generate energy (in their tiny cellular batteries called mitochondria) is exhausted, and cells become energy deprived. Chronic illness is a low-energy state. As such, most chronic illnesses are associated with some level of fatigue. In fact, one of the first signs of deteriorating health is loss of energy.

When cells are chronically stressed and energy deprived, they lose the ability to keep up with internal repairs. In other words, healing is impaired. *Low energy* and *impaired healing* are signature features of any chronic illness. If you're talking about cardiovascular disease, diabetes, multiple sclerosis or other autoimmune illnesses, dementia, or cancer, these two factors are always present.

The Genetic Factor

One of Anne's greatest fears was developing Parkinson's disease or dementia herself. She felt that it was her destiny because she was like her father in many ways. I reassured her that, while genetics may play a role in defining a person's *risk* of certain illnesses, it doesn't mean that person will actually ever get those illnesses.

We all have tendencies for certain illnesses as defined by our genes. It's a function of what we inherit from our distant ancestors. When it comes to risk, however, health habits matter more than genetics. Good health habits turn on favorable genes, and bad health habits turn on unfavorable genes. It means that you can dramatically influence your genetic risk of chronic illness and cancer simply by being smart about your health.

Even though Anne may have inherited genes that put her at increased risk of developing Parkinson's disease or dementia, she will only develop those illnesses if she's chronically exposed to the stress factors that tip the balance toward chronic symptoms. It was my job to keep that from happening.

Defining the Obstacles to Wellness

Chronic illness is a slow-moving disaster—it typically comes on gradually. Symptoms can start years before a person reports an issue to a health care provider, and it is often years after that before the patient receives a diagnosis for a specific illness (and often, multiple illnesses by that point).

Anne was at a point I refer to as *pre*-diagnosis. In other words, she had chronic symptoms, but didn't have a formal diagnosis. This is my favorite kind of patient to work with. If I can catch people at that point along the wellness-illness continuum, it's much easier to guide them back to the wellness end of the spectrum and help them stay there. Anyone at any point along the continuum can benefit, however.

When I do an evaluation, I'm looking for hidden stress factors that precipitated the person's symptoms and are holding them in place. In other words, I want to know what's stressing their cells. Sometimes cellular stressors are obvious; but more often, they are hidden or unrecognized. Symptoms don't just happen, however. There are always underlying causes that can be defined. I use the five categories of stress factors as my guide. Systematically, I go through each group: (1) poor diet, (2) toxic environment, (3) mental stress, (4) physical stress, and (5) microbial stress.

From this information, I can get a pretty good idea of how the patient's symptoms evolved and why they are persistent. It's the first step in the pathway back to wellness.

Stress Factor #1: Poor Diet

Overall, Anne's dietary habits were pretty good. She made vegetables a priority, didn't eat a lot of meat, and tried to limit high-calorie foods such as bread and pasta. That hadn't always been true, though. Donuts and cookies were once frequent distractions at the office. And during the stressful years, she had often resorted to fast food and packaged meals to make life a little easier.

Despite good intentions, most of us have room for some dietary improvement. The diet for many people in the modern world is heavy in grains, meat, and dairy. Brimming with calories, but sparse in plant fiber and nutrients, it's the exact opposite of what cells need to thrive. Our cells are designed to run lean. They are programmed as a result of the hundreds of thousands of years of our ancient ancestors eating wild plants and animals, which were lean in both carbohydrates and fats. When cells are chronically exposed to excess carbohydrates and fats, it causes energy overload, which stresses cells and causes them to burn out faster.

Excess dietary carbohydrates have another problem that hobbles cells and accelerates cellular aging. Most forms of carbohydrate (starches, sugars, fruit) are eventually converted to glucose by the liver. Glucose is a high-energy molecule that has a tendency to stick to other molecules, especially to proteins. This "protein-sticking effect", called glycation, adversely affects the functions of every cell in the body. It gums up the internal working parts of cells and prevents cells from functioning properly. Glycation also damages collagen in skin, eyes, and joints (think: wrinkles, impaired vision, and knees that crunch and crackle). It also damages blood vessels and sets the stage for plaque formation.

Overconsumption of carbohydrates is directly linked to obesity and diabetes. But, well before a person's blood sugar starts going up, the damaging effects of glycation weaken cells and make them more vulnerable to other stress factors. Chronic overconsumption of carbohydrates also disrupts insulin, the hormone that regulates blood sugar levels. Glycation and insulin resistance have both been linked with immune system dysfunction.

Dietary excesses of fat and carbohydrate also adversely affect the cardiovascular system. Every cell in the body depends on good blood flow to get nutrients and oxygen and also expel waste. Both excess fat and carbohydrate consumption have been directly linked to arterial plaque formation. Although Anne didn't have any well-defined dietary risk factors for cardiovascular disease, most people in America do.

Stress Factor #2: Toxic Environment

During my talk with Anne, I found no unusual exposure to toxic substances. She ate mostly organic food, had a water filter for her drinking water, and didn't have mold issues in her home. That's not always the case. Some people live or work in dwellings containing mold. Also, certain occupations, such as farmers having day-to-day contact with pesticides and herbicides or people who work with fiberglass or varnish, are associated with high exposure to toxic substances. These individuals are at higher risk of developing chronic health issues.

All of us, however, are exposed to higher than natural levels of toxic substances. Our use of fossil fuels for energy, plastics, and chemicals has silently saturated our surroundings (indoors and outdoors) with unnatural substances that are toxic to life. It's in our food, in the water we drink, and in the air we breathe. Every living creature on earth is being affected.

Low-grade exposure to toxic substances affects our cells in a variety of ways. Many toxic chemicals are potent free radicals that damage cells directly. Others inhibit or poison cellular functions, thereby weakening the ability of cells to do their jobs. These factors have been linked to cardiovascular disease, cancer, and most chronic illnesses. Many toxic chemicals mimic hormones in the body, such as estrogen, which has been specifically linked to increased risk of hormone-dependent cancers, such as breast and prostate cancer.

Of all the cells in the body, liver cells are the hardest hit. Liver cells have the tough job of neutralizing all toxic substances that come through the body. As we go through life, liver cells burn out from processing toxic substances and are replaced by fat cells. As our processing ability declines, toxic substances build up in tissues, which weakens cells and contributes to immune system dysfunction.

Liver cells are responsible for more than just processing toxic substances, however. They also play an important role in maintaining normal blood glucose levels and cholesterol levels. Increased blood cholesterol has been linked to non-alcoholic fatty liver disease (fatty liver not associated with drinking alcohol).[3] It is currently estimated that 25 percent of the world's population has non-alcoholic fatty liver disease.[4] The rise in Anne's blood cholesterol, which is typical for people her age, may be partially linked to gradual loss of functional liver cells that occurs over time.

The Aging Liver

For twenty years, I routinely did laparoscopic surgery, a minimally invasive surgical method that allows the surgeon to see the inside of the abdomen with a scope. During these procedures, I had a habit of visualizing the entire abdomen, including the liver. People in their twenties usually had a beefy red, healthy-looking liver. By age forty, however, it wasn't uncommon to see a mottled yellow liver, a sign that liver cells had burned out from processing toxic substances and had been replaced with fat cells. Loss of liver cells associated with fatty liver dramatically lowers a person's capacity to neutralize toxic substances and compromises the liver's ability to manage our blood sugar and cholesterol levels.

---

3   Malhotra P, Gill RK, Saksena S, and Alrefai WA. Disturbances in cholesterol homeostasis and non-alcoholic fatty liver diseases. *Front Med.* 7:467.

4   Mitra S, De A, Chowdhury A. Epidemiology of non-alcoholic and alcoholic fatty liver diseases. *Transl Gastroenterol Hepatol.* 2020;5:16.

Stress Factor #3: Mental Stress

Of all of Anne's stress factors, chronic mental stress was the most significant. The stress of dealing with her father's situation, along with juggling her CPA job, being a parent to teenagers, and all of life's other responsibilities had been unrelenting.

Constantly maintaining the body in high-alert mode drives cells harder and burns them out faster. It also disrupts the cellular communications in the body. Cells must talk to one another for the body to function as a unit. They depend on the nervous system, hormones, and other signaling agents to stay constantly connected. When these communication pathways are disrupted by chronic stress, coordination of functions in the body breaks down, and all cells suffer.

Most importantly, sleep suffers when the body is maintained in a constant state of high alert. Cells need the downtime provided by deep sleep to recover from the stress of the day. When that doesn't happen, cells stay chronically stressed, and healing is impaired. Chronic stress and poor sleep are well-recognized factors that contribute to immune dysfunction and chronic illness in general.

The fact that Anne was going through menopause at the time of all the other stress had compounded her problems (and hampered her recovery). Menopause disrupts central hormone pathways in the body, which not only causes the classic symptom of hot flashes but also poor sleep and a lower threshold for dealing with stress in general. The increased tension affected her blood pressure. This, along with the increase in her blood cholesterol, may have contributed to a future increased risk of cardiovascular illness.

Stress Factor #4: Physical Stress

Although human existence has historically been associated with excessive physical stress and strain, modern life is remarkably sedentary. The human body is designed to move, and if that doesn't happen, the body suffers. Regular physical activity enhances blood flow to cells and flushes debris and metabolic waste that has collected around cells. Good blood flow from being physically active reduces arterial plaque formation, which reduces risk of cardiovascular disease. Regular exercise normalizes blood glucose levels, which lowers risk of diabetes. Being physically active is one of the best things you can do to stay well.

Because of her sedentary job, Anne recognized the need for regular exercise, but it also was her primary outlet for relieving stress. Exercise offers release that equilibrates hormones associated with stress. It also increases endorphins, the chemical messengers that increase tolerance to pain, and balances neurotransmitters in the brain associated with thinking processes. As such, regular physical activity is associated with lower incidences of depression and anxiety and improved cognitive functions.

Another side of physical stress, however, is trauma. When Anne fell and broke her arm, it was the proverbial straw that broke the camel's back. It not only added another stress but it robbed her of exercise, her one outlet from stress and a key pathway to wellness. After the injury and the discomfort in her knees set in, she lost her incentive to exercise. When I saw her, she was walking and doing some yoga, but she was having trouble getting back into her regular routine.

Stress Factor #5: Microbial Stress

After Anne got the wound infection after the surgery to set her arm, the wound culture grew a bacteria called *Propionibacterium acnes* (*P. acnes*), along with other skin bacteria. *P. acnes* is a common skin bacteria associated with teenage acne. An infected wound is an open invitation for foreign bacteria to get into the bloodstream. If this happens, which isn't as uncommon as you might think, bacteria can end up anywhere in the body. *P. acnes* has been found in the brains of people with Alzheimer's disease,[5] atherosclerotic plaques in arteries,[6] degenerated spinal joints,[7] and even in prostate cancer.[8]

Taking antibiotics for six months was yet another factor that exacerbated Anne's condition. Prolonged antibiotic use disrupts the balance of bacteria in the gut, a condition called dysbiosis. This not only leads to intestinal dysfunction, but a 2015 study[9] showed that pathogens from the gut cross over into the bloodstream and end up in tissues throughout the body, even the brain. Disruption of the balance of microbes in the gut has been linked to an increased incidence of depression, anxiety, arthritis, Parkinson's disease, dementia, cardiovascular disease, autoimmune illnesses, and a range of other chronic illnesses.

---

5   Emery DC, Shoemark DK, Batstone TE, et al. 16S rRNA next generation sequencing analysis shows bacteria in Alzheimer's post-mortem brain. *Front Aging Neurosci.* 2017;9:195.

6   Lanter BB, Davies DG. *Propionibacterium acnes* recovered from atherosclerotic human carotid arteries undergoes biofilm dispersion and releases lipolytic and proteolytic enzymes in response to norepinephrine challenge *in vitro. Infect Immun.* 2015;83(10):3960-3971.

7   Capoor MN, Ruzicka F, Schmitz JE, et al. *Propionibacterium acnes* biofilm is present in intervertebral discs of patients undergoing microdiscectomy. *PLoS One.* 2017;12(4):e0174518.

8   Bae Y, Ito T, Iida T, et al. Intracellular *Propionibacterium acnes* infection in glandular epithelium and stromal macrophages of the prostate with or without cancer. *PLoS One.* 2014;9(2):e90324.

9   Potgieter M, Bester J, Kell DB, Pretorius E. The dormant blood microbiome in chronic, inflammatory diseases. *FEMS Microbiol Rev.* 2015;39(4):567-591.

I believe microbes provide the key to understanding why symptoms become chronic and sometimes worsen over time. The common denominator for all of the previously mentioned stress factors is cellular stress. Cells weakened by chronic stress are vulnerable to invasion by bacteria and other microbes. Each of these factors are also known to cause immune system dysfunction. Your immune system's biggest job is protecting your cells from microbes.

One of the greatest revelations of my journey is that life is marked by a running conflict with microbes, and many of them end up permanently in our tissues. As we go through life, bacteria, viruses, and other microbes find their way across barriers of the skin, sinuses, intestinal lining, and body openings to get to the bloodstream. Once they get to the bloodstream, they can become embedded in tissues throughout the body—brain, joints, muscles, heart—everywhere. Essentially, those microbes become part of us.

When immune system functions are disrupted, microbes in our tissues become active. The ongoing interaction between the microbes and the immune system increases cellular stress and precipitates symptoms in different parts of the body. Once this process is established, it becomes a self-perpetuating problem. I couldn't ignore the possibility that hidden microbes could be contributing to Anne's persistent symptoms—the arthritis, the low stamina, and possibly the cognitive dysfunction. Even after Anne was able to shed her stress and return to normal life, her symptoms had persisted. I knew that she would need more than improved health habits alone to shake the symptoms and return to a normal state of wellness.

Chapter Highlights

- Symptoms result when cells are stressed or injured.

- Healing results from the collective ability of cells to repair and regenerate.

- Symptoms become chronic only when stresses are ongoing and cells never have an opportunity to recover.

- The underlying stressors that promote all illnesses fall under five categories:

  - Poor diet

  - Toxic environment

  - Mental stress

  - Physical stress

  - Microbial stress

- The key to wellness is reducing those stress factors.

3

Microbes: A Dormant Danger

At this very moment, trillions of microorganisms are living *in* and *on* your body. Microorganisms, aka microbes, are microscopic, single-celled, living organisms that are invisible to the naked eye. The term *microbe* is very general. It includes mostly bacteria, but also protozoa and certain types of fungi. Although technically not cells, viruses are also considered microbes.

Because microbes are invisible, sometimes we forget how pervasive they really are. Microbes are everywhere—they thrive in every environment and colonize every living organism on earth.

The sum total of all the microbes that inhabit the body is called the microbiome. It includes somewhere between 20–40 thousand bacterial species, but scientists have just begun cataloging all the viruses. With an infinite number of different combinations, your microbiome is different from every other person's on the planet.

The balance of your microbiome is very dynamic. Everything that happens to you in life—what you eat, where you live and travel, your stress level, how active you are, and new microbes that you're exposed to—affects the balance of your microbiome. In turn, your microbes have a huge impact on your life—far more than most people realize. Microbes affect everything about you: your mood, your energy level, whether you will become chronically ill, what type of symptoms you might develop, and even how fast you will age.

To understand how microbes can affect your health, you have to consider what microbes want from you and how they go about getting it.

A Microbe's Mission

All microbes—no matter whether you're talking about bacteria, viruses, protozoa, or yeast—have only one purpose: to make more microbes. To reproduce, they need food. As long as nutrients and the right conditions are present, they're compelled to keep growing and expanding at the expense of all life around them.

If that sounds a bit threatening, it should.

The primary microbes that we interact with as we go through life are host dependent—they must get the nutrients they need from a living host to survive. In other words, they rely on us for food. Not surprisingly, the highest concentration of bacteria in the body is in the large intestine where there's a high density of freely available nutrients from partially digested food material that bacteria can live off of.

The availability of nutrients is the primary factor that limits growth of bacteria and other microbes that inhabit the body. Your bacteria depend on you eating to be able to continue growing. Most bacteria divide every two to twelve hours. Some are especially fast movers. For example, *E. coli* in the gut can divide every twenty minutes, which means after seven hours, one bacterium can become two million.[10] One of the biggest reasons for having a bowel movement every day is to expel bacteria that have built up throughout the day.

On the skin and body openings, growth of bacteria and other microbes is limited by the fact that nutrients are sparse. Skin bacteria survive off oils you naturally secrete to lubricate your skin. Because growth is restricted by the low availability of nutrients, the concentration of bacteria on the skin is much lower than in the gut.

Food material in the gut and oils on the skin, however, aren't the only sources of nutrients in the body. Bacteria and other microbes can use any organic matter as a food source—including the carbohydrates, fats, and proteins that your cells are made of. In other words, **the cells that make up the tissues of your body are also a potential food source for microbes**.

If that seems like a major conflict of interest, you're right on track.

Because your cells are such an exceptionally good food source for microbes, your body must maintain defenses to protect your cells and keep microbes out of your tissues. The three primary levels of defense include physical barriers, the immune system, and bacteria called normal flora. Without this protection, your tissues would quickly be overrun with microbes.

The first level of defense is physical barriers to keep microbes that inhabit your body separate from your tissues. Bacteria and other microbes are contained inside the gut by the intestinal lining. They are kept on the outer surface of the skin by the dense outer layer. Other

---

10 The Microbiology Society. Accessed February 26, 2022. microbiologysociety.org

microbe barriers include the linings of body openings, such as the mouth, sinuses, bronchial pathways, and bladder.

The second layer of defense is the immune system. The barriers of the body aren't as secure as you might hope. Bacteria and other microbes are constantly finding ways to sneak through barriers to get to tissues. To guard against this ongoing threat, the immune system places white blood cells as sentries at the borders of every barrier. Because the highest concentration of bacteria is in the gut, 70 percent of the immune system's cells surround the linings of the intestinal tract.

Even with these elaborate defenses, however, some bacteria and other microbes break through. For this reason, the immune system constantly circulates a variety of white blood cells that defend against different types of microbes in the bloodstream and throughout tissues of the body. Your immune system is constantly on guard, protecting your cells from every type of microbial threat.

A third part of the defense system is bacteria called normal flora. Normal flora are bacteria with which you share a mutually beneficial relationship. In trade for nutrients and resources, they secrete substances that suppress growth of other, more menacing microbes. Because the immune system has little reach into the insides of the gut or on the surface of the skin, you depend heavily on a healthy balance of normal flora to keep more threatening microbes in check.

Invaders from Outside

Of course, it's not just the microbes that already inhabit your body that you have to worry about. You also depend on the natural barriers of your body and your immune system to protect you (and your cells) from foreign invaders. Because the cells and tissues that make up your body are such a great food source, foreign bacteria and other microbes from the outside environment are constantly trying to cross barriers to get to them.

Most of us think of an infection in terms of the misery it causes. Medically speaking, an *infection* is a microbe (or microbes, as is often the case) breaking through the barriers of the body to get to your cells. A *pathogen* is a foreign microbe that invades the body and does harm by consuming cells.

Microbes are everywhere and they're constantly looking for opportunities to invade your body. Every time you have ever been nipped or scratched by a pet; scraped or cut your skin; put your fingers in your mouth or your nose; hugged another person; had intimate contact with another person; consumed any food or beverage that's been left out too long; taken a breath just after someone sneezed; or were bitten by a tick, mosquito, flea, or other biting insect, microbes have had an opportunity to enter your body.

Different microbes specialize in crossing different barriers. Influenza and SARS-CoV-2 (the viral cause of COVID-19) are defined as respiratory infections because the nasal passageways and lungs are the barriers where the microbes try to enter the body. Sexually transmitted infections, such as syphilis and gonorrhea (among many others), specialize in entering through the genital tract. A multitude of microbes use insects and ticks as vectors for entering the body.

The symptoms we feel with an infection are caused by a confrontation between the microbe and the immune system at the border crossing. For example, a flu virus encounter may morph into that scratchy-throat, runny-nose, achy-all-over feeling. Most insect-borne microbes work in stealth mode: they often don't cause much in the way of symptoms (except sometimes a rash around the bite) because the insect injects the microbes directly through the skin barrier, directly into the bloodstream. Often, we're not even aware that it happens.

Make no mistake, however, the entry point is *only* an entry point. All invading microbes want exactly the same thing—to get to the bloodstream—**because the bloodstream is the highway that provides access to all cells in the body**. Once inside, your cells offer a nearly infinite source of food and resources.

How severe an infection is depends less on the microbe than you might think because all foreign microbes are aggressive. What matters most is whether you have built-in immunity against the microbe. Built-in immunity is a function of past human exposure. The more our human ancestors were exposed to a particular microbe, the more built-in immunity we have to that microbe.

Ebola virus is deadly only because humans have rarely been exposed to it; therefore, we have no built-in immunity against it. When Ebola virus hits the bloodstream, there's nothing to stop it, and it's free to ravage cells throughout the body. The mortality associated with Ebola virus infection is 40–60 percent.

Fortunately, the human immune system is extraordinarily sophisticated. It evolved over millions of years of repetitive exposure to an enormous variety of different microbes. For every trick that microbes devised to get past immune system barriers, the immune system developed countermeasures to match. Redundant layers of protection are hardwired into your immune system for a countless number of microbial threats.

This means that you have at least some immunity against most of the microbes that you will encounter during your lifetime.

Occasionally, you might have an infection that's significant enough to get your attention, such as a cold or a bladder infection. Microbial encounters that put you in bed for days to weeks, such as a bad influenza or COVID-19, fortunately don't come along that often, especially if you're healthy. If you live in a developed country, the chances of encountering something truly life threatening, such as Ebola virus, are low.

Whether mild or severe, symptoms of an infection typically reach a peak and then gradually subside and resolve as the immune system gains the upper hand. In the acute phase, sometimes an antibiotic or antiviral (depending on the type of infection) can help knock down the numbers of microbes enough to help the immune system get a handle on things. Antibiotics, however, don't work by themselves. They only assist the immune system in doing its job.

Once symptoms resolve, you feel better and go on with your life. However, and this is important, **it doesn't necessarily mean that the microbes are gone**.

Microbe Persistence

One of the most important things that I learned from my encounter with chronic Lyme disease is that microbes have very sophisticated ways of persisting inside the body.

No matter how or where microbes enter the body, once they enter the bloodstream, it becomes a race. The microbes' mission is getting to the tissues of the body. The immune system's job is keeping them from getting there.

During the time that the microbes are coursing through the bloodstream, they are vulnerable—the immune system can take them out. They are also vulnerable to antibiotics. For most infections, the immune system does a valiant job of eliminating most of the microbes. Notice that I said most, but not 100 percent. All it takes is a few microbes to make it to tissues for the microbe's mission to be successful.

Once they get deep inside tissues, many microbes have adapted to enter and live inside cells. Cells not only offer nutrients for the microbe to reproduce, but they also offer protection. Once inside cells, the immune system can't get to them directly. They're shielded from antibiotics as well. In some cases, they can stay there for a *very long time*.

Many microbes have adapted to being able to live *inside cells* of the body. Microbes that have this ability are called **intracellular microbes**. Virtually all of the microbes that enter the bloodstream, including many types of bacteria, all viruses, and some protozoa and yeast, have the capacity to live inside cells.

I first became acquainted with the term *intracellular microbes* through my encounter with Lyme disease. The bacterium most associated with Lyme disease, *Borrelia burgdorferi*, is one such microbe. But, there are many others. As my journey progressed, I learned that intracellular microbes are quite common. Every living organism on earth—plants, animals, and even mushrooms—harbors intracellular microbes. The number of intracellular microbes that can infect humans ranges in the hundreds—and those are just the ones we know about.

When Normal Cells Become the Target

One question you might have is: Why doesn't the immune system clear out all the cells that have been infected with microbes from the body? The answer is that the penalty is too high. The immune system can target infected cells with antibodies, but in the process, it also inadvertently targets normal cells of the same tissues. You might recognize this as autoimmunity. It's kind of like dealing with criminals hiding out in a city. It's impossible to eradicate them completely, so the most practical strategy is controlling their activity. Likewise, your immune system lives with the presence of intracellular microbes in tissues, but it controls their activity and minimizes their potential for harm.

Although different intracellular microbes have a preference for different types of cells in the body, most microbes have the capacity to infect a variety of cells. It's important to note that it's never a full assault of microbes that make it to this point. It's more like a random sprinkling. Tissues throughout the body become peppered with microbes. If the immune system is healthy, it can keep them contained. The other important factor is that healthy cells can also repel invasion by microbes.

And the microbes seem perfectly fine with this arrangement. They don't need a huge presence to be successful. Food, safe harbor, and possible opportunities to spread to new hosts in the future are enough. That's not a bad existence by microbe standards!

Consider the possibility that this happens throughout your lifetime. With every microbe encounter, including both the ones that you're aware of and the ones you aren't, your tissues become peppered with a smattering of microbes. Many of the microbes that you picked up as a child, including the likes of Epstein-Barr virus (harbored by ninety-five percent of the world's population), Varicella zoster virus (chicken pox), *Mycoplasma pneumoniae* (a common childhood respiratory infection), human herpes 6 (roseola), and many others may be still quietly residing inside the cells of your body.

As long as you and your cells stay healthy, you'll never even know they're there. Interestingly, harboring microbes without being ill sometimes works out in the microbe's favor. It's been well documented that healthy people intermittently shed Epstein-Barr virus (EBV) and roseola virus (HHV-6) throughout their lives. This is why most people pick up these viruses during early childhood—they're around healthy adults who are actively shedding the viruses. Who knows what else we're actively passing around!

We *All* Have Microbes in Our Tissues

The idea that we have a wide spectrum of microbes buried in our tissues isn't just a theory. As researchers turn their eyes toward exploring possible connections between aging-associated diseases and intracellular microbes, they're finding microbes in surprising places.

Two studies from 2016 and 2017 especially caught my attention. In the first study, researchers were searching for bacteria in the brains of people with multiple sclerosis (MS).[11] It was followed by a similar, but independent study, searching for bacteria in the brains of people who had died of Alzheimer's disease.[12]

In both studies, diseased brain specimens were matched with an equal number of specimens from people who had died of something other than neurodegenerative disease (in other words, healthy brains).

The results were astonishing: **in *every* specimen studied, healthy and diseased brains alike, they found *hundreds* of species of bacteria.** It implies that the presence of bacteria in the brain is a normal state. This contradicts everything we've come to assume about our relationship with microbes. (Rather unsettling, isn't it?)

In both studies, the biggest difference between the diseased brains and the healthy brains was the **dominance of proinflammatory bacteria** (bacteria that promote inflammation) and **higher concentrations of bacteria in the diseased brains.** The types of bacteria present could be sourced internally to the gut, skin, and sinuses, but foreign bacteria were also found that originated from outside the body. In other words, they came in from all directions and across all barriers.

---

11 Branton WG, Lu JQ, Surette MG, et al. Brain microbiota disruption within inflammatory demyelinating lesions in multiple sclerosis. *Sci Rep*. 2016;6:37344.

12 Emery DC, Shoemark DK, Batstone TE, et al. 16S rRNA next generation sequencing analysis shows bacteria in Alzheimer's post-mortem brain. *Front Aging Neurosci*. 2017;9:195.

If microbes can make their way to your brain, you can bet that they're present in every tissue in the body. Indeed, other studies have verified the presence of bacteria in the heart, vascular system, lungs, kidneys, bladder, joints, muscles, and even the human placenta. Wherever you find bacteria, expect to find the full range of microbes, including viruses, protozoa, and fungi—and not just in people who are ill, but in all of us.

Connections to Chronic Illness

With the combined facts that **our cells and tissues are food for microbes** and **microbes keep growing and expanding as long as food is present**, the mere presence of any microbes in our tissues should be cause for great alarm. The potential connections to chronic illness should be obvious.

Healthy cells can repel invasion by microbes. When cells are weakened by a toxic lifestyle of poor food choices, chronic stress, inadequate sleep, and not getting enough exercise, they become vulnerable to invasion. These same factors disrupt immune system functions. If immune system functions become dysfunctional, the immune system can no longer keep a thumb on microbes buried inside cells, so microbes can emerge and infect cells that have been weakened by chronic stress. In a desperate struggle to maintain control, the immune system intensifies the war on infected cells, but normal cells get caught in the crossfire (a possible explanation for autoimmunity that is common to most chronic illnesses).

Cells become stressed and die, tissues become congested and inflamed, and symptoms occur. Not just at one location in the body, but throughout the body—brain, joints, muscles, heart, gut, everywhere. Possible symptoms include brain fog, joint pain, muscle pain, heart irregularities, odd neurological symptoms, digestive issues, and fatigue.

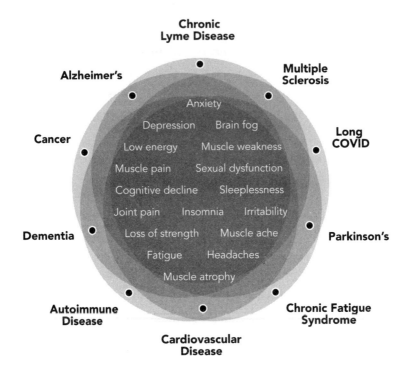

These symptoms are typical for fibromyalgia, chronic fatigue syndrome, chronic (long) COVID, chronic Lyme disease, and many autoimmune illnesses. Many of these symptoms, along with more specific symptoms, are also common with Alzheimer's dementia, Parkinson's disease, rheumatoid arthritis, osteoarthritis, and a range of other chronic illnesses.

Research into Lyme disease opened the door to understanding the connection between intracellular bacteria and chronic illnesses. *Borrelia burgdorferi*, the Lyme bacteria, has been found in association with dementia, Parkinson's disease, chronic arthritis, multiple sclerosis, and a variety of cancers. What's more, people diagnosed with the chronic form of Lyme disease are typically found to carry "coinfections" with other microbes, including various species of Bartonella, Babesia, Anaplasma, Ehrlichia, Rickettsia, Mycoplasma, and Chlamydia. Every year, as our ability to test for microbes has expanded, the list of possible coinfections grows longer. The list includes insect-borne bacteria, but also a range of other bacteria and viruses that aren't typically spread by insects. **All of them are intracellular microbes.**

With increased availability of testing, sufferers of fibromyalgia, chronic fatigue syndrome, autoimmune illnesses, and many other chronic illnesses are testing positive for one or more of these same microbes. The scientific journals are also becoming peppered with case reports and clinical studies linking these microbes (along with other intracellular microbes) to various chronic illnesses, including dementia, rheumatoid arthritis, osteoarthritis, Parkinson's disease, MS, amyotrophic lateral sclerosis (ALS), and autoimmune illnesses. (I find it hard to explain autoimmune illness without considering a microbe factor.)

In fact, I've been able to find links between intracellular microbes and almost every chronic illness. EBV alone has been linked to rheumatoid arthritis, lupus, Sjogren's syndrome, autoimmune thyroiditis, and MS. The most recent in a line of studies linking MS with EBV was published in *Science* in January 2022, which found a 32-fold increased incidence of MS after infection with EBV.[13]

Of course, there's still a lot we don't know. Everyone infected with EBV doesn't get MS, and not everyone with MS has been acutely infected with EBV. Other studies show just as strong a connection between MS and a bacteria called *Chlamydia pneumoniae*. Mycoplasma and Borrelia have also been linked to MS. It implies that different intracellular microbes could cause the same illness or that multiple microbes are at play in each case—which is likely, in my opinion.

C. pneumoniae is a respiratory bacteria responsible for at least 10% of community-acquired cases of pneumonia and bronchitis. Of course,

13   Bjornevik K, Cortese M, Healy BC, et al. Longitudinal analysis reveals high prevalence of Epstein-Barr virus associated with multiple sclerosis. *Science.* 2022;375(6578):296-301.

the lungs are just the entry point. Once it's disseminated through the body, it can maintain a chronic presence in tissues throughout the body. *C. pneumoniae* has been linked to a variety of chronic illnesses, including atherosclerosis.[14] The association was first made in 1988.[15] Since then, the bacteria have been found in artherosclerotic plaques in cerebral (brain) arteries, coronary arteries, and larger arteries in the legs.[16] Although *C. pneumoniae* has been implicated as a risk factor for stroke and heart attack, there are no medical therapies that address the issues; therefore, it is largely ignored.

It's not just foreign microbes from infections that you have to worry about either. Microbes from the gut, skin, and other body areas pass across barriers more freely than once thought. A study in 2015 found that bacteria in the gut can trickle across the gut-blood barrier and into the bloodstream, after which they can end up in tissues throughout the body, including the brain.[17] If the balance of gut bacteria becomes disrupted (a condition called dysbiosis) by antibiotics or poor eating habits, a trickle becomes a steady flow. That's called "leaky gut".

Chronic periodontitis and tooth decay (associated with over 700 species of bacteria) have been closely linked to everything from cardiovascular disease to prostate diseases. *Propionibacterium acnes* (*P. acnes*), the bacteria causally linked to teenage acne, was commonly found in the diseased brains in the Alzheimer's study previously mentioned. This was also the bacteria that grew out of Anne's wound from Chapter 2 that's been closely linked to numerous chronic illnesses.

14   Chen J, Zhu M, Ma G, Zhao Z, Sun Z. Chlamydia pneumoniae infection and cerebrovascular disease: a systematic review and meta-analysis. *BMC Neurol.* 2013;13:183.

15   Saikku P, Leinonen M, Mattila K, et al. Serological evidence of an association of a novel Chlamydia, TWAR, with chronic coronary heart disease and acute myocardial infarction. *Lancet.* 1988;2(8618):983-986.

16   Taylor-Robinson D, Thomas BJ. Chlamydia pneumoniae in atherosclerotic tissue. *J Infect Dis.* 2000;181(suppl 3):S437-S440.

17   Potgieter M, Bester J, Kell DB, Pretorius E. The dormant blood microbiome in chronic, inflammatory diseases. *FEMS Microbiol Rev.* 2015;39(4):567-591.

It strongly implies that our tissues aren't sterile, as once thought. Microbes of every variety are constantly trickling across barriers and circulating around inside your tissues.

Putting it all together, it's now hard for me to think about any chronic illness without considering the possibility of intracellular microbes being involved. **Now that I've seen the connections, I can't unsee them.** Microbes and chronic illness are firmly intertwined. Even symptoms that we commonly associate with aging, such as joint discomfort, might have a microbial component.

Because your personal assortment of microbes may be quite different from the next person's, it just makes sense that **microbes are likely the biggest wild card that determines what type of chronic illness a person might end up with.** It's like a time bomb in your tissues. When enough cellular stress adds up, it trips the fuse. How big an explosion you have depends on the types of microbes you've picked up during your life and how healthy you keep your cells.

Keeping your cells healthy is especially important as you age. A key feature of aging is that your cells become less functional. That includes the cells of your immune system. Your microbes, however, don't age in the same way that your cells age—they stay strong forever. It means that as you get older, you become more vulnerable to microbes.

The good news is that there are so many things you can do to keep your immune system in tip-top shape even as you add birthday candles. One of those things involves taking herbs every day. I've learned about the power of herbs to combat microbes lurking in tissues, and later in this book, I'm going to share strategies for incorporating herbs for health. As we age, that extra protection becomes increasingly important.

Chapter Highlights

- An infection occurs when invasive microbes break through our natural defenses.

- Once symptoms resolve, it doesn't mean that the microbes have been fully eradicated, as many microbes can maintain a presence inside our cells.

- In this way we all collect microbes throughout life.

- Healthy cells are more resistant to invasion by microbes. As long as immune system functions and cells are healthy, intracellular microbes in the body are kept in check and symptoms do not occur.

- When immune system functions are disrupted by stress factors, intracellular microbes throughout tissues of the body are able to emerge and cause chronic symptoms.

- There is now solid science linking many chronic illnesses to intracellular microbes.

4

The Aging Factor

It's not the inevitability of aging that bothers most people, it's the possibility of life being compromised with some type of chronic illness along the way. Dementia, cardiovascular disease, and cancer generally top the list of concerns. And it's true that as the years add up, it's all too easy to slip from wellness toward the chronic illness side of the spectrum.

The good news is that it doesn't have to be that way. After my struggle with illness, I was able to regain wellness and hold onto it, despite growing older. In fact, I've enjoyed better health in the latter third of my life than I did during midlife.

Beyond staying well, we all want to live as long as we can, but there are limits that can't be surpassed. Researchers who study aging speculate that the absolute ceiling of human life is approximately 120 years.[18] That's how long they estimate that the human body would last if all stress factors that could be controlled, were controlled. That figure is also consistent with actual human experience. The age of the longest-lived person ever recorded belongs to Jeanne Calment (1875–1997) of France, who made it to 122 years.[19] Though there are claims of 140 years, none have been officially verified.

While hitting that lofty goal might be elusive to most people, evidence suggests that living into your 80s or 90s *without* developing chronic illness is not only possible but also practical for most anyone. I can live with that.

In the early 2000s, a group of scientists headed by Dan Buettner—an explorer, journalist, and National Geographic fellow—set out to study the health and dietary habits of long-lived modern-day populations around the world. The project was dubbed "Blue Zones" because researchers used a blue highlighter to circle regions on the map where the study populations lived.

Their research defined five primary geographic hot spots of longevity where centenarians were common. The list included Sardinia, Italy; Ikaria, Greece; Okinawa, Japan; Nicoya, Costa Rica; and the Seventh-Day Adventist community in Loma Linda, California. These regions are not exclusive. Since the Blue Zones project, other countries have gained recognition for average lifespans stretching well into the 80s and even 90s. One is Iceland, which, despite its frigid temperatures and rugged terrain, recently held the record for longest average lifespan for men.

---

18   Beltrán-Sánchez H, Austad SN, Finch CE. Comment on "The plateau of human mortality: demography of longevity pioneers". *Science.* 2018;361(6409):eaav1200.

19   Robin-Champigneul F. Jeanne Calment's unique 122-year life span: facts and factors; longevity history in her genealogical tree. *Rejuvenation Res.* 2020;23(1):19-47.

What they found was that these populations consistently stay healthy and happy well into their 90s and beyond. Their rate of chronic illnesses, such as dementia, cancer, and autoimmune illness was negligible. By evaluating different populations from different geographic locations around the world, the studies also showed that living to an old age is not exclusively tied to genetics, race, or specific geographic regions. It's mostly about choices: what they ate, the air they breathed, and how they went about life. And they do it with far less money and resources than we use to keep people alive in the United States.

Although there is much we can learn from the Blue Zone investigations, I came away with two important conclusions. One, that life is finite—there are certain limits that can't be breached. The other is that it's possible for most people to reach the outer limit of aging without suffering from chronic symptoms. It implies that aging and chronic illness aren't necessarily connected.

Why We Age

Again, cells provide the answers. Simply put, we age because our cells age. As cells age, the body gradually runs out of functional cells. When the body reaches a critical point of not having enough functional cells, especially in vital organs such as the heart or brain, then life has reached the end. How fast you get to that endpoint and whether you develop chronic illness along the way are related to how well you take care of your cells. When cells are stressed, aging is accelerated and risk of chronic illness increases.

The process of body aging actually begins around age twenty. Up until that point, the body accumulates new cells in a cycle of growth that lasts all during childhood and throughout adolescence. When peak adulthood arrives, the bucket is filled to capacity and cell accumulation halts.

When you were twenty, you might remember feeling pretty invincible. With good reason. Your twenty-year-old body contained five to ten times more cells than you needed to survive.[20] What's more, those cells were at peak health. With the risk of childhood illnesses in the rearview mirror, your biggest threat was some sort of trauma or doing something foolish. At that point, your risk of becoming chronically ill was lower than at any other point in your life. After the peak, however, your biological clock started ticking: the number and functional quality of cells in your body began a slow but steady decline.[21]

Even though the body has a remarkable capacity for repairing and replacing cells, that capacity isn't unlimited. Eventually, every cell in the body loses its ability to repair itself and regenerate. The process of aging is defined not only by the loss of functional cells, but also by the loss of the body's ability to generate *new* cells.

It's All About Energy

One of the primary reasons that cells lose function is because they run out of energy. The energy that cells need to function is supplied by microscopic structures called mitochondria scattered inside each cell. The number of mitochondria present in a cell depends on the energy demands of the cell. A skin cell, which doesn't have to work very hard, contains only a few hundred mitochondria, whereas a heart cell, which needs lots of power, contains up to 5,000 mitochondria.

20   Bianconi E, Piovesan A, Facchin F, et al. An estimation of the number of cells in the human body. *Ann Hum Biol.* 2013;40(6):463-471.
21   Davidovic M, Sevo G, Svorcan P, Milosevic DP, Despotovic N, Erceg P. Old age as a privilege of the "selfish ones". *Aging Dis.* 2010;1(2):139-146.

The Cost of Generating Energy

Mitochondria function much like tiny batteries. Inside the mitochondria, carbohydrates and fats are burned to generate energy. That energy is stored in a high-energy molecule called adenosine triphosphate (ATP), which circulates throughout the cell, providing energy to power all cellular functions.

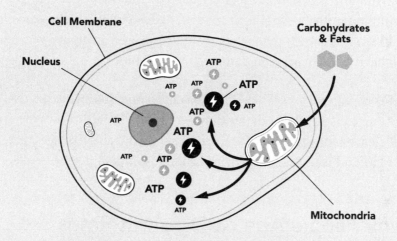

During the process of generating energy, potent free radicals are produced that damage mitochondria internally. Though mitochondria utilize specific antioxidants (vitamin C, vitamin E, glutathione, superoxide dismutase, alpha lipoic acid) to control the intensity of the energy-generation process, *eliminating all free radicals would snuff out the energy-generation process entirely*. Therefore, the mitochondria must sustain a certain amount of net damage in exchange for energy. Eventually, mitochondria burn out and lose the capacity to generate energy.

Because energy is so vital, cells continually monitor and manage all of their mitochondria. Mitochondria that have reached the end of their useful life are eliminated, and new ones are generated from remaining mitochondria as needed. "New" mitochondria, however, are only as good as the ones they come from and as life progresses, "good" mitochondria become more and more scarce. Gradually, all the cell's mitochondria are exhausted, and the cell runs out of energy.

As cells throughout the body gradually burn through their mitochondria, cell strength and stamina steadily decline. The loss of energy from dwindling mitochondria is the primary reason why a forty-year-old will have less energy than a twenty-year-old, and an eighty-year-old will have less strength than anyone in the room.

With waning energy, cells lose the capacity to function and, collectively, all functions in the body gradually decline. In addition, without sufficient energy, cells lose the ability to repair internal damage created by wear and tear. In other words, healing is impaired.

Why People Age At Different Rates

If it was possible to eliminate all cellular stress for everyone on the planet, the rate of aging would be about the same for everyone (assuming everyone started with the same supply of cells and mitochondria). Of course, we don't live in a perfect stress-free world. Each person's cells are uniquely exposed to varying types and degrees of stress throughout life. Even with the best of intentions, it's hard to escape all of it.

When cells are stressed, they work harder, consume more energy, and burn out their mitochondria faster. This, in turn, accelerates cell loss associated with aging. Accelerated cell loss is also a factor with any type of chronic illness. Because the types and degrees of stress that people are exposed to as they go through life are highly variable, people age at strikingly different rates.

Though scientists have identified "survivor genes" that give some people a better-than-average ability to tolerate certain stress factors, it is still that list of cell stressors that plays the biggest role in the acceleration of aging.[22]

Ultimately, taking care of your cells becomes increasingly important as you age. As cells lose energy and functional capacity, they become more susceptible to being stressed. The newly minted cells of a twenty-year-old are fairly stress-resistant, whereas the aged cells of an eighty-year-old are easily stressed. As cells lose stress resistance, risk of chronic illness and cancer goes up. With every year that passes, protecting your cells from being stressed becomes more imperative.

Tips from the Blue Zones

As you might guess, the traits common to long-lived populations revealed in the Blue Zone project line right up with the factors that promote wellness on the Wellness Diagram.

- They don't overeat. And although the diets varied among Blue Zones, they all tend to eat natural, whole foods, not carb-loaded processed food products.

- They live in places where the environment is clean—clean water, clean air, and clean food. Toxic substances not only stress cells, but many unnatural toxic substances damage mitochondria directly.

- They follow a low-stress lifestyle that is complemented by positive social interactions. Living with chronic stress increases energy demands on cells and accelerates burnout of mitochondria.

---

22   Passarino G, De Rango F, Montesanto A. Human longevity: genetics or lifestyle? It takes two to tango. *Immun Ageing*. 2016;13:12.

- Their lifestyle requires moderate physical activity throughout the day, but not excessive physical labor. Regular physical activity improves mitochondrial efficiency and reduces damaging free-radical production associated with metabolism. Regular exercise stimulates cells to generate new replacement mitochondria from the best of the best remaining mitochondria.

- The habits of Blue Zone populations included culinary and medicinal herbs. This gave their cells added protection against microbes and a range of other cell stressors. We'll explore the remarkable power of herbs in upcoming chapters.

This project reveals that longevity is closely tied to creating an internal environment that minimizes stress on your cells. When stress is reduced, energy demands go down and a cell's supply of mitochondria lasts longer. (Stay tuned for practical guidelines on how to make it happen in your life in Part Three.)

Recommended Reading:

Dan Buettner, *The Blue Zones, 2nd edition*: 9 Lessons for Living Longer From the People Who've Lived the Longest National Geographic Society, 2012

A fascinating public health research initiative exploring the common denominator health practices for the world's longest living cultures.

When Cells Reach Their Functional Limit

Sooner or later cells run out of energy and reach the end of their functional life. When a cell loses its capacity to function normally, there are a couple of different possibilities for what can happen next. The first is that the cell can undergo programmed cell death called *apoptosis* to make room for other more functional cells. A less desirable outcome is that the cell can become a senescent cell.

Senescent cells are cells that have reached the end of their useful life, but, for reasons that are yet unclear, don't undergo apoptosis. They are still metabolically active but are only marginally functional. They just hang around and take up valuable resources and space. As such, they're a weak link in the team of other more functional cells—it's like an employee who goofs off all day while everyone else is working. Not surprisingly, they've acquired the nickname "zombie cells".

Aging is marked, then, not only by the gradual loss of cells but also by the gradual accumulation of senescent cells, which are undesirable because they are still drawing resources from the body but not contributing anything. Zombie cells are undesirable because they collect throughout all tissues in the body, crowd out normal cells, and compromise functions. Zombie cells accumulate faster when cells of the body are chronically stressed. A healthful diet, clean environment, low stress, and regular activity all slow the rate of zombie cell accumulation.

Though accumulation of zombie cells doesn't directly cause illness, it may increase risk of chronic illness.[23] It also crowds out and steals resources from healthy cells. When healthy cells can't function optimally, all the other cells in the body suffer. Possibly most concerning, however, is how senescence affects the immune system, both directly and indirectly.

---

23   Burton DG. Cellular senescence, ageing and disease. *Age (Dordr)*. 2009;31(1):1-9.

Telomere Shortening

In anti-aging circles, you'll often hear about something called telomere shortening. Telomeres are structures within a cell that pull the cell apart during cell division into two cells. With each cell division, telomeres shorten until cell division is no longer possible and the cell reaches a state of senescence. The number of times a cell line can divide is limited to 40-60 divisions, variable depending on the cell type. One focus of anti-aging research is creating drugs that artificially lengthen telomeres. The idea being that if you can restore telomere length to cells throughout the body, then you can artificially extend cellular life and thereby increase longevity. This thinking, however, completely ignores the possibility that nature put this limit there for a reason. Limiting cell division by telomere shortening may be one mechanism that prevents cells from becoming cancerous.

Stem Cells to the Rescue

When it comes to staying alive, the body always keeps one ace in reserve. This ace is *pluripotent stem cells*. Stem cells are undifferentiated cells that have the potential to become any type of cell. Stem cells are distributed throughout the tissues in the body. They remain in a state of stasis, which means they do not divide until they are needed. When tissue is damaged, stem cells activate and differentiate into the cell types needed for repair. You've seen this in action when you've nicked your finger and then, a few days later, it is completely healed and looks like normal skin again.

While this might seem like a ticket to eternal life, the number of stem cells present in tissues is very limited. For any tissue to function, there has to be a much higher concentration of actively functioning cells over nonfunctioning stem cells. This leaves room for only enough stem cells in tissues to provide for basic repairs after injury. Therefore, regeneration of a new limb or an entire organ, such as the liver or heart, after a catastrophic injury does not occur spontaneously (unless you're a lizard and happen to lose your tail).

Gradually through life, the body uses up stem cells (and some simply atrophy over time). So, the process of aging is associated with a gradual decline in the concentration of stem cells in tissues. Therefore, you can't depend on stem cells alone to reverse the aging process.

That being said, stem cell therapy is one of the most promising areas of regenerative medicine. Stem cells can be extracted from fatty tissue around your abdomen (your "spare tire") and injected into the damaged parts of the body, such as worn-out knees or an injured spine. The injected stem cells convert into the types of cells needed to repair the damage. In the future, it may be possible to use stem cells to grow new tissue, such as insulin-producing cells of the pancreas to cure diabetes, or possibly even whole organs, such as a liver or kidneys.

How Senescence Affects the Immune System

All systems in the body accumulate senescent cells, including the immune system. The process of immune cells aging out and becoming immune zombie cells is called *immunosenescence*. As functional immune cells are replaced with zombie immune cells and the total number of healthy immune cells declines, the immune system is less capable of keeping up with its responsibilities of clearing debris from around cells and keeping microbes in check.

The problem is compounded by the fact that your microbes don't age like your cells age. Bacteria and viruses are very simple compared to your cells. When they replicate, completely new bacteria or viruses are formed. It means that viruses or bacteria currently replicating inside your body look and act the same as the bacteria or viruses that first entered your body. As such, they haven't lost any potential to be threatening. Your cells, on the other hand, undergo aging. They gradually burn out mitochondria, lose energy, and lose the ability to function. Even when they replicate to make replacement cells, any aging is passed along to the new cells formed. This happens to every cell in your body, including your immune cells.

This is where the conflict of interest between microbes in tissues and the immune system becomes a real issue. As immune cells age, they are less capable of keeping the lid on all the microbes in the body's tissues. As you remember, microbes have only one purpose: making more microbes. Throughout life, we continue to collect intracellular microbes in tissues. By the end of life, we've accumulated quite a collection. Some microbes are more threatening than others, of course, but they're all a greater threat as the functional capacity of your immune system declines with age.

The Microbe-Cancer Connection

The issue of latent microbes came closer to home when my father, who was in his early eighties at the time, developed blurriness and discomfort in his right eye. An ophthalmologist diagnosed him with an eye infection with toxoplasma and treated him with antibiotics. Although his symptoms resolved with antibiotics, I wasn't so sure that would be the end of it.

I knew about toxoplasma because it was one of the many intracellular microbes I'd been researching. Toxoplasma is a protozoan, a single-celled microbe one step more advanced than bacteria. It's commonly contracted from cats or by eating undercooked meat. In a person with a healthy immune system, toxoplasma typically stays dormant in tissues without causing any symptoms like many other intracellular microbes. In fact, about 60 percent of the world's population harbors toxoplasma without knowing it. If the immune system becomes disrupted, however, the microbe can cause illness. Toxoplasma has been linked to schizophrenia, depression, anxiety, and a range of other conditions.

As mentioned, eating undercooked meat is a common way that people pick up toxoplasma. Steak, often cooked rare, was a staple at my parents' dinner table. No doubt, my dad had picked up toxoplasma at some point during his life, and it had quietly remained in his tissues until his immune system started to fail with advancing age. The eyes are one place that this microbe can surface.

When my dad developed cloudiness in that same right eye several months later, it didn't come as a surprise. Antibiotics can lower the concentrations of intracellular microbes like toxoplasma enough to eliminate symptoms, but not enough to eradicate the microbes. I was surprised, however, when aspiration of the fluid from the eye revealed lymphoma, a cancer of the white blood cells.

I searched the scientific literature and immediately found a direct link between this particular type of lymphoma and toxoplasma.

My father's case provides a perfect example of what happens when the immune system begins to decline. In all likelihood, toxoplasma had been in his tissues for much of his life. It wasn't until the cells of his immune system started aging out that the toxoplasma emerged and caused illness.

After my dad's diagnosis, I started researching the connection between intracellular microbes and cancer. Scientists first began proposing links between microbes and cancer back in the 1800s; however, it wasn't until 1964 that researchers documented the first definitive cause-and-effect connection between a microbe and human cancer.

The microbe was Epstein-Barr virus (EBV). The cancer, Burkitt's lymphoma, was prevalent in the lymph nodes of children in a certain region of Africa where a particular strain of EBV was present. Since then, other strains of EBV have been linked to esophageal and gastric cancers, along with a variety of different lymphomas.

Other documented microbe-cancer links include:

- *Helicobacter pylori (H. pylori)* with cancer of the stomach

- *Salmonella typhi* with gallbladder cancer

- *Chlamydia pneumoniae* with lung cancer

- *Streptococcus bovis* with colon cancer

- A variety of species of mycoplasma with a variety of different cancers

- Multiple bacteria with oral cancers

This is only a partial list. In all, about **20 percent of human cancers have been directly linked to various microbes**, and with time, I predict that many more associations will be identified.[24]

---

24 Vedham V, Verma M, Mahabir S. Early-life exposures to infectious agents and later cancer development. *Cancer Med.* 2015;4(12):1908-1922.

HPV and Cervical Cancer

My earliest professional association with the microbe-cancer link was some thirty years ago when human papillomavirus (HPV) was associated with cervical cancer in women. It totally changed how we screen for cervical cancer. Women with HPV often develop a precancerous state called dysplasia, which in some cases progresses to cancer. Why do some women develop cervical cancer when others exposed to the same virus do not? It left me wondering if there might be cofactors involved, such as other microbes. Various mycoplasma and ureaplasma would be high on my suspect list because these tiny bacteria have been found to facilitate entry of viruses into cells. But the cancer link has not been proven thus far.

In the past several years, connections between intracellular microbes and cancer have been popping up everywhere. In a 2020 study[25] published in the journal *Science*, **researchers found a distinct "tumor microbiome" consisting of intracellular bacteria in each of 1,526 different tumor specimens**. The specimens were taken from seven different cancer types including breast, lung, ovarian, pancreatic, melanoma, bone, and brain cancers.

Not long after, an internationally recognized expert on Lyme disease, Eva Sapi, Ph.D., was featured in an article about **finding *Borrelia burgdorferi* in over 400 specimens of breast cancer tissue**.[26] Her

25 Nejman D, Livyatan I, Fuks G, et al. The human tumor microbiome is composed of tumor type-specific intracellular bacteria. *Science.* 2020;368(6494):973-980.
26 Chmiel R. University of New Haven Professor Makes Great Strides in Lyme Disease, Cancer Research. University of New Haven. September 15, 2020. https://www.newhaven.edu/news/blog/2020/eva-sapi-research.php. Accessed February 26, 2022.

team also found that Borrelia readily invaded breast cancer cells in the lab. The late Neil Spector, M.D., a friend and oncology researcher at Duke University, reported finding Bartonella, a bacteria common in all mammals, in cancer cells of a certain type of breast cancer (just before his untimely death tied to Lyme disease).

Does this mean that microbes such as Borrelia and Bartonella are the specific cause of breast cancer? No, but it does imply that **microbes play a key role in the process of cancer formation**. This role has actually been demonstrated experimentally.

Microbes' Role in Cancer Development

Our knowledge of the role intracellular microbes play in cancer was taken a step further by a 2018 study published in *Cancer Cell International*.[27] The study was significant because **researchers were able to experimentally induce cancer formation in eukaryotic cells (cells like ours) using intracellular bacteria.**

For the experiment, they used an algae species. They started by placing the algae cells in the dark, which weakened the cells. When the researchers exposed the cells to chemical carcinogens (toxic chemicals that promote cancer), the cells simply died, but when they exposed the weakened algae cells to an intracellular bacteria common to that species of algae, the cells became cancerous.

In every case, when the bacteria invaded the weakened cells, the cells took on the unrestricted growth common to bacteria and turned to cancer. They were also able to

27   Dong, Q., Xing, X. Cancer cells arise from bacteria. *Cancer Cell Int.* 2018;18:205.

demonstrate that the bacteria had inserted a segment of DNA into the cell's genome that turned on unrestricted growth in the host cell. The researchers proposed that this may be a primary mechanism for cancer cell formation.

It's a bit unnerving when you think about the fact that we all harbor microbes inside our cells that have the potential to adversely affect our cells. It's important to note, however, that it's the stressed cells that are vulnerable.

Aging Cells are Vulnerable Cells

As cells age, they are more easily stressed, which makes them more vulnerable to invasion by microbes. Beyond cancer, this may be a significant factor that increases the incidence of many chronic illnesses, especially neurodegenerative illnesses such as dementia, with age.

This means that keeping your cells healthy as you age is really important. Good health habits are part of the equation, but taking a regular daily regimen of herbs can provide a level of protection that surpasses good dietary and health habits alone. In the next chapter, we'll start exploring the remarkable benefits of herbs.

Chapter Highlights

- We age because our cells age.

- Cells age because they run out of functional mitochondria and therefore energy.

- Life is marked by gradual loss of cells.

- When cells are stressed, they burn out faster.

- Impaired immune cells are less capable of keeping microbes in tissues in check, which may be one reason why the incidence of chronic illness and cancer increases with aging.

- The key to slowing aging is taking really good care of your cells.

5

Charting a Pathway to Cellular Wellness

ircling back to my patient, Anne, she was struggling with a variety of seemingly unrelated and persistent symptoms, even though the stress in her life had largely resolved. I speculated that residual stress at the cellular level could be a factor holding her symptoms in place. Once cells become chronically stressed, restoring a normal state of wellness requires maintaining a very low-stress environment until healing is complete. That takes time, and often good health practices alone are not enough to make it happen.

I had a hunch that herbs could give her the extra edge she needed. **Herbs, in the form of concentrated standardized extracts like I had used, had the potential to help her in a way that medical therapies could not.** The benefits of conventional medical therapies are restricted to artificially blocking symptoms and slowing the progression of illness. While that can be valuable in certain situations, pharmaceuticals have little capacity to reduce cellular stress and promote healing. In contrast, herbs work specifically by countering cellular stress and promoting healing.

My confidence with herbs comes from well over a decade of using them in my practice and studying their mechanisms of action. In that time span, there's been an explosion of scientific research on herbs. As the world has reawakened to the remarkable benefits of plant medicines, researchers from across the globe have focused their efforts on verifying traditional uses of herbs and understanding exactly how herbs work.

What they've found is that all herbs contain *hundreds* of chemical substances called **phytochemicals** (phyto means "plant" in Greek). Phytochemicals serve the plant's needs in a variety of ways.

Phytochemicals: The Power Behind the Herbs

To us, phytochemicals give plants their intense colors, such as the orange of carrots, the yellow of the spicy herb called turmeric, and the deep purple of an eggplant or blackberries. Other phytochemicals give vegetables, such as kale and Brussels sprouts, their bitter tastes and give cinnamon and vanilla recognizable aromas. To the plant, however, phytochemicals are purely functional—they make up the plant's defense and regulatory systems.

The complex array of phytochemicals present in plants doesn't work randomly or individually. Plants are living organisms. Plants produce phytochemicals to serve a broad range of functions within the plant, ranging from signaling agents to protective properties. The plant's phytochemicals work in synergy to optimize the plant's ability to thrive. It's often referred to as the "innate intelligence" of the plant.

The purpose of many phytochemicals is protective. Plants are constantly confronted with a range of different threats, including free radicals, toxic chemicals, radiation, direct damage by physical stress, and being consumed by other living organisms, including insects and every variety of microbe. Phytochemicals are designed to protect the plant's cells from those threats.

When we consume phytochemicals from food plants or herbs, our cells gain extra protection against free radicals, toxic substances, radiation, and microbes including bacteria, viruses, protozoa, and fungi. When cells are protected from such a wide range of different stress factors, they remain less stressed and more functional. They also use less energy and last longer, which slows the cell loss associated with aging.

The Power of Phytochemicals

Two phytochemicals from familiar sources include *resveratrol*, found in grapes (also Japanese knotweed, a remarkable herb covered in Chapter 10) and *pterostilbene*, found in high concentrations in blueberries (but also other berries, cocoa, and the bark of certain trees). These substances are potent antioxidants, which protect the internal structures of cells from free-radical damage. They also protect mitochondria directly. Resveratrol and pterostilbene are known as "uncoupling agents". This means that when mitochondria are overstressed, these compounds uncouple the energy generators inside the mitochondria so that they spin freely, which reduces generation of free radicals and lowers mitochondrial damage when cells are overworked. As an added benefit, these phytochemicals provide antimicrobial properties.

A plant's phytochemical makeup also includes signaling agents that coordinate the plant's cellular defense efforts, along with the plant's cellular functions. The plant's signaling agents shift the plant's internal environment to match changes in the outside environment, such as temperature and light that vary between night and day and with the seasons. Interestingly, the chemical structures of many plant signaling phytochemicals are similar to or the same as our hormones and neurotransmitters.

For the human body to function as a unit, all cells in the body must be in continual communication with each other. The language they use is chemical. Cells communicate using hormones, neurotransmitters, peptides, and a vast array of different signaling agents. The brain constantly monitors changes in the environment outside the body and fine-tunes the cellular functions inside the body using these chemical messengers.

Many common stress factors, including insulin resistance associated with excessive carbohydrate consumption, toxic chemical substances, chronic emotional stress, and invasive microbes can disrupt the flow of chemical messengers that our cells use to communicate. Because plants use a chemical language that is similar to ours, many herbs have the effect of normalizing hormones and neurotransmitters that have been disrupted by any type of stress.

The complexity of phytochemicals is the key to understanding how herbs provide such a wide range of remarkable benefits. **By taking herbs, we adopt the plant's natural ability to protect itself against microbes, counteract a wide variety of stress factors, and maintain internal balance.** Instead of being targeted therapy like drugs, it's more like integrating the plant's survival intelligence and defense capabilities with that of our own. It has the effect of protecting cells that make up our tissues and normalizing communications in the body that have become disrupted by stress, which promotes wellness and lowers risk of chronic illnesses in general.

The Multifaceted Benefits of Herbal Phytochemicals

When I was a newbie to herbal therapy, I found it puzzling that any given herb might be used for a wide variety of applications. For example, turmeric, an herb from traditional medicine of India, has been used to treat arthritis, skin conditions, respiratory infections, cognitive dysfunction, stomach ulcers, and a range of other ailments. As I was more familiar with the narrow, targeted actions of drug therapy, such a range of benefits seemed a bit far-fetched.

Understanding chronic illness as chronically stressed cells, however, provides the answer. Instead of having targeted actions like a drug, herbs provide the full cellular defensive and regulatory properties of the plant's phytochemicals. By protecting cells of the body from stress factors and normalizing hormones disrupted by stress, herbal phytochemicals promote an environment in which cells can recover from stress. In other words, herbs promote healing. And when cells heal, symptoms resolve.

Interestingly, within the past decade, research has defined how phytochemicals from commonly used herbs and food plants **counteract each of the five categories of stress factors that promote illness**. The following are some of the documented phytochemical actions:

Poor Diet

- Inhibit the damaging effects of glycation to collagen and cellular structures[28]

- Normalize insulin[29] and provide antidiabetic properties[30]

- Protect cellular structures and mitochondria from oxidative stress caused by metabolism, which increases cellular longevity and optimizes cellular energy[31]

 # Toxic Environment

- Provide antioxidants that protect cells, tissues, and organs from free-radical damage associated with exposure to toxic substances[32]

- Optimize detoxification by promoting ideal levels of glutathione[33]

- Protect liver cells, which enables the liver to process higher levels and types of toxic substances[34]

---

28 Parveen A, Sultana R, Lee SM, Kim TH, Kim SY. Phytochemicals against anti-diabetic complications: targeting the advanced glycation end product signaling pathway. *Arch Pharm Res.* 2021;44(4):378-401.

29 Mahdavi A, Bagherniya M, Mirenayat MS, Atkin SL, Sahebkar A. Medicinal plants and phytochemicals regulating insulin resistance and glucose homeostasis in type 2 diabetic patients: a clinical review. *Adv Exp Med Biol.* 2021;1308:161-183.

30 Salehi B, Ata A, Anil Kumar NV, et al. Antidiabetic potential of medicinal plants and their active components. *Biomolecules.* 2019;9(10):551.

31 Zhang YJ, Gan RY, Li S, et al. Antioxidant phytochemicals for the prevention and treatment of chronic diseases. *Molecules.* 2015;20(12):21138-21156.

32 Forni C, Facchiano F, Bartoli M, et al. Beneficial role of phytochemicals on oxidative stress and age-related diseases. *Biomed Res Int.* 2019;2019:8748253.

33 Minich DM, Brown BI. A review of dietary (phyto)nutrients for glutathione support. *Nutrients.* 2019;11(9):2073.

34 Madrigal-Santillán E, Madrigal-Bujaidar E, Álvarez-González I, et al. Review of natural products with hepatoprotective effects. *World J Gastroenterol.* 2014;20(40):14787-14804.

Mental stress

- Restore homeostasis (balance) by normalizing hormones, neurotransmitters, and other signaling agents that have been disrupted by chronic stress[35]

- Protect cells from the damaging effects associated with overactivation of the sympathetic nervous system

 ## Physical stress

- Reduce inflammation associated with physical overexertion[36]

- Normalize the inflammatory response and optimize healing

 ## Microbial stress

- Suppress invasive microbes and balance the microbiome, which protects cells and reduces stress on the immune system[37]

- Modulate immune system functions, which allows the immune system to function more effectively and efficiently[38]

35 Panossian A. Understanding adaptogenic activity: specificity of the pharmacological action of adaptogens and other phytochemicals. *Ann N Y Acad Sci*. 2017;1401(1):49-64.

36 Saleh HA, Yousef MH, Abdelnaser A. The anti-inflammatory properties of phytochemicals and their effects on epigenetic mechanisms involved in TLR4/NF-κB-mediated inflammation. *Front Immunol*. 2021;12:606069.

37 Borges A, Saavedra MJ, Simões M. Insights on antimicrobial resistance, biofilms and the use of phytochemicals as new antimicrobial agents. *Curr Med Chem*. 2015;22(21):2590-2614.

38 Patel S. Phytochemicals for taming agitated immune-endocrine-neural axis. *Biomed Pharmacother*. 2017;91:767-775.

A 2015 landmark study published in the scientific journal *Molecules* summarized the health benefits of consuming phytochemicals from food plants and medicinal herbs for reducing the incidence of chronic illnesses including cardiovascular disease, diabetes, cancer, Alzheimer's disease, and inflammatory bowel disease.[39] This study detailed the protective actions of a wide variety of phytochemicals from vegetables, fruits, and medicinal herbs. It's a strong argument not only for eating plenty of vegetables and fruits but also for taking herbs every day to prevent chronic illness from ever happening.

Still, the concentration and diversity of phytochemicals found in herbs is much greater than in food plants. It's because herbs are wild plants. Plants in the wild are exposed to greater stress than plants cultivated for food and grown under controlled conditions, therefore they produce higher concentrations of protective phytochemicals.

It is interesting to note that every herb has a unique palette of phytochemicals. It's all a function of the stress factors present in the plant's natural environment and the phytochemical spectrum the plant uses to counteract those stressors. For example, cat's claw, an herb native to the warm, moist environment of the Amazonian jungle, has to deal with a high degree of microbial stress. Not surprisingly, it has strong antimicrobial properties. In contrast, the phytochemistry of rhodiola, a plant native to the northern reaches of Siberia, is aimed at protecting the plant from the harsh environment. As such, taking rhodiola is exceptionally good for increasing resiliency to intense physical stress.

---

39   Zhang YJ, Gan RY, Li S, et al. Antioxidant phytochemicals for the prevention and treatment of chronic diseases. *Molecules*. 2015;20(12):21138-21156.

Preserving Autophagy with Phytochemicals

One way that phytochemicals provide benefit is by preserving cellular *autophagy*. Autophagy is the process by which cells perform internal housekeeping. Cells continually break down misfolded proteins, burned-out mitochondria, damaged DNA, and worn-out parts and recycle them into new proteins and cell parts. It is also the mechanism by which cells expel many types of intracellular microbes. In this way, cells stay lean and strong.

Autophagy is impaired when cells are chronically stressed. Worn-out parts and damaged proteins accumulate inside the cell, which compromises the cell's ability to function properly. It also makes the cell more vulnerable to invading bacteria and other microbes. Impaired cellular autophagy has been linked to every imaginable chronic illness and many cancers.

Because herbal phytochemicals reduce cellular stress by counteracting free radicals, toxic substances, radiation, and microbes, it would be expected that taking herbs preserves cellular autophagy. Indeed, a 2021 study published in *Frontiers in Pharmacology* provided evidence for the exact mechanisms by which seventy different phytochemicals induce or preserve cellular autophagy. The phytochemicals were sourced from a range of different herbs; among these were Japanese knotweed, green tea, ginger, turmeric, wild celery, garlic, berries, maritime pine bark, and Chinese skullcap.[40]

40   Rahman MA, Hannan MA, Dash R, et al. Phytochemicals as a complement to cancer chemotherapy: pharmacological modulation of the autophagy-apoptosis pathway. *Front Pharmacol.* 2021;12:639628.

Using Herbs to Cultivate Wellness

The first thing I did for Anne was recommend a regimen of herbs. I knew the herbs would boost her recovery by suppressing threatening microbes, supporting immune system functions, and protecting her cells against a range of stress factors. Though all herbs share some similar protective properties, each herb is different in its own way. Combining herbs synergizes the benefits of each herb individually. To provide the highest potential for benefit, I recommended high-grade botanical extracts with concentrated phytochemicals.

The herbs were specifically chosen because they had low potential for toxicity and were free of drug-like effects. That would allow her to take them every day without concern. The list of herbs I recommended included Japanese knotweed, andrographis, cat's claw, garlic extract, reishi, and turmeric (full profiles on these herbs can be found in Chapters 9 and 10).

Though this regimen of herbs covered a lot of bases, there were other herbs and natural substances that could boost her recovery even faster. One of the biggest factors that precipitated Anne's symptoms was the unrelenting stress during the time of her father's illness and ultimate death. While that issue had resolved, she still had stress in her life. The simple fact that she was having to work full time, despite having low energy and cloudy mental functions, was stressful in itself.

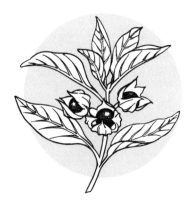

To balance her stress hormones and increase stamina, I recommended an herb called ashwagandha (pronounced, "ash-wah-gon´-dah"). Ashwagandha works exceptionally well for balancing hormones in the body that have been disrupted by any sort of chronic stress. It's also known to support cognitive function, which might help her think more clearly. In addition, it would help some of the lingering hot flashes from menopause several years prior.

Ashwagandha for Stress Support

The science is there to boost our confidence in ashwagandha. A rigorous study published in the journal *Medicine* in 2019 demonstrated that ashwagandha caused significant reduction in stress-related anxiety by balancing the HPA axis (hypothalamic-pituitary-adrenal axis—a central regulatory hormone pathway in the body associated with stress, stress control, reproductive hormone functions, and more).[41] Another study, published in *Sleep Medicine* in 2020, verified ashwagandha's ability to improve sleep quality.[42] Still other studies have documented ashwagandha's beneficial effects on cognitive functions[43], reduction of hot flashes associated with menopause[44], and thyroid function[45]. And all of those studies on ashwagandha noted a very low incidence of side effects. Use of ashwagandha isn't limited to women. In addition to improving tolerance for both physical and mental stress, ashwagandha has been shown to restore depressed testosterone levels in men to normal levels.[8]

41   Lopresti AL, Smith SJ, Malvi H, Kodgule R. An investigation into the stress-relieving and pharmacological actions of an ashwagandha (Withania somnifera) extract: a randomized, double-blind, placebo-controlled study. *Medicine (Baltimore)*. 2019;98(37):e17186.

42   Deshpande A, Irani N, Balkrishnan R, Benny IR. A randomized, double blind, placebo controlled study to evaluate the effects of ashwagandha (Withania somnifera) extract on sleep quality in healthy adults. *Sleep Med*. 2020;72:28-36.

43   Choudhary D, Bhattacharyya S, Bose S. Efficacy and safety of ashwagandha (Withania somnifera (L.) Dunal) root extract in improving memory and cognitive functions. *J Diet Suppl*. 2017;14(6):599-612.

44   Johnson A, Roberts L, Elkins G. Complementary and alternative medicine for menopause. *J Evid Based Integr Med*. 2019;24:2515690X19829380.

45   Sharma AK, Basu I, Singh S. Efficacy and safety of ashwagandha root extract in subclinical hypothyroid patients: a double-blind, randomized placebo-controlled trial. *J Altern Complement Med*. 2018;24(3):243-248.

For sleep, I recommended the calming herbs, passionflower and lemon balm, along with magnesium and low-dose melatonin. None of these substances is as strong as sleep medications, but they can help promote calm (and better sleep) without the risk of habituation or causing drug-like effects. I also talked to Anne about relaxation techniques and practicing good sleep hygiene in the evening.

Although Anne had already adopted a healthy diet and had been taking a probiotic for some time, she was still having persistent gastrointestinal symptoms of bloating, gas, and sometimes reflux. I suspected the culprit was slow motility and bacterial imbalances brought on by chronic stress and prolonged antibiotic use. Though the primary regimen of herbs I recommended would help restore balance in her gut microbiome, I had other recommendations to support normal gut function.

I encouraged her to take digestive enzymes with every meal to augment the digestive process. I also recommended an herbal preparation called slippery elm, which contains mucilage, a natural substance that protects the intestinal lining and allows it to heal. To promote normal bile flow and encourage intestinal motility, I recommended dandelion extract. She also asked about her current probiotic. I said it was okay to continue taking it, but that a good diet and herbs are often just as effective. An herbal substance called berberine is especially beneficial for suppressing abnormal growth of bacteria in the gut. Dandelion and berberine are bitter herbs—this provides added benefit, because bitter taste stimulates intestinal motility (more about restoring gut function in Chapter 21).

Lastly, for Anne's joint discomfort, I recommended a combination of turmeric, boswellia, and other nutrients to reduce inflammation and support joint health. Turmeric is also known to support brain health. I also suggested full-spectrum organic CBD oil to be used as needed for joint and muscle discomfort. It would also ease some of her anxiety and help her sleep better. I talked to her about not overdoing it with exercise and suggested starting with regular walking, gentle yoga, and qigong. She could progress to more vigorous physical activity as her body recovered (more on managing joint discomfort in Chapter 22).

At our six-week follow-up session, Anne was starting to see some improvement. Just seeing a change was her incentive to do more. By the time six months rolled around, her energy had rebounded, the joint discomfort was gone, her thinking was clear, and she felt like her life was returning to normal. Along with shedding the symptoms, her concern for developing Parkinson's disease and dementia was also eased. In the recovery process, she had established lifelong health habits that would help her maintain symptom-free health as she aged.

After Anne's wellness was restored, I shifted her to a daily regimen of herbs to be taken on an ongoing basis to maintain wellness. This regimen of herbs is thoroughly discussed in Chapter 9. It includes herbs such as rhodiola, which supports energy; reishi, which supports immune system functions; gotu kola, which supports brain function; milk thistle, which protects the liver; turmeric for reducing inflammation; and pine bark extract for supporting healthy cardiovascular function.

How Herbs and Drugs Can Work Together

At this point in my career, I typically leave the management of medications to other health care providers. My focus is teaching the person how to cultivate a state of wellness and maintain it throughout life. Even so, I recognize that drugs can be valuable in certain situations. In fact, herbs and drugs can be complementary.

Hypertension provides a good example of how herbs and drugs work differently but can complement each other. For a patient with a blood pressure elevated to 160/110, the risk of heart damage and having a stroke is very real. There is no herb (or combination of herbs) of which I am aware that can quickly bring the elevated blood pressure under control. So, for bringing blood pressure down out of the danger zone, antihypertensive medications are the right answer.

Drugs, however, have little capacity to restore the cardiovascular system back to normal. As the vascular changes that drive hypertension inevitably worsen, patients typically end up needing higher doses or additional medications over time. Because the actions of drugs are very specific, conventional medical treatment of cardiovascular disease may require one drug for lowering blood pressure, another drug to control cardiac arrhythmia (irregular heartbeat), and still another drug to lower blood cholesterol.

Though herbs don't have the capacity to lower blood pressure as quickly as drugs, herbs can do something that drugs can't do: **herbal extracts have the capacity to restore the integrity of the blood vessels.** When the functional capacity of the vascular system is restored, blood pressure naturally returns to normal. One herb that stands out for this purpose is hawthorn.

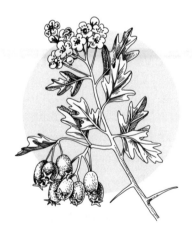

Hawthorn is a shrub in the rose family that grows throughout Europe and Asia. It's been used since the time of the Romans for every type of heart ailment. In traditional Chinese medicine, hawthorn is considered a heart tonic (a substance that invigorates the heart). Medicinal extracts can be made from all parts of the plant, including the leaves, flowers, berries, and bark, and the berries are often consumed as food. Traditional applications aren't isolated to the heart. It's also been used for digestive issues, kidney problems, and anxiety.

Hawthorn for Heart Health

Hawthorn's benefits have been well documented by Western science. A study published in 2018 revealed that taking hawthorn is associated with greater efficiency of heart contractions, reduction in irregular heartbeats, improved coronary artery blood flow, improved exercise tolerance, and normalization of blood pressure in hypertensive individuals without affecting blood pressure in people without hypertension.[46] Other documented benefits include protecting the stomach lining and supporting normal digestion, providing anti-inflammatory properties, and promoting calming effects on the nervous system.

Plus, you don't have to wait until you have symptoms to take hawthorn. In a 2013 study published in *Evidence-Based Complementary and Alternative Medicine*, researchers concluded that because the incidence of side effects, adverse reactions, and interactions with drugs were so remarkably low, hawthorn is ideally suited for prevention of cardiovascular illness.[47]

Personally, I've been taking 900 mg of standardized hawthorn extract on a daily basis for over a decade. When I first started the herb, it didn't immediately bring down my high blood pressure. However, over several years, my blood pressure gradually normalized and irregular heartbeats resolved. As a bonus, I didn't have any side effects. I'm grateful, because I never found a blood-pressure medicine that I could tolerate.

---

46   Orhan IE. Phytochemical and pharmacological activity profile of Crataegus oxyacantha L. (Hawthorn) - a cardiotonic herb. *Curr Med Chem.* 2018;25(37):4854-4865.

47   Wang J, Xiong X, Feng B. Effect of crataegus usage in cardiovascular disease prevention: an evidence-based approach. *Evid Based Complement Alternat Med.* 2013;2013:149363.

In my opinion, we should be carving out a niche for herbs like hawthorn in clinical practice. Cardiovascular disease is the leading cause of death for both men and women in the United States. It's also one of the most common concerns expressed by patients. And yet, herbs like hawthorn are being left out of the discussion in both the management and prevention of heart disease, heart attacks, and strokes (see discussion on cardiovascular health in Chapter 20). As a bonus, hawthorn has a nice calming effect.

In summary, the potency of herbs lies in their protective phytochemicals, which offer the power to promote healing and restore wellness. These herbal heroes help to protect your cells from stress factors that can lead to illness and cancer. Making herbs a part of your everyday life is one of the easiest—and also one of the most powerful—things you can do to protect your health as you age.

Chapter Highlights

- Plants produce a vast array of phytochemicals to serve a broad range of functions within the plant.

- When we consume phytochemicals from herbs or food plants, the benefits are transferred.

- Phytochemicals with protective properties reduce cellular stress by neutralizing free radicals, toxic substances, and damaging radiation, and by guarding against invasive bacteria, viruses, protozoa, and fungi.

- Phytochemicals with signaling properties affect cellular communication pathways. Many herbs normalize hormones and neurotransmitters that have been disrupted by stress.

- By reducing cellular stress, herbal phytochemicals have the capacity to reduce the incidence of chronic illness and cancer.

- Many commonly-used herbs have completely different mechanisms of action than drugs.

6

The Case of the Missing Phytochemicals

Now that I've made a case for the importance of phytochemicals, I have to inform you that the average American consumes a lower concentration of protective phytochemicals than ever before in human history. We're not getting enough of them in our food. We've traded medicinal herbs for drugs. We've lost an ancient connection—and we're suffering because of it.

We need phytochemicals because our cells are adapted to having them. Members of our species, *Homo sapiens*, have been wandering the planet for more than 200,000 years. For the vast majority of that time, high concentrations of dietary phytochemicals have been an integral part of human existence.

Our most ancient ancestors were hunter-gatherers. While that might induce imagery of people clad in animal skins gathered around a spit with rump of mastodon roasting over an open fire, that was likely the exception rather than the norm. Much of their diet came from wild plants, many of which would likely be classified as herbs today. This means that ancient humans unwittingly included high concentrations of phytochemicals in their diets on a daily basis.

Ancient life was dominated by finding something to eat. People lived a nomadic existence in which they followed the food as it changed through the seasons. The day's agenda included pulling edible leaves; stripping bark from certain trees; digging roots and tubers; and collecting wild fruit, berries, and mushrooms. Although humans relied heavily on plants, the foraged food menu also included bird and reptile eggs, insects, grubs, fish, shellfish, and wild game.

They didn't eat for pleasure, as much of their diet was likely bitter, not tasty. They ate purely for survival. In terms of calories, foraging was a break-even proposition: a full day of foraging brought in enough calories to survive another day. It's because wild plants don't provide nearly the concentration of calories found in modern food plants. Even wild fruits and berries, which offer the highest caloric content of all foraged foods, only offer a fraction of the calories found in their modern cultivated cousins.

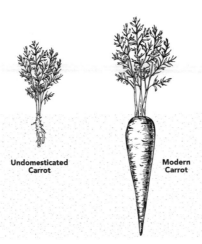

Undomesticated
Carrot

Modern
Carrot

Wild plants are a far cry from the foods we cultivate today.
Most of our crop plants have been selectively bred over many years to produce
larger fruiting and vegetative structures that provide more calories.

When humans did happen upon a bountiful source of calories—a slain wildebeest, a cache of honey, a fall salmon run, or a bush full of ripe berries—they gorged on it because it wouldn't last long. With no refrigeration, food spoiled rapidly. Also, there was a lot of competition in nature for calories. If you didn't eat it, something else would. This left humans with a nearly unstoppable urge to gorge on high-calorie foods whenever they could—which, back then, wasn't very frequently.

Often our undoing, this tendency persists in our modern times of caloric excess. Our programming still compels us to constantly seek high-calorie foods—namely foods loaded with carbohydrate and fat—though not from the forest floor but from the convenient aisles of the local grocery store or from a drive-through window. The bottom line is that we live in a fast-food era, but our genes—and our bodies—are still optimized for a hunter-gatherer lifestyle that is inconsistent with our new food supply.

Instead of power bars and tacos, the everyday staples of ancient life were the leaves, stems, roots, and bark of plants that were always available. Because the calorie yield of these food sources was sparse, ancient humans had to eat a lot of it to survive. Wild plants consist mostly of cellulose, the non-digestible fiber that adds some "bulk" to our diet and helps to keep intestinal contents moving along. Dietary fiber is also essential for cultivating a favorable balance of gut microbes. Although we don't digest dietary plant fiber, our gut bacteria do. They break it down into short-chain fatty acids for their own energy needs but importantly, those short-chain fatty acids also energize the cells lining our colon.

What the foraged food diet lacked in calories, it made up for with loads of fiber, vitamins, minerals, and *phytochemicals*. Ancient humans ate a wide diversity of wild plants. Each plant provided an array of protective phytochemicals that, when consumed, transferred to human cells and gave them an operational edge.

Today humans cultivate an estimated 150 of the roughly 30,0000 edible plants worldwide—and of those cultivated plants, the typical modern diet contains a mere 17 different plants consumed over the course of a whole year.[48] Compared to our ancient hunter-gatherer ancestors who ate as many as 500 different plants in a year, we have significantly narrowed the variety of protective phytochemicals we consume through these plants and thus diminished their ability to protect our health.

Ancient life was completely surrounded by nature and organic matter. In fact, to most of us today, it might have seemed a bit *too* organic—imagine a primitive camping trip that never ends. Being bitten by microbe-transmitting ticks, mosquitos, and flies was a common occurrence. People ate fermented fruits and soil-covered roots and drank from streams. As such, ancient humans had day-to-day exposure to high concentrations of bacteria and other microbes.

Even with such high microbe exposure, however, it's unlikely that they became ill from it. Although humans were exposed to a lot of microbes, they were the *same* microbes, year after year and generation after generation. They lived in small bands or tribes and had only limited contact with other humans. Even though they were nomadic, they actually didn't roam very far.[49] Because their living environment changed little, they developed immunity to most of the microbes in their environment.

In fact, it was such a cozy relationship that bacteria and other microbes from fermented foods, the dirt from the ground where they lived, other humans, and the environment at large populated their guts and skin and became their normal flora. Their normal flora, along with high intake of phytochemicals from food helped protect them when threats from foreign microbes did come along.

---

48 Shelef O, Weisberg PJ, Provenza FD. The Value of Native Plants and Local Production in an Era of Global Agriculture. *Front Plant Sci.* 2017;8:2069.

49 Our human ancestors spread out to cover the planet in small increments over tens of thousands of years, not in great leaps. It's estimated that for humans to spread across Europe and Asia, migration would have required moving only six miles per generation (Sapiens).

Modern-Day Foraging

Decades of research on the Hadza tribe in Tanzania, a modern-day population of people who subsist solely by foraging, can tell us a lot about our ancient ancestors. Only a few hundred of the remaining 1,300 tribe members live connected to the ancient past strictly as hunter-gatherers. Foraging keeps them physically active throughout the daytime hours, but they typically take more downtime than modern cultures. Hadza typically sleep nine hours a night.

Their diet consists of wild plants, particularly tubers but also including berries; baobab fruits and seeds; various leafy greens; marula nuts; and hunted meat from birds, porcupines, and other wild game (they do not keep livestock). Though sparse in calories, their diet is rich in fiber (150 grams per day compared to a paltry 15 grams per day for the average American), nutrients, and phytochemicals, which promotes high diversity of their gut microbiome—40% greater than the average American's. Remarkably, the foraging Hadza don't experience intestinal illnesses that plague modern society. In fact, chronic illnesses, such as autoimmune illnesses, skin conditions, and cancer are virtually unknown to them.

Of course, a high consumption of phytochemicals couldn't protect our ancient ancestors from everything. Life for early humans was often cut short by natural threats such as snake bites, falls, encounters with large animals, hunting accidents, conflicts with other humans, birth trauma, and exposure to harsh weather. But those types of threats couldn't be predicted, so the mental stress they caused occurred strictly at the time of the event—the classic fight-or-flight response. In other words, ancient stresses were very real but probably didn't cause much chronic worry because they couldn't be anticipated. Compared to today, our ancient ancestors lived "in the moment."

Transition to Farming

As humans gradually became more skilled at hunting and more efficient at gathering, populations gradually expanded to the point that they placed pressures on natural resources. That, more than anything else, incentivized farming. It's important to keep in mind, however, that agriculture is a relatively recent part of human history. Humans only started farming around 11,000 years ago. Put into perspective, if all of human history were condensed into a single day, the time that humans have been farming would account for less than an hour. And our current century would account for *less than a* minute.

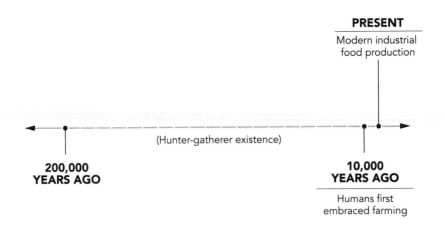

PRESENT

Modern industrial
food production

(Hunter-gatherer existence)

**200,000
YEARS AGO**

**10,000
YEARS AGO**

Humans first
embraced farming

The Dawn of Agriculture

Though cultivation of plants specifically for the purpose of providing food is thought to have occurred as far back as 20,000 to 30,000 years ago, agriculture didn't become established until around 11,000 years ago. The first recognized farming settlement was Ain Ghazal (Spring of the Gazelle), located in what is known as the Fertile Crescent, near the current city of Amman, Jordan. Archeological evidence has painted a picture of what that early agricultural community might have looked like (~7200-5000 B.C.).[50] The inhabitants of this small village of a thousand or so people lived in one- or two-room, mud-brick dwellings. They raised goats and other domesticated animals and were known for making small ceramic figures of animals and people to bury with the dead, which were sometimes laid to rest underneath the homes.

We also know what crops they farmed: mainly grains (barley and ancient species of wheat) and beans (peas, beans, lentils, and chickpeas), which are food sources that store fairly well and offer a reliable calorie source. The countryside around Ain Ghazal was forested and offered a wealth of additional food resources. Evidence at the site suggests that the inhabitants still ate a wide variety of foraged wild plants and hunted a range of small wild animals.

As agriculture gradually became established worldwide, wheat became the dominant grain in the Middle East and Europe, rice in Asia, millet in Africa, and corn (maize) in the Americas. It wasn't that grains and beans were necessarily better food than foraged food, but it was

50 Simmons AH, Köhler-Rollefson I, Rollefson GO, Mandel R, Kafafi Z. 'Ain ghazal: a major neolithic settlement in central jordan. *Science*. 1988;240(4848):35-39.

more reliable food. Grains and beans stored easily and could be fed to domesticated animals, which provided a reliable source of protein and milk products. As a bonus, grains could be easily fermented into alcohol—and the world would never be quite the same!

However, grains and beans were a big switch from the long-standing wild plant diet. They were packed with calories, for one thing. Another was that the fiber was different, which likely altered the balance of gut microbes and affected digestion. In addition, grains and beans contain high concentrations of certain proteins called lectins, which give some people digestive upset. (For the record, lectins are the reason grains must be cooked and beans must be soaked and boiled to be edible.)

Possibly the biggest change that came with the shift to these new foods was a loss in phytochemicals. Grains, beans, meat, and dairy are poor sources of protective phytochemicals as compared to the plants that made up the foraged diet. For a while, people supplemented their new grain-based diet by continuing to forage for wild plants, berries, and mushrooms. But as agriculture brought a surge in world population, people migrated to cities. This occurrence increased our dependence on grain-centric cultivated foods and further distanced us from our wild-plant roots.

Herb, Food, or Medicine?

Gradually, a concept of herb as distinct from food began to evolve. Plants that we now know as culinary herbs and spices became essential complements to food. Herbs with bitter phytochemicals were traditionally reserved as medicines. The traditional use of medicinal herbs and mushrooms dates back thousands of years and has been an integral part of human culture. In fact, all human cultures on earth have maintained herbal medicine traditions since the dawn of agriculture. Early practitioners of traditional medicine in both China and India used complex herbal formulas that were designed to not only relieve symptoms but also to promote wellness.

In Europe, things evolved a bit differently. University-trained physicians focused heavily on plants with strong drug-like properties (poisons); elemental chemicals such as antimony, lead, and mercury (more poisons); and bloodletting, which was performed by barbers. Herbal medicine was practiced by lay herbalists, who were typically illiterate women. The fact that the herbalists generally had better outcomes and were more popular among common folk didn't sit well with the physicians. For a period between the thirteenth and fifteenth centuries, lay herbalism was banned. Those who didn't comply were often labeled as witches and burned at the stake.

The Spice Trade

Beyond adding flavor, the natural antimicrobial and antioxidant properties found in herbs and spices retard food spoilage, which was a big problem in the days before refrigeration. Demand for this preservative effect was a huge driver in the development of the spice trade.

The demand for herbs and spices opened up trade between East and West to bring aromatics such as cinnamon, cardamom, ginger, pepper, nutmeg, star anise, clove, and turmeric to growing European civilizations. The flavors and aromas of spices are courtesy of certain phytochemicals that they contain. Other herbs were traded for use as perfumes and essential oils, such as frankincense and myrrh from the near East. Tea, coveted by the British, was initially brought into Europe from China and later from India, as well. The East-West trade also expanded the selection of herbs available as medicinal herbs from China and India.

The Story of the Four Thieves

During the Middle Ages, when the black plague was rampant, a story surfaced about a group of thieves who learned that dousing themselves with essential oils provided protection against the disease. This enabled them to rob the dead and dying without becoming ill. It was probably because it protected them from the fleas that were spreading the bacteria. Essential oils are derived from volatile oils that certain plants use to deter insects. The combination of oils they used has been immortalized in an essential oil formula, aptly named "Four Thieves", which contains clove, cinnamon, eucalyptus, rosemary, and lemon oils. Four Thieves oil is still used for a variety of purposes, including as an insect repellant.

Competition for better access to herbs and spices spurred Columbus to search for quicker routes to the East. Though he didn't find what he was looking for, his discovery opened up access not only to new lands but also to new herbs and spices. Herbal medicine traditions were already well established in native populations throughout North, Central, and South America when Europeans arrived. Medicines from the New World were found to be effective against some of the old European diseases. Bark from the cinchona tree, native to South America, was found to be an effective treatment for malaria. Much later, quinine was extracted from cinchona bark and made into a drug for malaria treatment.

Fast-Forward to Today

Because our modern food system prioritizes calories and taste over everything else, phytochemicals have largely been left behind. The bulk of the American diet comes from only a few food sources: wheat, corn, soybeans, and meat or dairy from animals that are fed corn and soybeans. It is the very opposite of our ancient food heritage.

Although all parts of a plant contain phytochemicals, seeds contain the very lowest phytochemical concentrations. This is because seeds are preferentially loaded with varying ratios of carbohydrates, fats, and proteins to nourish a new plant when the seed germinates. From a food point of view, this makes seeds—grains, beans, and nuts—an ideal source of calories but a poor source of protective phytochemicals. When seeds are processed into flour or refined oils (depending on which seed is used and how it is processed), the phytochemical concentration is further reduced.

This isn't in sync with our ancient food past. Our genes—and therefore our cells—were shaped mostly by foods common to the ancient pre-agricultural, pre-industrial world. Though we've made some adaptations to foods brought in by the agricultural age, our genes simply haven't had time to adjust to the high concentrations of fats and carbohydrates found in modern food products.

Adding more vegetables and fruit into your diet is a step in the right direction, but the phytochemical concentration of cultivated fruits and vegetables still doesn't come close to matching their wild counterparts. **Our modern food plants are cultivated to produce calories, not phytochemicals.** To maximize yield of carbohydrates, food plants are grown under strictly controlled conditions to reduce stress from insects, microbes, and competition with other plants. Because plants produce protective phytochemicals to counteract stress, when stress is controlled, the need for the plant to produce phytochemicals declines.

Reconnecting with Our Ancient Foraging Past

One of my favorite summertime activities is picking wild blueberries. In the North Carolina mountains, wild blueberry bushes surround exposed outcroppings of rocks along trails. Each year, I try to plan a hiking trip there in July when the berries reach peak ripeness. A wild blueberry is about a quarter the size of the grocery store variety and is tart in comparison, but loaded with protective phytochemicals. Nothing connects you with your ancient foraging roots like picking berries from a bush in the wild. When I pass people along the trail, I often ask if they are enjoying the blueberries. They invariably reply that they hadn't noticed them or ask if the berries are safe to eat. It just shows how far removed we are from our food roots.

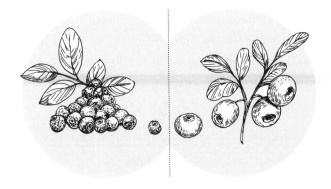

Smaller wild blueberries (*Vaccinium angustifolium*), which face a greater variety of environmental stressors, have higher amounts of protective phytochemicals when compared to larger domesticated blueberries (*Vaccinium corymbosum*). Wild blueberries typically have twice as many antioxidants and 33% more anthocyanins than domesticated blueberries.

When plants are cultivated under stress-controlled conditions for thousands of generations, as all our food plants have been, the plant loses much of its ability to produce protective phytochemicals. In short, our cultivated food plants have lost the ability to protect themselves. This is why the heavy use of herbicides and pesticides has become so common in modern agriculture.

Another factor is taste. Many phytochemicals present in wild plants are bitter. In fact, the taste of bitter was so prevalent in ancestral human diets that it became an important trigger for normal digestion. Bitter, however, isn't perceived as a pleasant sensation. Therefore, over the centuries, food plants were cultivated to have less and less bitterness. In the process, important protective phytochemicals were also lost.

It means that even the healthiest diet consisting of foods from a grocery store doesn't come close to matching the phytochemical concentration found in our ancestral diets. **In fact, if we were going to identify the most significant modern dietary deficiency, it would be protective phytochemicals, not vitamins and minerals as you might expect.**

Replacing What's Most Missing

When people look to supplements to replace what may be missing in their diet, they typically turn to vitamin supplements, which may not be money best spent.

Vitamins and minerals are *nutrients*—substances that cells need to function. Cells of the body require an enormous variety of nutrients to function optimally. Vitamins and minerals are cofactors for many chemical reactions inside cells, including energy production by mitochondria. Mitochondria require nutrients such as NAD/NADH, coenzyme Q10, L-carnitine, PQQ, and a variety of others for the energy generation process.

Carbohydrates, fats, and amino acids are also nutrients. Though cells use carbohydrates and fats to generate energy, they are used for several other functions as well. Amino acids are the building blocks of proteins and are also used as signalizing agents, such as neurotransmitters in the brain.

Nutrients—vitamins, minerals, amino acids, and all the rest—come from food. And while the body can readily make certain nutrients, such as L-carnitine and coenzyme Q10, on an as-needed basis, it still requires raw materials found in food. Supplements can be a source of nutrients, but it's not necessarily the most natural or best way to acquire them.

An important caveat about nutrients is that cells and mitochondria need a continual supply of them but only in amounts that can be immediately utilized. This is a problem with any nutrient supplement only dosed once or a few times each day. Cells become overloaded with the supplemented nutrients at the time of the dose, but because cells have no mechanism for storing excess vitamins and minerals, most of the dose is degraded or excreted in the urine. Vitamins and other nutrients acquired from food are slowly released as food is digested, which gives cells the continual supply they need.

Another problem with nutrient supplements is that cells of the body require a wide variety of nutrients, all of which work in synchrony. Supplementing with a few nutrients can offset the balance of other nutrients in the body and compromise chemical reactions necessary for biological functions. In addition, any given nutrient may exist in the body in a variety of different forms. Supplementing with one form of the vitamin or nutrient may offset the balance of other forms of that nutrient in the body.

The only time supplementing with various nutrients may be beneficial is when cells are stressed. Cellular stress can be caused by anything from bodybuilding to chronic illness. When cells are stressed, they work harder, generate more energy, and have a higher demand for nutrients. Even then, a healthy diet is important for supplying the wide range of nutrients cells need to function properly.

In comparison, herbal supplements provide an entirely different type of benefit. The phytochemicals found in food plants and herbs are *non-nutritive*. In other words, they *aren't* raw materials that are necessary for cells to function. What they *do* provide, however, is protection—against free radicals, radiation, toxic substances, and threats from different types of microbes. In other words, phytochemicals reduce cellular stress. When cells are less stressed, they don't work as hard, use less energy, and have lower nutrient demands—not just some nutrients, but all nutrients. This makes herbal supplements the better choice for optimizing cellular functions.

Protective phytochemicals have gone missing from our natural diet at a time when we need them the very most. The unique stresses of modern life—unnatural diet, chronic low-grade exposure to toxic substances, incessant daily stress, inactivity, and exposure to new and novel microbe threats—put undue pressure on cells. Phytochemicals are our cell's best protection, and without them, our cells are vulnerable.

The good news is that, beyond making healthy dietary choices, high-quality herbal supplements are widely available to fill the phytochemical void. Herbs are one of the richest sources of phytochemicals on the planet and can provide you with greater access to protective phytochemicals than any other source. In **Part Two**, we'll explore how to make herbs part of your life.

Chapter Highlights

- Our need for herbal phytochemicals is rooted in our ancestral foraging diet, which included a wide variety of plants.

- The human diet changed significantly with the rise of agriculture. Notably, herbal phytochemicals were largely phased out in our shift to a grain-based diet.

- Our physiology has not changed significantly over time. Our bodies still crave phytochemicals to operate at our full potential.

- Modern vegetables have been cultivated to taste good and be high in vitamins, but most do not offer phytochemical potency. In selectively breeding the bitter taste out of vegetables, we lost phytochemical potency.

- Taking herbs can be an important way for us to get more phytochemicals into our diets.

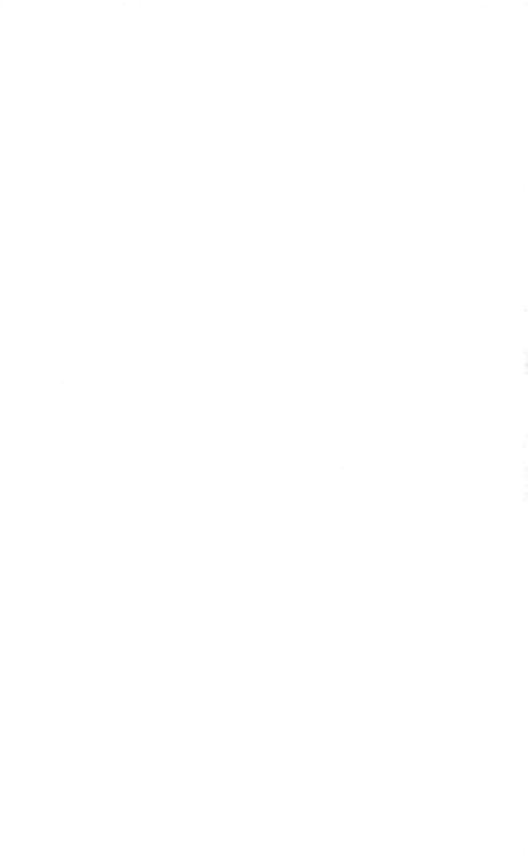

Part Two

Embracing Herbs

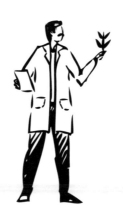

Making herbs a part of your life is a key strategy for optimizing cellular wellness. To gain full benefit from herbal phytochemicals, potency and consistency are key. In this section, we will explore the many ways to make herbs a part of your life. I'll teach you where to start with herbs and supplements—and introduce you to a range that you can build on and customize to your needs.

Here's what you'll learn in Part Two:

- Classifying herbs along a spectrum of therapeutic potential and safety

- Defining herbs for everyday use

- Understanding herbal preparations

- Herbal supplements versus vitamin supplements

- Featured regimen of herbs to take every day

- Herbs with antimicrobial properties and when to use them

7

Understanding the Spectrum of Herbs

When I was a newbie to the herbal supplement world, I found walking down the supplement aisles of a health food store to be quite intimidating. There were often dozens of bottles to choose from, each containing different combinations of herbs. The internet was even more dizzying; a single search might reveal hundreds of products.

Determined to master herbs, I spent years immersed in study. I attended herbal conferences around the country and devoured authoritative books on the different forms of traditional herbal medicine from around the world: traditional Chinese medicine; Ayurvedic medicine from India; and North American, European, and Amazonian medicine.

Frankly, it was a bit overwhelming (unnecessarily so, as I found out later). Each different herbal tradition uses a wide selection of herbs specific to one region of the world. Studying different traditions meant studying hundreds of unique herbs. Also, I found the methods used by these ancient herbal traditions for evaluating patients and defining therapies were complex and foreign to my medical training.

Fortunately, modern science has made understanding herbs quite a bit easier. What was missing was knowledge of phytochemicals and how phytochemicals interact with cells and communication pathways in the body to provide therapeutic benefits. Because many plants from around the world are related and share similar phytochemical makeup, they typically share similar therapeutic properties. It means that herbs from different places can be used for similar purposes.

In other words, you don't need a deep understanding of the world's herbal traditions to gain full benefit from taking herbs. Because so many herbs have overlapping properties, knowing about a dozen or so herbs is all you need. To start, you'll want a half-dozen herbs to take on a daily basis to promote wellness. Beyond that, it's handy to know about a few others for addressing specific issues, such as taming a viral illness or keeping your heart healthy as you age. By the end of this book, all the information you need to make herbs a functional part of your life will be right at your fingertips.

The Herbal Safety Spectrum

The first step in using herbs is defining what an herb is. That varies depending on who you talk to. To a botanist, an herb is any non-woody plant. To a chef, herbs refer to culinary herbs that add flavor to food. To a practicing herbalist, an herb is an edible plant used specifically for therapeutic benefits. Herbs used for therapeutic purposes can include the leaves, roots, flowers, berries of various wild plants, and the bark of certain trees (which is technically not an herb at all, according to botanists). Even defining an herb as a plant isn't absolute because certain edible mushrooms (which are fungi, not plants) are routinely used in herbal medicine right alongside herbs.

While the majority of commonly used herbs have a long history of human use and have a low potential to cause harm, there are exceptions. Some herbs contain phytochemicals with drug-like actions. Stronger drug-like actions are associated with a higher incidence of side effects and adverse reactions. For these herbs, caution is advised, and a few should be avoided altogether.

To help guide your choices, I created a chart to define the relative therapeutic and safety potential of various herbs. The farther you move toward the left side of the chart, the less specific the actions of the herb and thus a lower potential for side effects and adverse reactions. Toward the right are herbs with more specific and drug-like actions, where you would expect a greater potential for side effects and toxicity. Beyond the examples provided for each category on the chart, Appendix B categorizes a more extensive list of commonly used herbs.

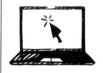

A printable, updated version of this list is available at **CellularWellness.com/Extras**

The Herbal Safety Spectrum

	The Green Zone			The Yellow Zone	The Red Zone
Vegetables	Reishi	Japanese Knotweed	Passionflower	Marijuana	Fox Glove
Food Plants	Everyday Herbs	Antimicrobial Herbs	Herbs with Targeted Actions	Cautionary Herbs	Potentially Harmful Plants

Food Plants

Starting at the far left are plants consumed primarily as foods. In other words, you eat them primarily to gain calories and not for therapeutic benefits. That being said, many food plants contain valuable phytochemicals. The phytochemicals found in food plants are mainly protective and don't cause specific physiologic actions in the body or drug-like effects. Not surprisingly, consumption of food plants is associated with a very low incidence of side effects and adverse reactions.

However, the margins between a food and an herb used for therapeutic benefits are not always distinct. Some food plants—broccoli, garlic, blueberries, acai and goji berries, and bitter melon, just to name a few—can be found with their phytochemicals concentrated into a supplement. And even though culinary herbs, such as oregano, basil, and rosemary, are best known for seasoning food, their therapeutic benefits rival any other herb.

Making the distinction between therapeutic herbs and food depends primarily on how a plant is used. For the purposes of this book, if a plant is consumed as part of a meal, it's placed in the food category. On the other hand, if a plant is consumed primarily for the benefits of its phytochemicals, it's placed in the therapeutic herb category. For example, fresh rosemary from the garden sprinkled into a sauté would put rosemary in the food category. Whereas taking a standardized extract of rosemary on a daily basis would put it in the therapeutic herb category (more on herbal preparations in Chapter 8).

Everyday Herbs

Just to the right of food plants is a sweet spot on the chart that I define as everyday herbs. As the heart of this book, these herbs are ideal candidates for anyone to take on a daily basis to promote or maintain wellness.

Consuming these herbs has low potential for side effects and adverse reactions. Overall, the risk associated with everyday herbs is no greater than that of most food plants. Their therapeutic actions are derived primarily from protecting our cells from a variety of stress factors and normalizing hormones that have been disrupted by stress. Because the phytochemicals of these herbs don't interfere with enzymes or hormone receptors in the body, their potential for causing drug-like effects is minimal.

Note that the absence of drug-like actions doesn't mean these herbs are "weak." In fact, some of the best herbs for promoting wellness and preventing chronic illness—the ones that brought me back to health—are found in this category. **As with many things in life, slow and steady wins the race.** While these herbs don't have an immediate drug-like effect, their power to cultivate long-term wellness at the cellular level should not be underestimated.

There are many wonderful herbs in the everyday category to choose from, with **turmeric**, **reishi mushroom**, and **rhodiola** being a few of my personal favorites. They each offer unique benefits that can be paired together for a synergistic effect. We will deep dive into this category of herbs in the next chapter.

Antimicrobial Herbs

Just beyond the "everyday" herbs are herbs with stronger antimicrobial properties. Historically, they were used to treat illnesses that we now know were caused by infections. Although these herbs are generally well tolerated, have a low incidence of drug-like effects or side effects, and can be taken for long durations when needed, I typically don't recommend them for individuals who aren't struggling with health issues. The reason is that people who are healthy just don't need that kind of antimicrobial power on an everyday basis. Save it for when you really need it. These herbs are useful to support recovery from many types of chronic symptoms, especially if there is a possible association with intracellular microbes. They are also useful for acute viral illnesses. (The proper use of antimicrobial herbs will be further covered in Chapter 10.)

It should be noted that **there are a few exceptions in the antimicrobial herb category, which do have potential for side effects**. Examples include *Stillingia sylvatica*, which can cause vomiting, skin rashes, fatigue, and sweating; **black walnut** (*Juglans nigra*), which can contain a toxic chemical called juglone; and **wormwood** (*Artemisia absinthium*), which contains a chemical called thujone that is toxic to kidneys and nerve tissue with prolonged use. These herbs sometimes show up in products promoted as natural antimicrobials, so it is something to be aware of. Not to say that these herbs shouldn't ever be used, but they fit into the cautionary category and should only be used for limited durations.

Herbs with Targeted Actions

A bit further to the right, you'll find herbs that offer more specific actions and benefits, but still have low potential for side effects and strong drug-like effects. This is due to the presence of phytochemicals in the herb that affects enzymes or hormone receptors, which causes a specific physiologic effect. Though all herbs in this category are beneficial to take long term, typically they are used for more targeted purposes, such as chronic stress or gut restoration.

A few examples include **passionflower** and **lemon balm**, which are both excellent herbs for promoting calm, but are free of drug-like effects and are generally safe to take on a regular basis. Another wonderful herb is **slippery elm**, which contains a substance called mucilage that protects irritated mucous membranes of nasal passageways and the intestinal tract. I commonly recommend this for mild reflux or during allergy season. And yet another is **bitter melon**, an herb that can help normalize blood sugar levels in individuals who have developed carbohydrate intolerance. More examples of herbs with targeted actions will be covered in Part Three and Part Four of this book.

The categories of herbs mentioned thus far fall into what I define as the *green zone*. These are herbs or food plants that have a low potential for side effects and toxicity. As a general rule, they can be taken on a regular basis. Note, however, that it's possible for anyone to have an unexpected severe reaction to any herb. When using a new herb or herbal product for the first time, it's advised to start with the lowest possible dose and wait 12 to 24 hours before taking another dose to see how your body will react to the herb. Please review the precautions in Chapter 8 before taking any herb on a regular or long-term basis.

For more information about common uses and key cautions for the *green zone* herbs mentioned in this book, visit **CellularWellness.com/Extras**

Just inside the *green zone*, I specifically want to call your attention to **CBD oil** (cannabidiol oil) from hemp. This herbal substance has been the subject of much controversy because it is from a plant strain that has close kinship to one commonly called marijuana. Hemp is a variety of *Cannabis sativa*. Unlike marijuana, hemp does NOT contain significant amounts of tetrahydrocannabinol (THC), the chemical that causes euphoria. Studies have shown that CBD oil can be effective for relieving mild anxiety, sleep dysfunction, and mild pain, but will not cause euphoria or habituation. (See Chapter 14 for more information on CBD oil.)

Defining Safety of Herbs

If you randomly collected plants and mushrooms from any natural area in the world, chances are that you'd end up with a few plants and mushrooms that could harm you. The phytochemical makeup of some plants just isn't compatible with our biochemistry. Some are even poisonous. Humans, however, learned to be selective a very long time ago.

There's little doubt that some of the wild plants and mushrooms defined as herbs today were part of that ancient foraged diet. As humans moved beyond foraging to farming, some plants were carried forward as culinary and medicinal herbs. The fact that the traditional use of medicinal herbs and mushrooms has been an integral part of every human culture on earth strongly suggests that the safety of commonly used herbs and medicinal mushrooms can reasonably be assumed. Honestly, it's a bit baffling that some people have more confidence in a drug that may have only been on the market for a few years than in an herb that has been used for more than a thousand years.

In the last few decades, science has turned its attention toward verifying the safety and efficacy of herbs traditionally used around the world. Both animal and human toxicology studies have shown that the incidence of toxicity and side effects associated with many commonly used herbs is remarkably low. This includes all of the herbs I've categorized as *green zone* herbs. Once you move outside of the *green zone*, the potential for toxicity goes up.

Cautionary Herbs

As we move toward the right side of the chart into the *yellow zone*, the incidence of potential side effects, interactions with drugs, and adverse reactions goes up. It's because these herbs contain phytochemicals that are potentially toxic. Though many of them have excellent therapeutic value and are sometimes a better choice than a drug with similar therapeutic actions, it's wise to seek advice from a practicing herbalist to gain the best results. If you are taking prescription medications, check with your health care provider before starting these herbs.

One example of an herb that's best to consult an herbalist before using is **St. John's wort**. This is especially true if you are taking medications. St. John's wort has well-known antidepressant properties. It works by inhibiting the breakdown of serotonin in the brain. Serotonin is a mood elevator. This is exactly the same mechanism by which many antidepressants, such as Prozac˚ and Zoloft˚, work. The drug-like actions of St. John's wort can interfere with the actions of other drugs. It also carries a higher incidence of side effects than many other herbs. Therefore, it should be used with caution.

Licorice is a well-known herb that should come with a recommendation for caution. It provides a range of benefits, including balancing underactive adrenal functions, but prolonged use of licorice extracts can overstimulate adrenal functions. For this reason, use of therapeutic doses of standardized licorice extract should be guided by a professional (low doses of licorice found in herbal tea are okay).

Other examples of herbs that require caution include **valerian** and **kava**. Kava is an herb with sedative properties from the South Pacific, where it is used in rituals. It is widely available as an herbal supplement and is commonly used to reduce anxiety and promote sleep. In high doses, however, it can cause intoxication and is habituating if used regularly. Generally, this one is best taken under the supervision of a professional. The same goes for valerian, which is also commonly found in products promoted for sleep. It has a relatively high incidence of side effects and can be mildly habituating.

Further to the right, at the outer margin of the *yellow zone*, you'll find **marijuana**. Marijuana is hemp's alter ego. Though it shares commonality in species, it comes from a completely different variety of *Cannabis sativa* than hemp. The primary difference is that marijuana contains significant concentrations of THC, while hemp does not. Although marijuana is best known for its recreational use to induce euphoria, it has valuable therapeutic properties for pain relief and conditions such as PTSD. Unlike opioids (narcotics and heroin), medical marijuana cannot cause death by overdose. It is habituating, but the withdrawal is much less severe than with opioids. This makes it safer for long-term pain management than any other choice, but it's still a medicinal herb that should only be used under supervision.

Size Matters When It Comes to Toxicity

When insects chomp down on tobacco leaves, *nicotine* and other chemicals are released. Nicotine is lethal to an insect's nervous system. Yet for a human who is using tobacco products, it provides a mild buzz that stimulates release of dopamine, a "feel-good" hormone. Tobacco use is highly habituating because the accompanying release of dopamine is associated with feelings of pleasure and satisfaction. Many herbs contain phytochemicals that are toxic to insects and microbes, but fortunately, most are not toxic to us and don't cause drug-like effects.

Potentially Harmful Plants

Moving into the *red zone* at the far right are plant substances that have strong drug-like properties but aren't regulated and are potentially harmful. These plant substances are best avoided completely. One example is **kratom**, a plant derivative with narcotic properties that can be addictive. The fact that it is unregulated by the Food and Drug Administration (FDA), but not defined as illegal by the United States Drug Enforcement Administration (DEA), makes it all the more concerning. Another is **ephedra** (ma huang in traditional Chinese medicine), a potent stimulant once used in weight loss and responsible for many deaths from overdose. Though it was banned from sale as a dietary supplement in 2006, ephedra (and ephedra look-alikes) still show up for sale on the internet.

At the very far right side of the chart, you'll find pharmaceuticals. Most people don't realize that over 70% of drugs originally came from plant sources. Many others come from synthetic drugs that also originally came from a plant or some other natural source. Drugs, however, typically don't come from plants defined as herbs. Most drugs are derived from plants that are considered poisonous. In the world of pharmaceuticals, poisons can sometimes be valuable. When used at a carefully controlled, therapeutic dose, this effect can be used to block symptoms or slow the progression of an illness in some way.

Unlike herbs, pharmaceuticals are derived from a *single* phytochemical isolated from a plant. Typically, these isolated chemical substances have very specific actions. They work by turning on or off specific enzymes or mimicking different signaling agents in the body. Therapeutically, this can have the effect of modifying or blocking processes in the body that have become dysfunctional. In the process of selecting single phytochemicals with specific actions, however, the natural intelligence inherent to the full spectrum of the plant's phytochemicals is lost. Therefore, the potential to protect cells and promote healing is also lost.

Once a phytochemical with drug-like properties is isolated from a plant, it's often chemically manipulated to further increase its potency, and then it is synthetically produced on a mass scale. Synthetic manipulation makes the chemical more foreign to us and thus more difficult for the liver to metabolize. This makes it all the more toxic. Because drugs have such a high potential for toxicity, anything beyond the narrow therapeutic dose can shut the whole body down. People typically respect this; everyone knows that taking a greater-than-prescribed dose of *any* drug can lead to serious consequences. It's for good reason that you should put a lock on your medicine cabinet.

One example of a drug that comes from a poisonous plant is digitalis, a medication used for heart failure. Digitalis comes from a phytochemical in **foxglove**, a common ornamental plant that graces many summer gardens. Digitalis works by blocking an enzyme in a way that leads to increased contraction of the heart muscle. But in anything but very low and carefully controlled doses, it stops the heart from beating altogether. Digoxin, the synthetic version of digitalis, is still used in hospitals today.

Another valuable drug that comes from a poisonous plant is Taxol,[51] which is derived from a phytochemical found in the bark of the **Pacific**

---

51   National Cancer Institute. Success Story: Taxol (NSC 125973). https://dtp.cancer.gov/timeline/flash/success_stories/s2_taxol.htm. Accessed February 28, 2022.

yew tree, *Taxus brevifolia*. Specifically, it's highly toxic to rapidly growing cells (in other words, cancer cells). It was first discovered in 1962, but it wasn't until 1992 that the FDA approved it for treating ovarian cancer. Two years later, it was approved for treating breast cancer. Since then, it has also been found to be effective in treating cases of Kaposi's sarcoma and certain forms of lung cancer.

Despite their toxicity, the world would be at a loss without pharmaceuticals. We need drugs that treat heart failure, treat cancer, act as anesthesia agents, block runaway inflammation, and more. However, relying exclusively on drugs to treat illness while doing little to prevent illness is shortsighted. That's a place where herbs could make a real difference because herbs can help to keep our immune system strong.

Getting to Know the Herbs Around You

I'm an avid walker and my favorite walks are in natural areas. I've always wanted to know more about the plants around me. However, that's challenging because there are so many plants, and I don't routinely carry a guidebook. This problem was recently solved for me by an inexpensive smartphone app called *PictureThis*. With a click of the camera, it compares the plant in question against an enormous database of known plants. It's opened up a whole new world for me. What was a "green wall" of unknown species is now becoming more familiar. By a wide margin, I've found that most plants are non-poisonous, and a surprising number have been used by humans as therapeutic herbs. You have to be careful, though: there are always a few deadly poisonous plants scattered about and they often resemble nonpoisonous ones.

Defining Herbs for Everyday Use

Although taking herbs every day specifically to promote health and longevity is just catching on in Western culture, the idea isn't new. Asian and Middle Eastern herbal traditions have long recognized the value of taking herbs with restorative or rejuvenating powers on a daily basis. In traditional Chinese medicine, the use of tonics (herbal substances that invigorate the body and restore tone), dates back thousands of years. In Ayurvedic medicine, the traditional medicine of India, herbs with properties of lengthening lifespan and invigorating the body are categorized as rasayana.

Our newfound Western appreciation for using herbs on a daily basis to protect wellness can be credited to a Soviet researcher, Dr. Nikolai Lazarev, who coined the term *adaptogen* in 1958. Adaptogens are now recognized as herbs that contribute to longer life by strengthening and invigorating different organs and systems throughout the body.

Dr. Lazarev was searching for substances that could improve human tolerance to stress. His definition of an adaptogen included three primary criteria:

- **Counteract a range of different stress factors**—including toxic chemicals, radiation, temperature extremes, undue physical stress, microbes, and even chronic mental stress.

- **Have nonspecific actions**—that is, full-body benefit with no drug-like effects.

- **Have low toxicity**—do not cause harm or alter normal functions of the body.

Trained as a pharmacist, Dr. Lazarev's initial search was for a drug that met the criteria of an adaptogen. He quickly found that all known drugs have very specific actions and significant potential for side effects. He had more success when he turned his attention toward plant substances used in traditional forms of medicine. Lazarev was eventually joined by other researchers who ultimately identified a half-dozen plants that fit the primary criteria for an adaptogen. Among the list of original adaptogens were **schisandra** (*Schisandra chinensis*); **Asian ginseng** (*Panax ginseng*); **eleuthero**, often called **Siberian ginseng** (*Eleutherococcus senticosus*); **rhodiola** (*Rhodiola rosea*); and **rhaponticum** (*Rhaponticum carthamoides*).

Adaptogens quickly became popular among Soviet Union leaders, military personnel, polar explorers, pilots, athletes, and virtually anyone who had to work under mentally or physically demanding conditions. Adaptogens were found to improve stamina and resilience while in stressful conditions—working in extreme cold or at high altitudes, exposure to radiation, intense physical labor, sleep deprivation, and mental stress. When the Iron Curtain came down in 1989, data that Soviet scientists had been collecting for years defining the efficacy and safety of adaptogenic herbs became available to the world at large.

A key feature of adaptogens is their safety. They are well tolerated by most adults and have a low rate of interaction with other herbs or most drugs. Because herbs with adaptogenic properties are generally free of side effects, they are well suited to be taken on a daily basis to maintain wellness.

Further refinements in the definition of adaptogen include these details:

- All adaptogens help modulate and/or enhance the immune system. By protecting cells from stress, adaptogens reduce the workload on the immune system, allowing it to function better.

- All adaptogens have antistress qualities that help provide stabilizing effects on the neuroendocrine system, especially the central hormone pathway in the body called the HPA axis (hypothalamic-pituitary-adrenal axis). In other words, adaptogens rebalance hormones that have been disrupted by stress.

- All adaptogens inhibit dysfunction in mitochondria. They do this primarily by reducing cellular stress, which decreases energy demands on mitochondria.

In the years since the concept of adaptogen was first introduced, herbs with adaptogenic properties have been widely accepted by herbal circles in both the East and West. Not surprisingly, dozens of other herbs, already recognized by other herbal traditions as having restorative properties, have been found to fit the criteria for adaptogens.

Not all herbs that fit into the everyday category are considered adaptogens, however. There are plenty of herbs that protect cells from stress factors, are safe for everyday use, and are free of drug-like effects, but don't directly affect stress hormones. For example, ashwagandha, mentioned above, is defined as an adaptogen because it balances the HPA axis. Hawthorn, however, does not, and therefore it is not considered an adaptogen, though it does meet all the other criteria and is an excellent herb to take for everyday use to promote wellness and prevent chronic illness.

The same would be true for turmeric, an excellent everyday herb for reducing inflammation. In India, turmeric is liberally used in most of their flavorful curries. Its anti-inflammatory properties may be one reason the people of India experience very low rates of dementia and cancer. We can't be sure whether turmeric can be given all the credit, but because dementia is on the rise in the U.S., why not enjoy some curry and hedge your bets? For even more protection, take a high-grade turmeric supplement.

In formal circles, turmeric and hawthorn are referred to as adaptogen companions, but you don't need to get hung up on definitions to enjoy the benefits. I encourage you to get all the protective phytochemicals you can from your diet and expand that by taking herbal supplements that fit the category of everyday herbs. In Chapter 9, I'll provide a basic list of everyday herbs that work together to protect your health.

Recommended Reading:

Two American herbalists, David Winston and Donald Yance, have been particularly instrumental in increasing awareness of the value of adaptogenic herbs. Both are pioneers in herbal medicine and have played a key role in the resurgence of herbalism in the past several decades.

David Winston's *Adaptogens, Herbs for Strength, Stamina, and Stress Relief* (co-written with Steven Maimes), details 25 different herbs defined as adaptogens. The monographs include traditional uses of the herbs alongside evidence-based scientific verification and safety information. In addition to providing a comprehensive introduction to herbal medicine, David's 2019 2nd edition unveils new research detailing the function of adaptogens at the cellular level.

In *Adaptogens in Medical Herbalism*, Donald Yance provides a detailed history of research on adaptogens, including the original Soviet investigations. He recognizes three categories of restorative herbs: primary adaptogens (herbs which fit the strict criteria of an adaptogen as validated by scientific investigations), secondary adaptogens (herbs that may not fit all criteria of primary adaptogens but offer value), and adaptogen companions (restorative herbs and supplements that are not technically adaptogens but enhance the actions of other adaptogens). Yance's book has a strong focus on the anticancer and longevity-promoting properties of various herbs.

Chapter Highlights

- You don't need a deep understanding of the world's herbal traditions to gain the full benefits of taking herbs.

- Because so many herbs have overlapping properties, knowing about a dozen or so herbs is all you need.

- **The Herbal Safety Spectrum** is a chart you can use to help define the relative therapeutic and safety potential of various herbs. See Appendix B for more than 200 herbs rated on the Herbal Safety Spectrum or visit **CellularWellness.com/Extras** for the extended list as well as periodic chart updates and additions

- Everyday herbs, such as adaptogens, turmeric, hawthorn, and others, are the heart of this book and ideal for anyone to take on a daily basis to promote or maintain wellness.

- Everyday herbs work by having a gentle, restorative effect on your cells and promoting balance at the cellular level with consistent use.

8

Making Herbs Part of Your Life

Given the stress factors we're all up against—and the fact that it's just plain impossible to eradicate stress entirely from modern life—it makes sense to give your body all the extra help it can get. That's where protective phytochemicals come in.

And the more the better. No doubt, a well-rounded diet weighted toward vegetables and fruits is a good start. For example, cooked tomatoes are high in lycopene, a potent phytochemical cell protector that has been associated with reduced prostate cancer risk in men. Lutein and zeaxanthin, phytochemicals that give summer squash and carrots their bright colors, protect eyes and skin from sun damage. Kale, spinach, and pasture-raised eggs are also a good source of these protective phytochemicals. And the blue in blueberries comes from phytochemicals called anthocyanins, which are potent antioxidants that protect everything from your vision to your vascular system.

Even a diet heavily weighted toward fresh vegetables and fruits, however, doesn't come close to matching the phytochemical concentrations found in herbs. As discussed in Chapter 6, we've largely bred phytochemicals out of our food plants to make way for calories and better taste. In contrast, herbs are plants that remain in a wild state. As such, their phytochemical concentration is much greater than any food plant. This is also true of cultivated herbs, which are grown under conditions to maximize yield of beneficial phytochemicals.

You may already be consuming some herbs without recognizing it. Black pepper, the ubiquitous companion to salt present in almost every kitchen in the world, is actually an herb that provides significant health benefits. The phytochemicals present in black pepper offer antioxidant, antimicrobial, and stomach-protective properties. Piperine, the most active phytochemical in black pepper, is also known to increase intestinal absorption of other healthful phytochemicals.

Black pepper, of course, is just one of many herbs that fall into the category of culinary herbs that we should use liberally and often to enhance our cooking. Just a few examples of common culinary herbs include basil, oregano, thyme, rosemary, turmeric, ginger, garlic, cinnamon, cumin, cardamom, and nutmeg.

Beyond infusing robust flavor into food, culinary herbs provide profound health benefits. All herbs are loaded with phytochemicals that provide anti-inflammatory properties, potent antioxidants, and protection against a variety of microbial threats. Ounce for ounce, turmeric, cinnamon, ginger, and oregano have ten times the antioxidant power of blueberries.[52] These phytochemical substances were built to protect the plant's cells, but they also protect your cells.

---

52   Halvorsen BL, Carlsen MH, Phillips KM, et al. Content of redox-active compounds (ie, antioxidants) in foods consumed in the United States. *Am J Clin Nutr.* 2006;84(1):95-135.

Spice It Up!

Dust off your spice shelf and make room to try something new! Spices can turn a "same old" dish into something special. The next time you're at the grocery store, pick out an herb that you've never used before. Do an internet search to look up a few recipes featuring that herb. You may also want to look up the herb's history and origins. It may become a regular addition to your cooking.

If you've never had an herb garden, consider starting one. Herbs are easy to grow because they are naturally pest resistant. Herbs can be grown from seed, but most garden centers offer seedlings in the spring, which makes it extra easy to get your garden growing. Common offerings include sweet basil (my personal favorite), thyme, oregano, dill, rosemary, sage, cilantro, and chives.

Another herb you know is tea. Whether referring to black tea popular in the West or green tea common in the East, the beverage tea comes from leaves of the plant called *Camellia sinensis* (a cousin of the showy flowering camellia). Tea leaves are actually the world's most commonly consumed herb. Green tea, prepared from fresh leaves that are steamed and dried, has a mellow flavor. When the same leaves are, instead, crushed and allowed to oxidize in the sun while drying, it gives them a deeper color and a slightly bitter taste.

Beyond flavor, the most sought-after benefit of drinking tea is the stimulating effect provided by caffeine. Caffeine is actually just one of a family of phytochemicals found in coffee, tea, cacao, and a few other plants. It gives us that boost we all love by blocking hormones associated with sleep and mimicking excitatory neurotransmitters. Tea made from camellia leaves also contains a range of other phytochemicals that have protective effects on our cells. One example is *catechins*, potent antioxidants that slow aging and prevent chronic illness by protecting cells from damaging free radicals.

Reading the Tea Leaves

A study in the *Proceedings of the National Academy of Sciences* journal found that drinking five cups of black tea a day seems to supercharge T cells (a type of white blood cell that plays a key role in the immune response).[53] After two weeks of drinking the tea, the cells produced ten times more *interferon*, a chemical that actively fights viruses and helps stop them from replicating. If you prefer green tea, it contains about three times the catechin concentration of black tea, along with a range of other protective phytochemicals. Green tea also contains L-theanine,[54] an amino acid that research shows may work with other polyphenols to give your immune system a boost. It also moderates some of the stimulating effects of caffeine.

Though it isn't thought of as such, tea from *Camellia sinensis* leaves is technically an herbal tea. Of course, there are many other herbal teas that can be prepared from fresh or dried herbs. Enjoying a cup

---

53 Kamath, Arati B. et al. Antigens in tea-beverage prime human Vγ2Vδ2 T cells in vitro and in vivo for memory and nonmemory antibacterial cytokine responses. *Proc Natl Acad Sci U S A*. 2003;100(10):6009-6014.

54 Li C, Tong H, Yan Q, et al. L-theanine improves immunity by altering TH2/TH1 cytokine balance, brain neurotransmitters, and expression of phospholipase C in rat hearts. *Med Sci Monit*. 2016;22:662-669.

of herbal tea with calming properties, such as chamomile or lemon balm, is a great way to ease into a good night's sleep. Drinking hibiscus tea is good for your cardiovascular system, and peppermint tea can soothe an upset stomach. You don't have to have a specific reason to drink herbal tea, however. They can be enjoyed simply for the flavor they provide and as a way to boost your daily quota of phytochemicals.

Getting Started with Herbal Supplements

Though culinary herbs and herbal teas can make up some of the difference in our modern phytochemical deficiency, it still doesn't approximate the phytochemical concentration found in our ancestral foraged-food diet. The most practical way to fill that void, I've found, is by taking herbal supplements. Herbal supplements provide the highest concentrations of phytochemicals to be found anywhere. They are an outstanding option for supplementing the herbal phytochemicals we are missing in our modern diets and lifestyles.

Keep in mind that there's a distinct difference between herbal supplements and vitamin supplements. Herbs are a high-potency source of phytochemicals, but not a concentrated source of vitamins and minerals. Look to a healthy diet as your best source of vitamins and minerals and herbal supplements as the best way to top off your daily phytochemical quota.

While wild harvesting or growing herbs and then making your own herbal preparations is an option, it's time intensive and not very practical for the pace of life of most people. Besides that, you'll also miss out on the benefits of great herbs that may not grow in your area. This is where commercial herbal preparations can be of great value.

Qualifications for Quality

I often have people tell me that they'd like to take herbs, but they're concerned about finding quality products. With thousands of herbal products on the market, making those initial choices can be quite intimidating. Don't worry; by the time you finish reading this section of the book, you'll have the confidence you need to find herbal products that meet your expectations.

The place to begin is defining what makes a quality herbal product. The primary considerations to keep in mind when choosing an herbal product include **potency**, **purity**, and **synergy**.

Potency

The potency of an herbal product is defined by its concentration of phytochemicals, which can vary quite a bit based on how the product is prepared. The three most common preparations of herbs include **powdered whole herb**, **liquid extractions**, and **powdered extractions**.

Herbal preparations can come from different parts of the plant including the leaves, bark, stems, roots, flowers, and fruit. The highest concentration of phytochemicals can vary depending on the plant; it may be concentrated in the leaves and stems of one herb and the roots or rhizomes of another.

Powdered whole herb products are made by drying the parts of the plant being used and crushing the dried plant into a fine powder. The powder can be put into capsules, formed into tablets, or sold as loose powder. The biggest disadvantage of whole herb powders is that the concentration of phytochemicals is often low, as the bulk of the powder is inert plant fiber. Although whole herb powders are often inexpensive, you get what you pay for.

Another herbal preparation method is **liquid extractions**, also known as *herbal tinctures*. To make an extraction, the desired parts of the plant are soaked in a liquid, typically water and alcohol, to extract the phytochemicals from the plant. After the extraction is complete, the plant parts are discarded. The potency of a tincture is defined by how much of the plant is used in the extraction. Quality tinctures will state the ratio of the liquid to the plant parts. A tincture with a 1:5 ratio is made with 1 oz of dried plant to 5 oz of liquid.

The advantage of herbal tinctures is higher concentrations of phytochemicals over whole herb powder. The disadvantage, of course, is that many highly beneficial herbs are extremely bitter. People often find tinctures to be unpleasant in taste and therefore hard to take consistently. Also, if you're taking several herbs, the amount of alcohol consumed is not insignificant. Although there are "alcohol-free" tinctures made with glycerite, these products tend to be lower in phytochemical concentration.

A **powdered extract** is my favorite preparation method, as it offers maximum phytochemical potency. A powdered extract is made by spraying a liquid extraction onto a surface and evaporating the liquid, leaving a powder consisting of pure phytochemicals. Powdered extracts are typically many times more potent than a whole herb powder. For example, 100 mg of powdered extract may contain the same phytochemical concentration as 1000 mg of whole herb powder.

Verification of potency is typically conveyed by a process called **standardization**. An extract is standardized by measuring key chemical constituents present in the herb. The potency of the extract is conveyed by the percentage of that phytochemical. For example, an ashwagandha extract standardized to 10% withanolides is significantly more potent than an ashwagandha extract standardized to 1% withanolides.

Standardized powdered extracts make up the majority of the herbal supplements I use. They are my go-to for gaining a full quota of daily phytochemicals. I use herbal tinctures when I can't find a particular herb in a powdered extract or when I'm trying a new individual herb and want to experience its unique taste. Tinctures also have an advantage for an individual who easily reacts to new substances because they can be dosed a drop at a time. I use whole herb powders only for certain herbs. For example, during my recovery, I used an herb with antimicrobial properties from the Amazon called anamu. Anamu is only available as a whole herb powder. It's typically dosed as 1200 mg twice daily.

Purity

Potency is the first indication of a quality herbal product, but purity can matter just as much. Purity is defined by several parameters. One is having the desired species of plant. Sometimes less expensive products contain related species of plants that are more common (therefore cheaper to obtain), but have less active phytochemicals.

Even more important, however, is the absence of impurities. Chemical impurities, heavy metals, and microbial contamination have obvious concerns. Even an herb harvested from the wild or grown under organic conditions can contain contaminants. Some plants readily pick up toxic substances from the soil or air. For example, a wild herb harvested from along roadsides may contain high concentrations of toxic substances from automobile exhaust. Chemical impurities can also be introduced by the extraction process. Some extracts are made using harsh chemicals that damage the phytochemicals and leave chemical residues in the final product.

Reputable supplement companies know where their herbs come from and perform independent, third-party testing of ingredients to ensure quality. This involves testing each batch of herbal extract for proper identification (verifying the plant species), potency, and purity; additional testing detects any organic toxins or heavy metal contaminants.

Typically, the more transparent a company is about their testing standards, the higher the quality of the products. At the end of the day, you want a product made by people with an appreciation for product purity and a deep understanding of herbal testing. While it's not practical or expected for you, as the consumer, to review lab test reports, you should do your homework on the quality standards and practices of any herbal brand you purchase from. The time you invest in choosing quality products will pay dividends for your health.

Synergy

As discussed in previous chapters, it's not the phytochemicals in an herb acting independently that make the difference. It's the phytochemicals working in synergy as a functional system that provides all the remarkable benefits. Therefore, quality herbal products contain the full spectrum of phytochemicals from the plant, as opposed to individual phytochemicals isolated from the herb. Only in rare cases, such as use of the phytochemical berberine for intestinal dysfunction, are single phytochemicals as useful as the full-spectrum herb.

Synergy also refers to the complementary effect of taking multiple herbs together. Phytochemicals from one herb can potentiate the value of other herbs by increasing absorption of other phytochemicals or by complementing the beneficial properties of phytochemicals in some way.

Two Herbs Are Better Than One

The turmeric in Indian curry dishes is felt to be one of the reasons why the rate of cancer and Alzheimer's is so low in India. However, the phytochemicals in turmeric aren't well absorbed. Interestingly, Indian curries also typically contain black pepper. Studies have shown that the addition of black pepper increases the bioavailability of the beneficial phytochemicals in turmeric (curcuminoids) by 1000%![55] This effect is an example of synergy: when herbs are combined, the overall effect is greater than that of the individual herbs.

You can think of it like an orchestra. In an orchestra, you don't hear the sound of each instrument—you hear the sound of all of the instruments playing in synergy. It's the harmony that makes the music come alive. Similarly, a blend of herbs amplifies the unique properties of each herb to create synergy in which the sum of all the herbs is more powerful than each herb individually.

Combining multiple herbs for synergy is a common practice in herbal medicine. Personally, I prefer to limit formulas to no more than six herbs to prevent diluting out the benefits of any one herb.

Delivery Methods

To gain the benefits of phytochemicals, you must, of course, get them inside your body. For that, there are a variety of different delivery

---

55   Shoba G, Joy D, Joseph T, Majeed M, Rajendran R, Srinivas PS. Influence of piperine on the pharmacokinetics of curcumin in animals and human volunteers. *Planta Med.* 1998;64(4):353-356.

methods, each with its own advantages and disadvantages. As someone who has been taking supplements for many years, I'll walk you through the practicality of each option. Keep in mind the importance of finding a delivery format that works well for you, based on your lifestyle and preferences, so that you can take the herbs consistently enough to see benefit.

For many people, the most practical way to take herbs is in a capsule. Both whole herb powders and powdered herbal extracts are available in capsules. Note that, because the potency is so much higher with extracts, it typically takes several large capsules of whole herb powder to equal the phytochemical concentration of one medium-sized capsule containing powdered herbal extract. Whenever possible, I look for standardized extracts to minimize the number of capsules required.

Capsule

Pros:

- Bypasses bitter taste
- One capsule of extract contains many times the potency of bulk whole herb powder
- Standardized dosing makes this the best option for achieving a therapeutic effect
- Ability to combine extract and whole herb for maximum synergistic benefit
- Portable and easy to take
- Has a long shelf life

Cons:

- Quality extracts are generally more expensive

- Sometimes requires taking many capsules

Some people prefer tinctures. Herbal tinctures can be dosed by the drop, which is ideal for someone who is very sensitive to chemical substances. Also, if you want to experience the taste of the herb, tinctures are the way to go. Keep in mind that many tinctures are very bitter in taste, which is their biggest drawback.

Tincture

Pros:

- Potent

- Well absorbed and fast acting

- Affordable

- Offers flexible dosing (can take by the drop)

- Has a long shelf life

Cons:

- Often unpleasantly bitter

- Involves consuming alcohol (unless glycerin based), sometimes in significant quantities if taking multiple tinctures at once

- More challenging for an on-the-go lifestyle

- Less ideal for traveling, especially with the limitations on bottle size with airline travel

Whole herb powders and powdered extracts can also be found in shake and smoothie mixes. Another popular delivery format is gummies or candies that contain herbal extracts. While these options can make getting your daily herbs more pleasant, they do have limitations. The biggest is that some of the most beneficial herbs are quite bitter and therefore are not ideal for smoothie mixes and gummies.

Drink Mix

Pros:

- Good option for consuming large quantities of mild (less bitter) herbs

- Allows you to make herbs a pleasant part of your day

Cons:

- Many wonderful herbs are not found in drink mixes due to their bitter taste

- In general, drink mixes offer far less potency than capsules or tinctures

- Most powdered herbs are whole herb powders, which are much lower in potency than standardized extracts.

Gummies/Candies

Pros:

- A way to consume herbs without taking capsules

- Some products do a nice job of hiding the taste

- Occasionally, can be a nice treat for consuming mild (less bitter) herbs

Cons:

- Low potency and concentration of phytochemicals

- The herbs that can be used in these products are limited

- High sugar-to-herb ratio

- Short shelf life; delivery form does not protect herb

- Most expensive option per dose of herbs

- Not recommended as a primary delivery form for herbs

Essential Oils

Although herbal products and essential oils both come from plants, they are not the same. The phytochemicals found in herbal extracts are used by the plant for protecting cells and coordinating internal functions. Essential oils, on the other hand, are used by plants specifically to deter insects and microbes. They are composed of volatile chemical substances called terpenes. Because these substances are potentially toxic to the plant's cells, they are contained within sacs located in the stems and leaves. When insects munch on a leaf, the noxious oils are released to chase the insect away.

Beyond deterring insects, terpenes have potent anti-inflammatory, antioxidant, and antimicrobial properties. Different plants have different spectrums of terpenes, giving them varying properties and benefits. In general, however, essential oils have a higher potential for toxicity than herbal products, a fact that should be respected.

The terpenes are removed from the plant by steam distillation. The final product is called an essential oil. Essential oils are extremely potent and generally only dosed a few drops at a time. They are most often used as aromatherapy. The oil is placed in a diffuser that sprays it into the air as a fine mist. Frankincense (of biblical fame) is a lovely mood elevator that you can use in a diffuser. Or you can simply put a few drops on your wrists, feet, or on your pillow. A few drops of lavender oil on your pillow at night can help ease you into sleep. The terpenes that make up essential oils are volatile, meaning that they evaporate completely and will not leave a stain on clothing or surfaces.

Certain essential oils such as frankincense, orange, turmeric, and lavender, can be used topically on skin but they are typically diluted with a carrier oil (usually grapeseed oil or jojoba oil). Topical uses for essential oils include rubs for sore muscles and joints or soothing dry and irritated skin (note that carrier oils do not evaporate and will stain clothing). Some essential oils, such as clove, thyme, and cinnamon, should not be used topically because they irritate skin.

Tea tree oil is a useful remedy for a wide range of ailments, including toenail fungus, though it may take persistence over many months. When greatly diluted (two drops stirred into one cup of water), it can be gargled as an antiseptic for sore throats. Don't swallow it; spit it out.

Neem oil can also be used for toenail fungus. I love neem oil because it has low toxicity as compared to some other essential oils, but it has very good antifungal properties. For folks who have mouth issues (canker sores, irritated gums, thrush), there are mouthwashes and toothpastes available with neem oil. My wife even uses neem oil (diluted, two tablespoons per gallon of water) to spray on plants suffering from powdery mildew or aphids.

Certain essential oils, including oregano oil, neem oil, and black cumin seed oil, are available in gel caps to use orally, typically for antimicrobial purposes, but this is generally not advised because of the high potential for any essential oil to irritate the stomach and intestinal lining. Oral essential oils should only be used under the guidance of a naturopath or herbalist.

Finding Quality Herbal Products

There can be a huge range in the quality (and price) of herbal supplements, and it can be overwhelming to know where to start. Quality matters when it comes to achieving the desired results. Bearing in mind that quality in herbs relates to their potency, purity and synergy, here are a few recommendations for choosing an herbal product. While this list is not exhaustive, it will serve as a good starting point.

The ingredient label on the bottle is the first place to look for quality. The more details listed on the label, the higher the potential for quality of the product. Beyond the milligram quantity of each herb in the supplement, look for the standardization or extraction ratio to be stated. This tells you the herb is an extract and not whole herb powder. In addition, I like to see the scientific name stated on the ingredient label or product website, but note this is not necessary in all cases.

Here's a comparative example of the same herb from two different products:

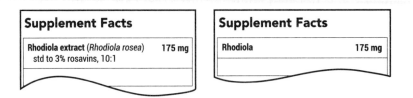

Supplement Facts	
Rhodiola extract (*Rhodiola rosea*) std to 3% rosavins, 10:1	**175 mg**

Supplement Facts	
Rhodiola	**175 mg**

In this case, the first ingredient is a standardized extract and you should assume that the second is a whole herb powder because no other information is provided. In terms of potency and quality, the first ingredient wins hands down. You might need to take ten times more of the second ingredient to gain the same level of benefit as the first.

The product webpage is also a source of information about quality. Information about supplement ingredients and company standards for quality should be easy to find. Companies producing high quality products are transparent about sharing ingredient information. If you have to go digging for what's in the product, assume the ingredients are of low quality or not adequately dosed.

Proprietary blends often contain low quality ingredients. It's not uncommon to find herbal supplements containing multiple herbs, but instead of providing the quantity of each herb, only the milligram quantity of all the herbs together is listed as a proprietary blend. Though this is meant to convey exclusivity, it's often a mechanism of hiding low quality ingredients. Generally, you're not getting good value for your money.

Price can be an indicator of quality, but not always. It is true that quality products cost more to produce, but expensive herbal supplements are not necessarily of high quality. All too often, marketing hype is used to sell low-quality ingredients for a premium price. Know what you're buying. Over the years, I've noticed a dramatic difference in the results achieved by patients who take premium-grade supplements as opposed to those who take less expensive herbal supplements. Investing in quality products will ultimately pay dividends for your health.

Do your homework to find brands with a strong track record that are willing to share details of their quality-control processes. There is no "one size fits all" quality indicator that covers every supplement. For example, what is important in measuring the quality of a vitamin product can be much different than for an herbal product. But the more information and transparency a brand is willing to offer about their ingredients, quality-assurance processes, sustainability practices, and third-party testing, the better. At the end of the day, it's the people and practices behind a brand that deliver quality products. If a company is not transparent about their team, mission, location, and quality commitments, then keep searching.

Recommended Reading:

Joe & Terry Graedon, *Spice Up Your Health: How Everyday Kitchen Herbs & Spices Can Lengthen & Strengthen Your Life*, 2016

An excellent guide to understanding the unique health benefits of common culinary herbs and spices, this book lays out simple and accessible options for making herbs a part of your everyday life—starting with your garden and spice rack. Complete with recipes and step-by-step explanations, you'll discover easy (and tasty) ways to boost your herbal intake.

Rosemary Gladstar, *Rosemary Gladstar's Medicinal Herbs: A Beginners Guide*, 2012

A great introduction to folk herbalism basics by the "godmother" of American herbalism. Rosemary has a deep love for plants and a delightful way of making herbs and holistic health approachable and fun. This fun book is full of recipes and instructions for growing, making, and using your own at-home herbal remedies.

David Hoffmann, FNIMH, AHG, *Medical Herbalism, the Science and Practice of Herbal Medicine*, 2003

This book is a classic herbal reference. It provides a comprehensive foundation on the principles and practice of clinical herbalism including phytochemistry, pharmacology, treatment approaches by body system, herbal actions, and a comprehensive selection of herbal monographs.

Chapter Highlights

- Protective phytochemicals give your body extra support to combat everyday stress.

- Herbal supplements provide the highest concentrations of phytochemicals and help fill the void found in our modern diets.

- When choosing an herbal product, factor in **potency**, **purity**, and **synergy** to get the highest quality.

- A variety of delivery methods exist for herbs, and the key to remaining consistent is finding one that works for you.

- Remember: The more details listed on an ingredient label, the higher the potential for the quality of the product.

9

Foundational Herbs for Every Day

While there are many choices for everyday herbs, I've narrowed it down to a list of favorites that I've used for years. I picked these herbs specifically because they are well known and well studied, are associated with very low potential for side effects and toxicity, and are free of drug-like effects. They provide foundational support for optimizing cellular health and counteracting the stress factors that promote chronic illness and accelerate aging.

You can start with one at a time or combine multiple herbs. The advantage of taking multiple herbs together is that you gain synergy (the benefits of the herbs are accentuated). These everyday herbs can be safely taken along with other herbs, a multivitamin, or other supplements such as fish oil.

As you'll discover in their individual profiles, these everyday herbs cover a lot of bases. They have the potential to increase your stamina, reduce inflammation in your body, balance hormones that have been disrupted by stress, and protect all of your organs (including your heart, liver, and brain). They do this by protecting your cells from stress.

"What about microbes?" you may ask. Although these particular herbs are best known for properties other than antimicrobial protection, each of them has been found by scientific studies to have antimicrobial properties. As I stated before, all plants produce antimicrobial phytochemicals— it's a necessity of survival. If you have certain health issues, however, you may elect to bring in herbs with stronger antimicrobial power. (Antimicrobial herbs are discussed in Chapter 10.)

While all the herbs listed below share many common benefits, each shines in its own way. Rhodiola is revered for increasing stamina and tolerance to physical stress. Reishi is an excellent immune system modulator. Turmeric is well known for its anti-inflammatory properties. Gotu kola has been treasured as a brain revitalizer in its native India for centuries. Shilajit is valued most for boosting energy and promoting optimal gut function. And milk thistle is liver protective (in a toxic world, we all need that). Combined, they give you a broad spectrum of coverage.

I am highlighting my favorite everyday herbs here, but keep in mind that there are many great herbs in the everyday category that can be added or substituted. For example, if daily stress is your issue, you may want to add ashwagandha, a previously mentioned adaptogen, to your daily regimen (it is also covered in Chapter 13). Or, you may want extra coverage for your cardiovascular system, and for that, there's no better herb than hawthorn (covered in Chapter 20).

Profiles of My Favorite Everyday Herbs

Rhodiola (*Rhodiola rosea*)

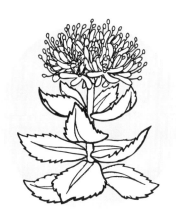

Rhodiola is a hardy perennial plant that grows in subarctic, high-altitude areas mainly in Europe and Asia, but it's also been found in the Appalachian mountains of the United States. The fact that rhodiola thrives in one of the harshest environments on earth is a testament to its adaptability. When we consume the phytochemicals that give rhodiola its powerful ability to endure, those traits are passed along.

When rhodiola was first defined as an adaptogen by modern scientists, it quickly became a favorite of Russian athletes and workers for improving stamina, supporting normal cardiovascular function, and maintaining alertness. The plant's ability to promote hardiness and stress resistance, however, was discovered ages ago. The documented use of rhodiola as a medicinal plant dates back almost 3,000 years in Siberia, China, and Tibet. Dioscorides, a Greek physician, described its use 2,000 years ago. There have even been suggestions that the Vikings used it to promote endurance and physical strength.[56]

Rhodiola enhances cardiovascular function and protects nerve and brain tissue. Traditionally, rhodiola was used to improve work tolerance at high altitudes; **research suggests that it may increase oxygen delivery to tissues, especially the heart.** Rhodiola is energizing and it also boosts mood, counteracts depression, and promotes restful sleep.

---

56   Ishaque S, Shamseer L, Bukutu C, Vohra S. Rhodiola rosea for physical and mental fatigue: a systematic review. *BMC Complement Altern Med.* 2012;12:70.

Rhodiola is a potent immunomodulator. This means it calms overactive portions of the immune system associated with destructive inflammation, but, at the same time, boosts the immune system's ability to fight off infections.

A 2016 review concluded that rhodiola helped improve mild stress-induced depression, most likely due to its role in regulating cellular response to stress, including in the neuroendocrine, neurotransmitter receptor, and molecular networks.[57] Other research has documented rhodiola's ability to enhance the oxygenation of tissues, balance blood glucose and insulin, reduce menopause symptoms, improve mood, improve learning and memory, and promote strength and sexual vigor.

Though rhodiola isn't typically recognized for its antimicrobial properties, two independent studies in 2018 and 2020 documented the antimicrobial activity of rhodiola's phytochemicals for a wide range of bacteria, many of which are potential pathogens, including various species of staphylococcus, streptococcus, and salmonella.[58]

An Adaptogenic Experience

Rhodiola is my first choice among all the adaptogens. I take rhodiola on a daily basis, but it became a favorite years ago on a skiing trip. The first day out on the slopes, we were at an elevation of up to 11,000 feet. I live at sea level, so that kind of altitude change is a recipe for altitude sickness. I had read about rhodiola's ability to increase tolerance to altitude, so I started taking it several days before the trip. I dosed up that morning before hitting the slopes. Not only did I not get altitude sickness, I was also able to keep up with the group!

---

57   Amsterdam JD, Panossian AG. Rhodiola rosea L. as a putative botanical antidepressant. *Phytomedicine*. 2016;23(7):770-783.

58   Kosakowska O, Bączek K, Przybył JL, et al. Antioxidant and antibacterial activity of roseroot (Rhodiola rosea L.) dry extracts. *Molecules*. 2018;23(7):1767.

Benefits of rhodiola:

- Reduces fatigue and restores energy

- Nervous system tonic

- Improves stress tolerance

- Promotes strength and endurance

- Promotes sexual vigor

- Modulates and balances immune system functions

- Enhances cardiovascular function and is heart protective

- Protects nerve and brain tissue

- Has antidepressant properties (increases serotonin and dopamine in the brain)

Suggested dosing: Rhodiola is available as a tincture or powdered extract. Typical dosage for a standardized powdered extract is 200-400 mg, one to three times daily. Make sure to use an extract, rather than the whole herbs (otherwise you'll need to use much more). If using a tincture, typical dosing ranges are 1-3 mL, two to four times daily.

Potential side effects and precautions: While rhodiola is generally well tolerated, it can be mildly stimulating for some people; therefore, avoid taking rhodiola late in the day to prevent potential interference with sleep. There are no known significant interactions with drugs.

Reishi (*Ganoderma lucidum*)

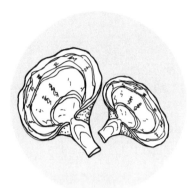

Reishi is a shelf mushroom that grows on the sides of trees. It looks somewhat like a fan with reddish-brown rainbow stripes. If you've ever taken a walk in a hardwood forest, you've probably come upon one. While different species of reishi mushrooms grow all over the world, *G. lucidum*, an Asian species, is the most studied for health benefits.

Reishi is best known for exceptional immunomodulating and antiviral properties. In other words, reishi helps to regulate and improve the immune system. **Reishi essentially directs the immune system to reduce harmful inflammation while increasing action against threatening microbes and cancer cells.** It also has direct antiviral and antimicrobial properties. The mushroom's power is due in part to its beta-glucans, polysaccharides found in fungi cell walls that are well known for their immune-enhancing ability.

In Asia, reishi is commonly used in conjunction with traditional cancer therapies. And, a growing body of research suggests the mushroom extract may help ramp up the body's defenses against the disease. A study in the journal *Nutrients*, for example, showed that the **extract helped prevent cancer cells' viability and blocked the release of inflammatory compounds in melanoma and breast cancer cells** while also blocking the release of inflammatory compounds.[59]

I am not suggesting that someone with cancer should forgo conventional treatment, but it's important to keep rethinking the way we look at

59   Barbieri A, Quagliariello V, Del Vecchio V, et al. Anticancer and anti-Inflammatory properties of Ganoderma lucidum extract effects on melanoma and triple-negative breast cancer treatment. *Nutrients*. 2017;9(3):210.

illness. This new viewpoint allows us to use tools such as reishi and other herbs to help mitigate the problem as early in the process as possible. Reishi has been extensively studied in Japan for potential anticancer properties and has been found to contain numerous potential cancer-fighting substances. So, taking it as part of a daily ongoing regimen to stay well and promote longevity makes a lot of sense.

Like rhodiola, reishi is an adaptogen, meaning it improves stamina during aerobic activity, boosts stress tolerance, reduces fatigue, restores normal adrenal-cortical function, and promotes calm and focus during stressful conditions. It offers significant cardiovascular benefits and has been used to prevent and treat altitude sickness, suggesting that it may also increase oxygenation of tissues. Reishi is neuro-supportive and promotes healthy liver function.

And there's another way reishi helps the body combat aging-accelerating stressors: it improves sleep. It helps to promote calm, a key step toward reducing high stress levels.

Benefits of reishi:

- Immunomodulating

- Anti-inflammatory

- Antiviral properties

- Anticancer properties

- Calming and restores normal sleep

- Anti-fatigue/adrenal support

- Increases resistance to stress

- Supports normal cardiovascular function

- Liver protective

Suggested dosing: Although reishi mushrooms are edible, they are hard (like cork) when dried, and that's not ideal for cooking. Reishi is most often purchased as powdered mushroom or extract. It has a slight chocolaty taste. I often mix some powdered reishi into smoothies, along with a banana or blueberries. You can also take it in capsule form at a dose of 200-400 mg, one to three times daily or in tincture form 3-5 mL, two to four times daily. As an indicator of potency, look for products with at least 7% beta-glucans.

Potential side effects and precautions: Well tolerated with rare side effects and no known long-term toxicity.

Herbs Are All around You

I was surprised to find that several of my favorite herbs known from distant herbal traditions grow right here in my home state of North Carolina. Gotu kola (*Centella asiatica*), an herb from Ayurvedic medicine of India, grows naturally along our coast. It's thought to be native and not transplanted. Though it hasn't been used commercially (thus far), the phytochemistry is the same as the species from India. Gotu kola is a calming herb that can be taken every day to promote optimal cognitive function.

Another favorite herb is *Rhodiola rosea*, which is native to Siberia and has been used through the ages to promote physical resilience. A very close relative with similar properties has been found growing at the higher altitudes of the Appalachian mountains.

If you take a jaunt through any woodlands, you may spy fan-shaped shelf mushrooms with brown rainbow streaks growing at the bases of older trees. These are reishi mushrooms. They are very close relatives of *Ganoderma lucidum*, the Asian species of reishi, which has been extensively studied for its antiviral, immune-enhancing, and anticancer properties.

Turmeric (*Curcuma longa*)

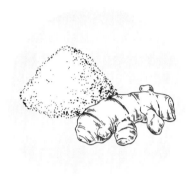

With its natural bright yellow color, turmeric is the spice that defines an Indian curry. Beyond adding flavor to food, turmeric also offers potent anti-inflammatory properties. It may be one of the reasons why the people of India experience lower than average levels of Alzheimer's disease and cancer.

Although turmeric can't take all the credit for those lower disease rates, most researchers acknowledge that the herb likely plays a key role. Indeed, lab studies show that curcumin, one of turmeric's primary phytochemicals, could **directly help protect against neurodegenerative changes, including those that lead to Alzheimer's and Parkinson's diseases.**[60] Other research has found it may enhance and protect cognitive function and memory as people age.[61]

Research has likewise found that turmeric could help lower your risk of cancer, specifically of the colon, stomach, and skin. And it may even play a role in directly fighting cancer cells.[62] The anti-inflammatory powerhouse also seems to be a **promising therapeutic agent for easing and preventing arthritis and other joint and back pain,** according to a review and meta-analysis in the *Journal of Medicinal Food.*[63]

60   Lee W-H, Loo C-Y, Bebawy M, Luk F, Mason RS, Rohanizadeh R. Curcumin and its derivatives: their application in neuropharmacology and neuroscience in the 21st century. *Curr Neuropharmacol.* 2013; 11(4):338-378.

61   Ng T-P, Chiam P-C, Lee T, Chua H-C, Lim L, Kua E-H. Curry consumption and cognitive function in the elderly. *Am J Epidemiol.* 2006;164(9):898-906.

62   Hutchins-Wolfbrandt A, Mistry AM. Dietary turmeric potentially reduces the risk of cancer. *Asian Pac J Cancer Prev.* 2011;12(12):3169-3173.

63   Daily JW, Yang M, Park S. Efficacy of turmeric extracts and curcumin for alleviating the symptoms of joint arthritis: a systematic review and meta-analysis of randomized clinical trials. *J Med Food.* 2016; 19(8):717-729.

One mechanism by which phytochemicals found in turmeric reduce inflammation is by affecting an enzyme in the body called COX-2. COX-2 generates inflammatory messengers in the prostaglandin family. This is the same enzyme affected by nonsteroidal anti-inflammatory drugs (NSAIDs), such as ibuprofen and naproxen. NSAIDs directly block COX-2. Turmeric is slower acting than NSAIDs because it inhibits *formation* of COX-2.

Not only does turmeric have antioxidant and anti-inflammatory properties, it also promotes healing of stomach ulcers (unlike anti-inflammatory drugs). Part of the ulcer-healing properties may be because turmeric has been found to have strong inhibitory properties against *Helicobacter pylori (H. pylori)*, a bacteria commonly associated with stomach ulcers.[64] Turmeric has also been shown to have antimicrobial properties against other common bacteria, including staphylococcus, and a range of viruses, including herpes viruses and strains of human papilloma virus (HPV) that have been associated with throat and cervical cancer (HPV 16 and 18).[65] In my opinion, discovering these links between microbes and cancer makes it important to look to herbs such as turmeric, which may be part of the solution.

Benefits of turmeric:

- Useful for arthritis and arthritic conditions

- Reduces risk of dementia

- Protects liver cells

- Promotes healing of stomach ulcers

---

64   Moghadamtousi SZ, Kadir HA, Hassandarvish P, Tajik H, Abubakar S, Zandi K. A review on antibacterial, antiviral, and antifungal activity of curcumin. *Biomed Res Int.* 2014;2014:186864.

65   Divya CS, Pillai MR. Antitumor action of curcumin in human papillomavirus associated cells involves downregulation of viral oncogenes, prevention of NFkB and AP-1 translocation, and modulation of apoptosis. *Mol Carcinog.* 2006;45(5):320-332.

- Antimicrobial properties

- Reduces gastrointestinal inflammation

- Aids digestion and enhances normal bowel movements

Curcumin is a phytochemical found in turmeric that was once thought to be almost solely responsible for turmeric's vast array of benefits. Continued research into the matter has shown that curcumin is just one of three main curcuminoids found in turmeric, along with a host of other phytochemicals that have their own complementary and therapeutic value. Those have been shown to increase absorption of curcumin. Isolated curcumin products are notoriously poorly absorbed and quickly excreted by the body. Therefore many curcumin products also contain black pepper (or phosphatidylcholine) added to increase absorption. While isolated curcumin does have potent benefits on its own, I recommend taking a full-spectrum extract of turmeric for maximum benefit.

Suggested dosing: Turmeric is available as a spice as well as a powdered extract (most concentrated), tincture (less concentrated) and tea (least concentrated). I use turmeric liberally in all forms. If you love curries, you already know the unique aroma of turmeric. Turmeric makes refreshing and colorful lattes and can be added to smoothies. If using a powdered extract, I generally recommend 200-500 mg, one to two times daily or 2-4 mL, one to two times daily.

Potential side effects and precautions: Turmeric has a very long history of human use. Side effects are rare. Taking large amounts of isolated curcumin should be avoided in people with low iron levels, as curcumin chelates (holds onto) iron. Full-spectrum turmeric extracts are less problematic, but iron levels should be checked periodically in individuals with low iron levels.

Gotu Kola (*Centella asiatica*)

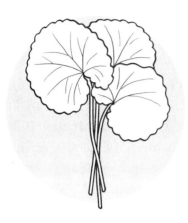

Native to India, gotu kola is an herb from the parsley family. In Ayurvedic medicine, a traditional medicine of India, gotu kola is considered a rasayana, a general tonic for increasing longevity. Classically, however, it's best known as a brain revitalizer. **It helps balance and calm the brain while also encouraging alertness and supporting brain function**, which are especially important as you age.

Research suggests it works by revitalizing and balancing the central nervous system and nerve function, promoting the production of GABA (a neurotransmitter that plays a role in mood regulation), and inhibiting excitatory neurons among other actions. It also helps support healthy cognition and memory. One study in the journal *Evidence-Based Complementary and Alternative Medicine*, for example, found that it was effective at improving cognitive function in patients who had experienced stroke.[66]

Beyond its effect on the brain, **gotu kola is an immunomodulator, helping the immune system manage stress**. Recognized traditionally as a blood purifier, gotu kola also promotes healthy circulation, including preventing or easing fluid retention and swelling, and is known for positive effects on skin and connective tissue.

Gotu kola also offers general adaptogenic properties including increasing stamina, improving stress resistance, and positively modulating immune

---

66   Farhana KM, Malueka RG, Wibowo S, Gofir A. Effectiveness of gotu kola extract 750 mg and 1000 mg compared with folic acid 3 mg in improving vascular cognitive impairment after stroke. *Evid Based Complement Alternat Med*. 2016;2016:2795915.

function. It does this by reducing overactive immune function and enhancing the ability of the immune system to manage threats. In addition, when used topically, gotu kola promotes wound healing and traditionally has been used for a wide range of skin afflictions.

Benefits of gotu kola:

- Brain revitalizer

- Anti-inflammatory

- Mild antimicrobial activity

- Immunomodulator

- Supports healthy skin

- Antihyperglycemic (lowers blood glucose), protecting cells against glycation[67]

Suggested dosing: General dosing for gotu kola is 200-400 mg, one to two times a day for standardized powdered extract capsules or 1-3 mL, one to two times daily for a tincture.

Potential side effects and precautions: Gotu kola is generally well tolerated and has low potential for side effects. Individuals taking medications to lower blood glucose (such as metformin) should be aware that gotu kola also helps to lower blood glucose in individuals with elevated blood sugar. However, it will not lower blood sugar in people with normal blood sugar—herbs are normalizers. Blood sugar levels should be monitored and dosages adjusted to avoid hypoglycemia. Also, because the herb promotes blood flow and stimulates menses, it is best to consult your health care provider if using during pregnancy.

---

67   Kabir AU, Samad MB, D'Costa NM, Akhter F, Ahmed A, Hannan JMA. Anti-hyperglycemic activity of Centella asiatica is partly mediated by carbohydrase inhibition and glucose-fiber binding. *BMC Complement Altern Med.* 2014;14:31.

Shilajit

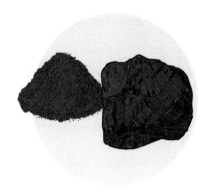

Shilajit isn't actually a plant; instead, it's a super-concentrated mix of phytochemicals and minerals from plants fermented by soil microbes. It's found in crevices around rocks in high-altitude environments. While that may sound a bit odd, it has been revered for promoting general health and longevity by civilizations surrounding the Himalayas for over 3,000 years.

Shilajit offers something that other herbs don't. It's rich in fulvic acid, a substance produced by soil bacteria. Fulvic acid is another important substance that was likely integral to the ancient foraged diet. Foraged roots and tubers carried soil with them and were high in fulvic acid. Because we thoroughly clean root vegetables before we eat them, fulvic acid is sparse in the modern diet. It's specifically why I added shilajit to the daily list.

Fulvic acid has been found to have both anti-inflammatory and antioxidant properties for protecting cells throughout the body. It's especially valuable for the gut, however. Fulvic acid promotes a healthy balance of gut flora, enhances absorption of nutrients, enhances production of digestive enzymes, and reduces gut inflammation.[68] It also has antidiabetic properties.

Shilajit has significant adaptogenic activity against a variety of behavioral, biochemical, and physiological factors caused by unpredictable stress. It works by providing a stabilizing effect on the neuroendocrine system via the HPA axis as well as by helping preserve mitochondrial function and integrity.

---

68   Winkler J, Ghosh S. Therapeutic potential of fulvic acid in chronic inflammatory diseases and diabetes. *J Diabetes Res.* 2018;2018:5391014.

In terms of healthy aging, shilajit has been shown in human clinical trials to increase energy and endurance (by reducing cellular stress and protecting mitochondrial functions), restore sexual vitality in men and women, promote optimal blood flow in skin, support bone health, and boost collagen synthesis.

Shilajit has proven antiviral activity against a wide range of different viruses, including herpes viruses and respiratory syncytial virus (RSV), a highly contagious respiratory virus that occasionally causes severe illness.[69]

Shilajit is considered a synergist, a substance that amplifies the benefits of other herbs by increasing absorption and enhancing bioavailability of phytochemicals from other herbs.

Benefits of shilajit:

- Supports optimal gut functions and balanced gut flora

- Improves skin health by stimulating collagen synthesis

- Supports overall fitness and endurance

- Supports a healthy inflammatory response

- Mitochondrial energy booster

- Normalizes natural testosterone secretion

- Supports healthy brain and heart functions

- Supports immune system functions

- Documented antiviral properties

---

69   Cagno V, Donalisio M, Civra A, Cagliero C, Rubiolo P, Lembo D. In vitro evaluation of the antiviral properties of Shilajit and investigation of its mechanisms of action. *J Ethnopharmacol.* 2015;166:129-134.

Suggested dosing: 200-1000 mg daily of shilajit standardized to a minimum of 20% fulvic acid.

Potential side effects and precautions: Because the composition of shilajit can vary, sourcing is extra important. One of the most reliable sources of shilajit is PrimaVie®, a purified GRAS-approved brand of shilajit standardized to >50% fulvic acid.[70] PrimaVie® was used in a placebo-controlled clinical study showing increased muscle strength and reduced fatigue post-exercise compared to placebo.[71]

Milk Thistle (*Silybum marianum*)

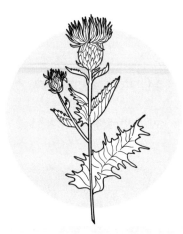

The modern world is a toxic place—over 200,000 man-made toxic substances are present in the environment that weren't here a hundred years ago. The liver, as the primary processing center for toxic substances in the body, takes a real beating. After years of chronic exposure to toxins, liver cells burn out and are replaced with fat cells, a condition known as fatty liver. Loss of liver cells not only reduces the body's ability to process toxic substances, but it also reduces the liver's ability to manage cholesterol, which may be a primary reason why blood cholesterol tends to rise with aging.

Although many herbs protect liver function, milk thistle is one of the best. Milk thistle, native to southern Europe and North Africa, has been

---

70 Generally Recognized As Safe (GRAS) is a designation given to any substance that has been defined as being as safe for consumption as any food product.

71 Keller JL, Housh TJ, Hill EC, Smith CM, Schmidt RJ, Johnson GO. The effects of Shilajit supplementation on fatigue-induced decreases in muscular strength and serum hydroxyproline levels. *J Int Soc Sports Nutr.* 2019;16(1):3.

used to treat jaundice and other liver conditions for thousands of years. *Silymarin*, the primary active component of milk thistle, offers potent antioxidant protection for liver cells. It also increases natural antioxidants (glutathione) found in liver cells.[72] Milk thistle has been found to induce regeneration of liver cells in patients with nonalcoholic fatty liver disease.[73] It is the most widely researched of all hepatoprotective (liver-protective) herbs and is well known for its low toxicity and high safety profile.

Milk thistle is also useful to promote normal digestion. In a 2015 study, silymarin was found to promote healing and maintain remission in patients with ulcerative colitis.[74] Interestingly, milk thistle has been used to protect and help repair the liver from chemotherapy-induced damage and could play a supportive role in a holistic approach to cancer treatment.[75]

Beyond the intestinal tract, silymarin was found to be neuroprotective— it provided antioxidant protection to neurons in the brain and was associated with reduced buildup of amyloid beta.[76]

Benefits of milk thistle:

- Potent liver support and protection

- Supports healthy glutathione and other antioxidant levels in liver cells

---

72 Vargas-Mendoza N, Madrigal-Santillán E, Morales-González A, et al. Hepatoprotective effect of silymarin. *World J Hepatol.* 2014;6(3):144-149.

73 Aller R, Izaola O, Gómez S, et al. Effect of silymarin plus vitamin E in patients with non-alcoholic fatty liver disease. A randomized clinical pilot study. *Eur Rev Med Pharmacol Sci.* 2015;19(16):3118-3124.

74 Rastegarpanah M, Malekzadeh R, Vahedi H, et al. A randomized, double blinded, placebo-controlled clinical trial of silymarin in ulcerative colitis. *Chin J Integr Med.* 2015;21(12):902-906.

75 Ramasamy K, Agarwal R. Multitargeted therapy of cancer by silymarin. *Cancer Lett.* 2008;269(2):352-362.

76 Borah A, Paul R, Choudhury S, et al. Neuroprotective potential of silymarin against CNS disorders: insight into the pathways and molecular mechanisms of action. *CNS Neurosci Ther.* 2013;19(11):847-853.

- Promotes bile flow

- Aids digestion

- Protects the kidneys

- Anti-inflammatory

Suggested dosing: General dosing recommendations are 200-300 mg, one to three times daily of a powdered extract or 2-3 mL, two to three times daily of a tincture. Much research has been done showing that silymarin is likely the most therapeutic phytochemical present in milk thistle. So, look for an extract of the seed standardized to at least 70% silymarin for maximum potency.

Potential side effects and precautions: Milk thistle is extremely well tolerated. Adverse reactions are rare.

Establishing a Routine

Once you obtain your herbal products, you'll want to organize them so that they are easy to use. Consistency is key. You'll want to take them every day to reach maximum benefit.

Most herbal preparations are best taken with a meal, especially if you have a sensitive stomach. Be sure to drink enough liquid to ensure that the capsules go all the way down your esophagus and into your stomach. Usually a full 8-oz glass will be enough. Drink an ounce or two after the last capsule just to make sure that it goes all the way to the stomach. If the capsule dissolves while inside your esophagus, it can cause discomfort. Capsules go down especially well with a viscous liquid such as coconut milk or a smoothie. (My wife swears that chocolate helps her swallow herb capsules, but I don't think there's been a study on that.)

What to Expect

Note that you probably won't feel an immediate effect from taking the herbs. You might even wonder if they're doing anything. Know that the herbs are subtly increasing your cellular resilience. The benefits accrue over time; the longer you take the herbs, the more benefit you'll notice. It might be a little more energy. Nagging symptoms that have been accepted as a part of life, such as joint discomfort or intestinal dysfunction, may start to ease. Your ability to navigate through problems that pop up through the day might get a bit easier. Whether you have symptoms or not, knowing that the herbs are counteracting the forces that contribute to illness may be the most important thing of all.

Side effects and adverse reactions with herbs in the *green zone* are uncommon, but they can occur. Become aware of your body in order to note any changes. If you develop hives, itching, or other symptoms of sensitivities, discontinue use. Though this is uncommon, it can happen. If it does, take a break from the herbs for several days to a week, and then start over at a lower dose.

Nausea and stomach discomfort are also possible, but fortunately are not very common. Taking herbal supplements with meals reduces this potential side effect. If it occurs, you can try skipping a day between doses or lowering the dosage. You can also add an herb called slippery elm with your regular supplements. Slippery elm protects the lining of the esophagus, stomach, and intestinal tract (see Chapter 21 for a complete profile on slippery elm).

Occasionally, people find certain herbs to be either too stimulating or too sedating. The same herb can affect two people in different ways because we all have unique chemistries. For the everyday herbs list included in this chapter, I've chosen herbs that are fairly neutral (neither excessively sedating nor stimulating for the majority of people).

General Precautions for Taking Herbs

While the herbs mentioned in this book have an excellent safety profile when used in recommended doses, there are certain precautions to be aware of that apply to any herb or natural substance.

- As with any plant-based substance, including foods, some people may have an allergy to a particular herb. For this reason, proceed with caution when you are first trying a new herb. Start with the lowest practical dose and work up to a full dose over several days. For capsules, that may require opening the capsule and only taking a small amount of the powder initially if you have a high potential for allergic reactions.

- Many herbs and natural substances have blood-thinning properties. If you are taking prescription blood thinners, have a history of coagulation problems, or have had a heart valve replacement or other mechanical heart modification, you should have a discussion with your health care provider or a practicing herbalist before taking herbs or other natural supplements. If you experience easy bruising, stop taking herbs and speak with your health care provider.

- Discontinue herbal supplements several days to a week before having major surgery (because of their natural blood-thinning tendency). They can generally be resumed the day after surgery unless otherwise defined by a health care provider.

- If you take immunosuppressive drugs, you should use caution and consult your health care provider before using any type of herbal therapy. Many herbs have immunomodulating or immunostimulating properties, which could theoretically promote organ rejection by the immune system.

- Use caution with herbal therapy while pregnant or breastfeeding. Though most herbs pose less risk to pregnancy than drugs, it's advisable to consult a practicing herbalist before using any herb during pregnancy or breastfeeding.

- Avoid high doses of any herb if you have compromised liver function. Though many herbs protect liver cells, the phytochemicals must still be processed by the liver. If you have a history of liver disease, having your liver functions tested by a health care provider every 3-6 months is a good practice.

- Individuals who retain iron (hemochromatosis) should use caution with certain herbs such as ashwagandha and shilajit because they contain low levels of iron. I have noted these cautions in the individual herbal profiles in the following chapters.

- Taking herbs or natural substances with the potential to cause sedation, such as passionflower, lemon balm, L-theanine, melatonin, GABA, magnesium glycinate, or CBD oil, should be avoided prior to driving or operating heavy machinery. Herbs or natural substances with calming properties may compound the effects of sedative drugs.

Going Beyond the Basics

If your health is good and you follow a healthy lifestyle, a core of everyday herbs may be all you need to protect your cells from the stresses of everyday life. As previously outlined, you can consider adding on a multivitamin or omega-3 fatty acid supplement. Alongside a healthful diet and lifestyle, this baseline regimen will offer terrific everyday coverage.

In Part Three, you'll learn about other supplements and herbs that will allow you to individualize your daily supplement protocol. For example, if your morning commute exposes you to smog-filled air every day, you may want to take an extra dose of milk thistle each day.

In the next chapter, you'll learn about herbs with stronger antimicrobial properties. Though these herbs are safe to take every day, they are better reserved for when you really need them.

Chapter Highlights

- The list of foundational everyday herbs is chosen because of the low potential for side effects and wide range of benefits.

- Though all the herbs share common benefits, they each shine in their own way.

  - Rhodiola—increased stamina and tolerance to physical stress

  - Reishi—excellent immune system modulator

  - Turmeric—well known for providing anti-inflammatory properties

  - Gotu kola—treasured as a brain revitalizer

  - Shilajit—revered for boosting energy and promoting optimal gut function

  - Milk thistle—protects and promotes regeneration of liver cells

- Everyday herbs work by protecting cells and increasing cellular resilience. The benefits accrue over time. The longer and more consistently you take them, the greater the outcome.

10

Antimicrobial Properties of Herbs

O f the many benefits that herbs offer, the antimicrobial properties of phytochemicals have me the most intrigued. While we depend on an immune system that uses different types of immune cells to keep our microbes in check and protect us from new microbial threats, plants accomplish these same goals with an equally complex defense system composed of phytochemicals.

The plant microbial defense system is made up of hundreds of phytochemicals that inhibit microbes in a variety of ways. When we consume a food plant or an herb loaded with phytochemicals, we basically borrow the plant's microbial defense system to enhance our own defenses. This isn't a new or novel idea. Humans have been doing it for a very long time.

Our ancient ancestors most certainly benefited from the extra antimicrobial protection found in the phytochemistry of wild foraged plants. Even after our foraging days were over, phytochemicals in herbs were used to treat a range of different illnesses that we now know are caused by infections with threatening microbes.

Plants, however, aren't the only way we borrow from nature to enhance our defenses.

Bacteria also produce chemical substances to inhibit competing bacteria, fungi, and threatening viruses. Similarly, fungi use chemical defenses to fend off bacteria and viruses. We depend on favorable bacteria and yeast (fungi) in the gut and on the skin to suppress growth of more threatening bacteria, yeast (such as candida), and viruses. It makes up a critical part of our defense system.

In recent history, we've adopted modern technology to borrow from these natural sources in more specific ways.

The Blessing and Curse of Modern Antibiotics

Modern antibiotics come from natural sources, chiefly a fungus or bacteria, but sometimes a plant. Instead of containing the full spectrum of chemicals making up the organism's defense system, however, antibiotics are made from a single isolated chemical compound found to have antimicrobial activity. After being extracted from the natural source, the compound is chemically tweaked for greater killing power and then produced synthetically.

The Accidental Discovery of Antibiotics

Penicillin, the first major antibiotic, was found by accident. In 1928, Alexander Fleming, a biologist working at St. Mary's Hospital in London, returned from a vacation to find a fungus invading a culture plate growing bacteria. The fungus, *Penicillium notatum*, had completely inhibited growth of bacteria on the plate. It took another decade for the penicillin compound to be isolated from the fungus, and not until the 1940s, for it to be approved for human use. That simple connection, however, changed the world.

What's gained is potency. Sometimes that's really important. For example, if you have an acute infection with high concentrations of fast-growing bacteria invading tissues, such as with a bacterial pneumonia or a bladder infection, synthetic antibiotics are the right choice. Within days, the antibiotics will usually knock down the numbers of bacteria enough for the immune system to gain control over the situation. Herbs typically don't work that quickly.

Synthetic antibiotics, however, have significant limitations. They not only kill pathogenic bacteria, but they also kill normal flora in the gut and on the skin. In fact, normal flora are especially sensitive to antibiotics. When normal flora are inhibited by antibiotics, harmful bacteria are able to flourish. All it takes is ten days of use of *any* synthetic antibiotic to cause significant and sometimes irreparable harm to the balance of bacteria in the body.

Messing up the gut microbiome with antibiotics can have far-reaching consequences. A study[77] published in 2022 found that menopausal age women who had greater than two months of midlife exposure to antibiotics had significantly lower cognitive scores later in life. This adds to the evidence linking gut microbiome imbalances to a growing list of chronic illnesses, including Alzheimer's disease, Parkinson's disease, depression, behavioral disorders, obesity, type 2 diabetes, cardiovascular disease, autoimmune illnesses, and inflammatory bowel disease.[78]

This is one place where herbs have an enormous advantage. The antimicrobial properties of herbs do not disrupt the balance of bacteria in the body. In fact, herbal phytochemicals with antimicrobial properties suppress pathogens in the gut and on the skin while promoting growth of normal flora.

It makes sense when you think about it. A plant's phytochemical defense system must distinguish between friend and foe, just like our immune system. Antimicrobial phytochemicals selectively target potential pathogens, but spare nonthreatening bacteria that might provide benefits to the plant. In addition, plants produce phytochemicals that act as signaling agents to attract favorable microorganisms.

The fact that the antimicrobial phytochemicals of herbs are *selective*— meaning they affect pathogens without harming normal flora—is fascinating. My personal experience, along with thousands of patients with whom I've worked, is that herbs with antimicrobial properties can be taken for years without disrupting the balance of flora in the gut and skin.

---

77   Mehta RS, Lochhead P, Wang Y, et al. Association of midlife antibiotic use with subsequent cognitive function in women. *PLoS One.* 2022;17(3):e0264649.

78   Durack J, Lynch SV. The gut microbiome: Relationships with disease and opportunities for therapy. *J Exp Med.* 2019;216(1):20-40.

The Selective Properties of Herbs

Herbal phytochemicals are the only known substances on earth that have the capacity to suppress pathogens without disrupting normal flora or causing side effects. This was documented in a study published in the October 2019 issue of *Biomedicine & Pharmacotherapy*, in which researchers detailed how phytochemicals from a variety of different herbs had a favorable effect on the balance of bacteria in the gut.[79] Herbal phytochemicals promoted growth of favorable species of bacteria, while suppressing growth of potential pathogens. What's more, they found that the bacteria metabolized the phytochemicals into smaller active chemical compounds that were more easily absorbed, which enhanced the health benefits of the herbs.

A further advantage of having the herb's full defense system is covering a wide range of microbe threats. Antibiotics kill bacteria but typically don't have any effect on viral, protozoal, and fungal infections. Different drugs are required for those types of microbes altogether. In contrast, the phytochemical defense system of herbs inhibits a full range of pathogens that includes different types of bacteria, viruses, protozoa, and fungi.

Another huge problem with antibiotics is bacterial resistance.[80] Almost immediately after penicillin was introduced in the 1940s, bacteria started becoming resistant to it. Bacterial resistance has occurred with every antibiotic that has ever been produced. The last major class of new antibiotics, the fluoroquinolones (Cipro, Levaquin) was

---

79   An X, Bao Q, Di S, et al. The interaction between the gut Microbiota and herbal medicines. *Biomed Pharmacother.* 2019t;118:109252.
80   Davies J, Davies D. Origins and evolution of antibiotic resistance. *Microbiol Mol Biol Rev.* 2010;74(3):417-433.

introduced when I was in medical school in the 1980s. Although pharmaceutical companies advertised fluoroquinolones as being immune to resistance, resistance started showing up within just years of their debut. Since then, the pharmaceutical industry hasn't made significant investments in developing new antibiotics.

Decades of steady antibiotic use has us at the point where antibiotic resistance is now a major medical issue. The CDC estimates that 35,000 Americans die of complications from antimicrobial resistance every year—that's about one person dying every 15 minutes. Overall, 2.8 million people in the U.S. contract infections caused by resistant bacteria each year. Overprescribing in both adults and children is a significant part of the problem. However, resistance can also be driven by antibiotic use in the livestock industry. Antibiotics used on the farm or ranch or dairy operation, including antibiotics added to animal feed (to reduce infections and increase productivity) account for 70% of all antibiotic use in the U.S.

In contrast, bacterial resistance to herbs has never been documented. It's probably due to that "combo" effect (recall that an herb has many chemicals, not just one), which makes it impossible for microbes to develop a "run-around". Several studies have documented antimicrobial activity of various herbs against a range of different antibiotic-resistant bacteria, including methicillin-resistant *Staphylococcus aureus* (MRSA).[81,82]

MRSA, harbored by somewhere between 1% and 24% of populations around the world, has been associated with chronic skin infections, sinus infections, pneumonias, bone infections, and infections of heart valves. It's extremely common in hospitals, where it increases

81   Walusansa A, Asiimwe S, Nakavuma JL, et al. Antibiotic-resistance in medically important bacteria isolated from commercial herbal medicines in Africa from 2000 to 2021: a systematic review and meta-analysis. *Antimicrob Resist Infect Control*. 2022;11:11.

82   Arshad N, Mehreen A, Liaqat I, Arshad M, Afrasiab H. In vivo screening and evaluation of four herbs against MRSA infections. *BMC Complement Altern Med*. 2017;17(1):498.

morbidity and mortality of all illnesses being treated. Hospital-acquired, antibiotic-resistant infections are a huge problem where herbs might be able to help.

In fact, in a world with the growing threat of resistant bacteria from antibiotic overuse, herbs may be our best hope.

The Herbal Antimicrobial Advantage

While herbs might not be the best choice for an acute bacterial pneumonia, they are especially good for increasing your daily resistance to threatening microbes. Low-grade microbial threats are coming at us all the time. Not only that, we have potential pathogens lurking in our gut, on our skin, and as recent evidence shows, even inside cells in tissues throughout the body. They're all waiting for an opportunity. All it takes is accumulation of enough stress, either acutely or chronically, to cause a downturn in immune system functions and give them that opportunity. The possible link to a wide range of chronic illnesses is not something that should be ignored.

One of the best ways to support your natural microbial defenses is by taking herbs. Because the antimicrobial properties of herbs don't generate bacterial resistance or disrupt normal flora, you can take them every day. You can even think of it as adding back something that's been missing from your life.

All of the herbs mentioned thus far—rhodiola,[83] hawthorn, ashwagandha, turmeric, and others on the everyday herb list—have documented antimicrobial properties. Though these herbs are typically recognized more for their general health benefits than fighting off microbes, they still provide a basic level of antimicrobial support.

---

83   Kosakowska O, Bączek K, Przybył JL, et al. Antioxidant and antibacterial activity of roseroot (Rhodiola rosea L.) dry extracts. *Molecules*. 2018;23(7):1767.

Many herbs are recognized specifically for their antimicrobial properties. We know more than you might expect about the antimicrobial properties of herbs because traditionally, many herbs were used to treat illnesses that we now know are infectious. Although microorganisms have only been recognized as a cause of illness for a few hundred years, microorganisms have been making people sick since the beginning of time—and herbs have been helping them to get well.

The "First" Antimicrobial Herb

When the Spanish colonized South America starting in the early 1500s, they brought malaria with them—but they also found a cure. The native populations in Peru were already using a variety of plant substances to treat illnesses now recognized as infectious. They found that one of them, bark from the cinchona tree, was effective against this new illness that had invaded their land. The Spanish took cinchona bark back to Europe, where it was recognized as the first effective treatment against malaria.

Early in the twentieth century, scientists isolated quinine from cinchona bark. Quinine was assumed to be the chemical substance that gave the plant its antimalarial properties. It was produced synthetically and distributed around the world to fight malaria. Within a relatively short period of time, however, malaria became resistant to quinine. Interestingly, cinchona bark extracts are effective against quinine-resistant malaria, demonstrating that the complex phytochemistry of the whole plant is a lot more sophisticated than one isolated phytochemical.

Herbs with recognized antimicrobial properties each offer a slightly different spectrum of antimicrobial coverage and other complementary disease-fighting benefits. All herbs positively affect the immune system, but in different ways. Some herbs, such as echinacea and elderberry, are known to stimulate immune system functions. While this can be beneficial for fighting off an acute viral illness, it's not ideal for long-term use because of the potential for immune overstimulation.

Many antimicrobial herbs, however, are immunomodulators, meaning they calm overactive parts of the immune system while stimulating underactive parts of the immune system. In other words, they balance immune system functions that have become disrupted by stress and microbes. This makes them more ideal for long-term use.

I've personally been using antimicrobial herbs with immunomodulating properties as part of my daily regimen of herbs for over a decade. I haven't suffered any harmful effects. In fact, I've only seen benefits. I also use them in my practice and have followed thousands of people who have used these types of herbs on a long-term basis to overcome chronic conditions. Reports of side effects and adverse reactions are remarkably low.

That being said, I don't think that everyone needs to take herbs with stronger antimicrobial properties on a daily basis. I generally recommend reserving them for specific indications. They are ideally suited for recovery from chronic illnesses that may be connected with overgrowth of intracellular microbes in tissues. For people struggling with chronic illnesses such as fibromyalgia, chronic fatigue syndrome, chronic Lyme disease, long COVID, and autoimmune illnesses, they are an ideal complement to any other therapies. For these situations, taking a full complement of three to five antimicrobial herbs, along with the core everyday herbs, is a good strategy.

For other situations, such as osteoarthritis, or concerns such as increased risk of dementia or cardiovascular illness, adding one or two antimicrobial herbs to the core everyday herbs can expand the spectrum of benefits. For example, traditional uses of *cat's claw* included both protecting cognitive functions and relieving arthritis. Japanese knotweed contains resveratrol, known to provide exceptional benefits to the cardiovascular system. Garlic extracts have well-documented antimicrobial properties, but garlic is also well known for providing cardiovascular benefits. Garlic extracts also suppress candida (yeast) in the gut, along with other gut pathogens. Similarly, andrographis suppresses gut pathogens, stimulates bile flow, and protects liver cells.

My Favorite Antimicrobial Herbs List

Though there are many herbs with documented antimicrobial properties, I have several favorites. I've used these herbs, both personally and in my practice, for many years. As you will see, beyond offering exceptional antimicrobial properties, they also offer a wide spectrum of health benefits that have been documented by scientific studies. I also chose them because they are immunomodulators, as opposed to immune stimulants, and because they are free of drug-like effects.

Note that these herbs have a lot of range. While they are ideal for addressing chronic conditions, they all have significant antiviral properties, making them beneficial for reducing the length and severity of common viral infections. This topic will be covered in Chapter 15.

Japanese Knotweed (*Polygonum cuspidatum*)

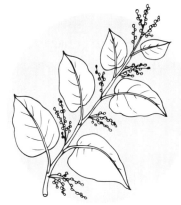

A good word to describe Japanese knotweed is tenacious. Native to Japan and China, it was carried to Great Britain for use as a garden ornamental. From there to Canada, the United States and New Zealand, where it is now considered a rapidly expanding invasive. Japanese knotweed is an attractive plant that looks something like bamboo, but with broad leaves. Once planted, the rhizome (root) expands rapidly, pushing out any other plants in the vicinity.

While horticulturists have declared war on this invasive, herbalists are celebrating. Those tenacious rhizomes contain potent bioactive substances. In its native countries, Japanese knotweed has been used for centuries for treating everything from respiratory ailments to rheumatism (arthritis).

Truly a wonder substance, Japanese knotweed offers exceptional antimicrobial activity, including activity against a wide range of bacteria, viruses, protozoa, and yeast. JKW is a systemic antimicrobial that crosses the blood-brain barrier, and it is protective of the central nervous system. It's also anti-inflammatory and supports immune function. Recognized as an immunomodulator, Japanese knotweed balances immune system functions that have been disrupted by chronic stress and microbes.

Beyond well-documented antimicrobial properties, Japanese knotweed is an excellent source of resveratrol, the age-defying, life-enhancing chemical compound also found in grapes—except Japanese knotweed contains high concentrations of *trans*-resveratrol, the active form of the compound most useful to the body.

Resveratrol offers significant cardiovascular benefits including support of optimal heart function, enhanced blood flow from dilation of blood vessels, enhanced integrity of blood vessels, and reduced blood viscosity (thickness). It is also a potent antioxidant with anti-inflammatory properties, and it offers protection to the brain, nervous system, and liver.

Benefits of Japanese knotweed:

- Cardiovascular

  - Cardiogenic (improves heart function)

  - Dilates blood vessels and improves blood flow (normalizes blood pressure)

  - Improves the integrity of blood vessel walls

  - Inhibits platelet aggregation (blood clotting)

- Potent antioxidant properties

- Anti-inflammatory

- Protects nerve tissue

- Protects liver function

- Immunomodulator

Dosing: The suggested dosage is 200-800 mg Japanese knotweed (standardized to 50% trans-resveratrol) two to three times daily.

Potential side effects and precautions: Rare with low potential for toxicity, Japanese knotweed has been used in traditional forms of Asian medicine for thousands of years and offers a high level of safety. Caution is advised if also taking anticoagulants because resveratrol has blood-thinning properties.

Andrographis (*Andrographis paniculata*)

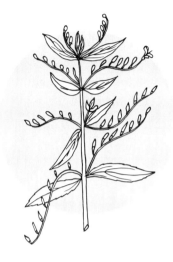

Andrographis has a wide range of benefits, mostly related to antimicrobial and immunomodulating properties. Native to India, traditional use has primarily included treating respiratory infections and influenza. Andrographis was credited for reducing the death rate in India during the great flu epidemic of 1918. During the twentieth century, use of andrographis spread outside India to Europe and beyond. Several studies have documented the ability of andrographis to reduce the duration and severity of viral illnesses.

Unlike conventional antibiotics, which are hard on the gastrointestinal system, andrographis offers many positive benefits. Andrographis has been used for dysentery and shows activity against pathogenic strains of *E. coli*. It is also active against common roundworms and tapeworms. In a 2011 study, andrographis was found to be as effective for treating ulcerative colitis as a commonly used drug.[84] Most of these benefits are related to the herb's ability to restore normal balance in bacterial flora of the gut.

One factor causing aging and disease is gradual decline in liver function, and andrographis offers significant liver protection. It also enhances bile flow, which reduces hepatic (liver) stagnation, improves digestion, and enhances detoxification of the body. This remarkable herb has also shown activity against viral hepatitis B and C. Most recently, andrographis

---

84   Tang T, Targan SR, Li Z-S, Xu C, Byers VS, Sandborn WJl. Randomised clinical trial: herbal extract HMPL-004 in active ulcerative colitis – a double-blind comparison with sustained release mesalazine. *Aliment Pharmacol Ther*. 2011;33(2):194-202.

was found to have significant activity against SARS-CoV-2 virus, the causative agent of COVID-19.[85]

Other benefits documented by studies published in peer-reviewed journals included decreased cytotoxicity of lung cells, antidiabetic properties, anticancer properties, reduction of joint pain in rheumatoid arthritis, and reduction of fatigue in multiple sclerosis.

Additional benefits include:

- Antiviral properties with activity against common viral illnesses and influenza

- Enhanced immune function

- Restoration of normal bacterial flora of the gut

- Possible benefit for intestinal disorders such as ulcerative colitis

- Protection of liver function

- Enhanced bile flow and restoration of normal liver function

Dosing: The suggested dosage is 200-800 mg, extract standardized to 10% to 30% andrographolides two to three times daily.

Potential side effects and precautions: About 1% of people who take andrographis develop an allergic reaction with whole-body hives and itching skin. The reaction will resolve gradually over several weeks after stopping use of the herb. The Ayurvedic name for andrographis translates to "king of bitters", therefore, this is one herb best taken in capsule form. When taken in capsules, the bitterness is not a factor.

85   Murugan NA, Pandian CJ, Jeyakanthan J. Computational investigation on *Andrographis paniculata* phytochemicals to evaluate their potency against SARS-CoV-2 in comparison to known antiviral compounds in drug trials [published online ahead of print, 2020 Jun 16]. *J Biomol Struct Dyn.* 2020;1-12.

Cat's Claw (*Uncaria tomentosa*)

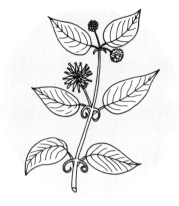

Cat's claw has been used for thousands of years by indigenous people of the Amazon for treating a variety of inflammatory conditions. Not surprisingly, the name is from the shape of the thorns on the woody vine from which the medicine comes. The medicine is derived from the inner bark of the vine. Common traditional uses included age-related cognitive issues, rheumatism, asthma, stomach problems, and tumors. It was also one of the pre-antibiotic treatments for syphilis.

The traditional uses of cat's claw have been documented by modern science. Numerous studies have documented the anti-inflammatory properties of cat's claw and its phytochemical constituents. Studies have demonstrated benefit from cat's claw for both osteoarthritis and rheumatoid arthritis.[86]

Cat's claw is a common addition to treatment protocols for chronic Lyme disease. Efficacy for treatment of Lyme disease is documented in a study from Johns Hopkins University detailed later in this chapter. Other independent studies have shown broad-spectrum antimicrobial coverage for a wide range of bacteria and viruses.

Cat's claw is a strong immunomodulator, meaning it calms an overactive immune system. It has been found to support healthy levels of white blood cells, including B and T lymphocytes, natural killer (NK) cells, and granulocytes.

---

86   Ahmed S, Anuntiyo J, Malemud CJ, Haqqi TM. Biological basis for the use of botanicals in osteoarthritis and rheumatoid arthritis: a review. *Evid Based Complement Alternat Med*. 2005;2(3):301-308.

The ability of cat's claw to support cognitive function and prevent dementia was demonstrated by a study from 2019 that defined *Uncaria tomentosa* as a "potent plaque and tangle inhibitor" for reducing these manifestations of Alzheimer's disease and brain aging.[87]

Several studies have also detailed *Uncaria tomentosa*'s anticancer properties and the ability to reduce tumor formation for a variety of cancers.

Benefits of cat's claw:

- Anti-inflammatory and antimicrobial properties

- Beneficial healing properties for the intestinal tract

- Promotes healing of stomach ulcers

- Enhances DNA repair and prevents cells from mutating

- Potent antioxidant properties

- Dilates blood vessels and normalizes blood pressure

- May reduce amyloid deposition associated with cognitive decline

Dosing: The suggested dosage is 400-800 mg (inner bark standardized to 3% alkaloids or 10:1 concentrate inner bark is preferred) two to three times daily. It is especially important to take this herb with food, as it is activated by stomach acid.

Potential side effects and precautions: Occasional stomach upset can occur, but it's generally well tolerated.

---

87   Snow AD, Castillo GM, Nguyen BP, et al. The Amazon rainforest plant Uncaria tomentosa (cat's claw) and its specific proanthocyanidin constituents are potent inhibitors and reducers of both brain plaques and tangles. *Sci Rep.* 2019;9(1):561.

Chinese Skullcap (*Scutellaria baicalensis*)

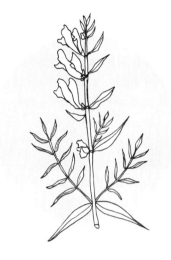

Chinese skullcap is a potent synergist, meaning it increases absorption of bioavailability of other herbal phytochemicals. Having at least one synergist is important when choosing herbs for a supplement regimen. Chinese skullcap is strongly antiviral against a range of different viruses.[88] It also offers antibacterial and antifungal properties documented by scientific studies.

Chinese skullcap has been found to have antiviral activity against reactivated Epstein-Barr virus, herpes viruses in general, and SARS-CoV-2 that causes COVID-19.

Chinese skullcap has mild sedative properties. It is also strongly protective of nerve tissue and liver function. Immunomodulating properties associated with the herb include anti-inflammatory, anti-allergenic (reduces allergic reactions), and anti-autoimmune. Another documented benefit is the protection of the cardiovascular system.

A review study from 2016 noted that Chinese skullcap extract was cytotoxic to brain cancer cells, prostate cancer cells, and head and neck cancer cells.[89] It induced cell death and suppressed growth of lymphoma and myeloma cells.

---

88   Li K, Liang Y, Cheng A, et al. Antiviral properties of baicalin: a concise review. *Rev Bras Farmacogn.* 2021;31(4):408-419.

89   Zhao Q, Chen XY, Martin C. *Scutellaria baicalensis*, the golden herb from the garden of Chinese medicinal plants. *Sci Bull (Beijing).* 2016;61(18):1391-1398.

Benefits of Chinese skullcap:

- Immunomodulator

- Antiviral, antibacterial

- Anti-inflammatory

- Antitumor

- Liver protective

- Neuroprotective

Dosing: The suggested dosage is 400-1000 mg, two to three times daily. Root extract, preferably a three-year-old plant with pronounced yellow color, standardized to >30% baicalin is preferred. (American skullcap does not offer the same antimicrobial properties and should not be substituted.)

Potential side effects and precautions: Side effects are uncommon and are mostly gastrointestinal.

Garlic (*Allium sativum*)

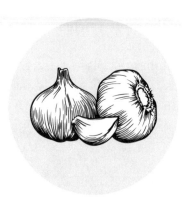

Beyond being a flavorful addition to any culinary experience, the health benefits of garlic have been recognized since the beginning of recorded history. Garlic contains a variety of beneficial phytochemicals, but the most well studied is a sulfuric compound called allicin.

Allicin has been shown to have potent broad-spectrum activity against gram-positive and gram-negative bacteria. It also has antiviral, antifungal, and antiparasitic properties. It is highly beneficial for chronic fungal infections and has shown activity against MRSA infections. It also has activity against SARS-CoV-2. Garlic has even been found to reduce the length and severity of the common cold.[90]

Eating garlic has been shown to slow growth of foodborne bacteria. Garlic has also been shown to balance the gut microbiome by suppressing pathogens, such as candida (yeast) and promoting growth of healthy flora.[91] Garlic has been found to specifically suppress *H. pylori*[92] and promotes healing of ulcers.

Garlic's well-known cardiovascular benefits include reduced cholesterol, inhibition of platelet aggregation (stickiness), improved blood flow, reduced blood pressure, and direct cardiogenic effects.[93]

Prostate cancer and gastrointestinal cancers have been shown to be less common among individuals who eat more garlic.[94] A study of men in Shanghai, China found that high intake of allium vegetables (garlic, onions, and scallions) was associated with a 53% decreased overall reduction in prostate cancer risk.[95]

Garlic can help ease the inflammation associated with arthritis. A study in the journal *Arthritis Research & Therapy* found that garlic reduces inflammatory cytokines and regulates the immune response.[96]

90   Lissiman E, Bhasale AL, Cohen M. Garlic for the common cold. *Cochrane Database Syst Rev.* 2014;2014(11):CD006206.
91   Chen K, Xie K, Liu Z, et al. Preventive effects and mechanisms of garlic on dyslipidemia and gut microbiome dysbiosis. *Nutrients.* 2019;11(6):1225.
92   Zardast M, Namakin K, Esmaelian Kaho J, Hashemi SS. Assessment of antibacterial effect of garlic in patients infected with *Helicobacter pylori* using urease breath test. *Avicenna J Phytomed.* 2016;6(5):495-501.
93   Chan JY-Y, Yeun AC-Y, Chan RY-K, Chan S-W. A review of the cardiovascular benefits and antioxidant properties of allicin. *Phytother Res.* 2013;27(5):637-646.
94   Nicastro HL, Ross SA, Milner JA. Garlic and onions: their cancer prevention properties. *Cancer Prev Res (Phila).* 2015;8(3):181-189.
95   Hsing AW, Chokkalingam AP, Gao Y-T, et al. Allium vegetables and risk of prostate cancer: a population-based study. *J Natl Cancer Inst.* 2002;94(21):1648-1651.
96   Ban JO, Oh JH, Kim TM, et al. Anti-inflammatory and arthritic effects of thiacremonone, a novel sulfur compound isolated from garlic via inhibition of NF-kappaB. *Arthritis Res Ther.* 2009;11(5):R145.

Benefits of garlic:

- Broad-spectrum antimicrobial against a wide range of bacteria, viruses, protozoa, and fungi

- Balances gut microbiome

- Wide-ranging cardiovascular benefits

- Anti-inflammatory

- Anticancer

The limitation of eating garlic for gaining health benefits is that allicin is very volatile. It exists inside the garlic bulb as a chemical compound called alliin. Alliin is tasteless and has no medicinal properties. As soon as garlic is crushed, the alliin is enzymatically converted to allicin, which breaks down as soon as it is released. Less than 1% of allicin from consumed garlic is absorbed. Encapsulated garlic extracts dramatically increase allicin yield by dehydrating garlic under low heat to preserve the alliin and then encapsulating it, such that the allicin is not released until the capsule dissolves in the intestinal tract.

Dosing: The suggested dosage is 180-1200 mg garlic (allicin), two to three times daily. The dosage is dependent on the garlic preparation used.

Potential side effects and precautions: Well tolerated. Raw garlic can cause stomach upset, but encapsulated garlic extracts are generally well tolerated. Garlic also has blood-thinning properties.

The Evidence for Herbs

In recent decades, the antimicrobial properties of most of the commonly used herbs have been documented by scientific studies. This not only includes in vitro (test tube) studies that show the ability of herbal phytochemicals to directly inhibit bacteria and other microbes, but also the mechanisms of action for different phytochemicals and how phytochemicals work in synergy in living models.

When searching for evidence that antimicrobial herbs can make a difference for chronic illnesses, chronic Lyme disease serves as a model. Many thousands of people struggling with chronic Lyme disease have reported benefit from using herbal therapy. Symptoms of chronic Lyme disease closely overlap with other chronic conditions, including fibromyalgia, chronic fatigue syndrome, multiple sclerosis and autoimmune illnesses, and, most recently, long COVID. Many people with these conditions have also reported benefits from taking herbs with antimicrobial properties. It suggests that all of these illnesses are closely related and have an intracellular microbe component.

In 2020 and 2021, researchers at Johns Hopkins University took notice. They found that several herbs commonly used to treat chronic Lyme disease—Chinese skullcap, Japanese knotweed, and cat's claw were on the list—had greater activity against Borrelia than conventional antibiotics.[97] In other studies, Chinese skullcap, Japanese knotweed, and andrographis were found to have equally impressive activity against Bartonella[98] and Babesia[99] (an intracellular protozoa). Even more interesting, these same herbs (along with garlic and ginger) were found to have activity against viruses, including SARS-CoV-2, influenza, and Epstein Barr virus (along with many others).

---

97 Feng J, Leone J, Schweig S, Zhang Y. Evaluation of natural and botanical medicines for activity against growing and non-growing forms of B. burgdorferi. *Front Med (Lausanne)*. 2020;7:6.

98 Ma X, Leone J, Schweig S, Zhang Y. Botanical medicines with activity against stationary phase *Bartonella henselae*. *Infect Microbes Dis*. 2021.

99 Zhang Y, Alvarez-Manzo H, Leone J, Schweig S, Zhang Y. Botanical medicines cryptolepis sanguinolenta, Artemisia annua, Scutellaria baicalensis, Polygonum cuspidatum, and Alchornea cordifolia demonstrate inhibitory activity against Babesia duncani. *Front Cell Infect Microbiol*. 2021;11:624745.

While this is good news for anyone trying to overcome chronic illness, it also supports the idea of taking herbs to reduce risk of chronic illness. All herbs—including both antimicrobial herbs and the everyday herbs—contain protective phytochemicals that help to keep your cells strong and healthy. Healthy cells are less vulnerable to microbes. Keeping your cells healthy is especially critical as you age. It's possibly the most compelling reason to make herbs part of your life.

Recommended Reading:

No one can be credited more for forwarding our knowledge of the antimicrobial properties of herbs than **Stephen Harrod Buhner** in his books, *Herbal Antibiotics*, **2012** and *Herbal Antivirals*, **2013**. These books offer a wealth of information, not only about the antimicrobial properties of herbal phytochemicals, but also the remarkable benefits of herbs in general. In *Healing Lyme*, **second edition, 2015** and other books in that series, Stephen Buhner starts to make the connection between microbes and chronic illness.

The Amazon basin of South America is a powerhouse of herbal phytochemical benefits, many of which have documented antimicrobial properties. In *The Healing Power of Rainforest Herbs*, **Leslie Taylor, ND** provides detailed evidence-based information about the most commonly used herbs in that region. A total of 92 herbs are profiled in depth, along with charts for how to best use the herbs.

Chapter Highlights

- Conventional antibiotics are ideally suited for acute infections with extracellular bacteria such as pneumococcal pneumonia.

- Limitations of conventional antibiotics include:

  ○ Disruption of the balance of normal flora

  ○ Bacterial resistance

  ○ Potential disruption of immune system functions

- Advantages of antimicrobial herbs include:

  ○ Suppress pathogens without disrupting the balance of the microbiome

  ○ Do not promote bacterial resistance

  ○ Modulate immune system functions

  ○ Low potential for toxicity

  ○ Offer a range of additional benefits

- Antimicrobial herbs are ideally suited for protecting cells of the body against everyday microbe threats and chronic conditions that may be associated with increased tissue activity of intracellular microbes.

Part Three
Staying Well & Living Well

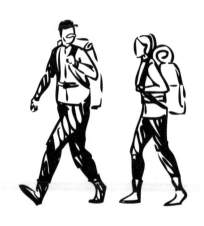

This section of the book is dedicated to simple, sustainable lifestyle habits that are central to promoting cellular wellness. While herbs have a remarkable potential to boost your health, the more you can build a foundation of good health habits, the better herbs can work for you. The next part of the book provides guidelines on how to nourish your body optimally, steer clear of toxins, be more active, balance stress, and defend yourself against microbial threats. These **five elements of wellness** reflect the model I follow myself and have used with patients for many years.

Here's what you'll learn in Part Three:

- **Nourish**: What to eat in order to nourish your body and reduce inflammation

- **Purify**: Where toxic substances lurk in the environment and how to minimize your exposure

- **Calm**: Key strategies for balancing the demands of modern life with the need for rest and rejuvenation

- **Move**: How to make physical activity a priority, no matter your age or physical ability

- **Defend**: Ways to reduce your exposure to microbes and support your immune system

11

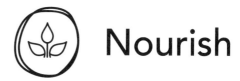 Nourish

Growing up in the early days of the fast food revolution, nutrition was the last thing on my mind. My diet, like that of most teenagers, was ruled by cheeseburgers and fries.

By the time I was a young physician in my thirties, I recognized that kind of eating was unsustainable, and I started adopting what I thought were healthy eating habits. Nutritional wisdom of the time suggested that whole grains were the key. I was fine with that idea, and my new dietary norm became whole grain breakfast bars, whole grain cereal, sandwiches for lunch, and pasta with garlic bread for supper. I even started baking my own bread.

My expanding waistline—along with digestive dysfunction evidenced as chronic reflux, gas, and a constant struggle with constipation—should have alerted me to the fact that it wasn't so fine, but I didn't know better at the time. Incorrectly assuming that not getting enough fiber was my problem, I poured myself king-sized bowls of bran cereal every morning and ate bran muffins at every opportunity.

As my health deteriorated through my forties, I began to question the nutritional status quo of the time. Though whole grain food products have more fiber than refined flour products, they are still loaded with carbohydrates and refined fats. And grain fiber doesn't necessarily promote a healthy balance of bacteria in the gut either.

Others were also questioning the wisdom of eating so much grain-sourced carbohydrates. That included voicing concerns about wheat gluten. Following that trend, I made my first major dietary adjustment: I cut out bread. Soon to follow, I eliminated pasta, as well as other products made from wheat flour. I don't know whether it was reducing the carbs or giving up gluten, but I started feeling better immediately, and gradually returned to a normal weight for me.

Recognizing the importance of food to health, I started exploring the question of what constitutes a healthy diet more deeply. Though we often allow our taste buds to dictate what we eat, foods that properly nourish the cells of our bodies and support normal digestion should be what guides our dietary choices. That, of course, is heavily influenced by what our ancient ancestors ate.

Following that angle, one dietary trend called the Paleo Diet seeks to mimic the pre-agricultural foraged food diet. The key feature of the Paleo diet is avoidance of *any* foods derived from grains and beans, including grain-fed meats and dairy. Unquestionably, eating fewer carbohydrates and fewer calories is more in line with our ancient food heritage and better health. However, I wrestled with just how restrictive it needs to be. Do you need to cut out all grains and beans to be healthy? Study of various populations around the world suggests not.

In Japan, people who follow a traditional diet have a low incidence of chronic illnesses and high life expectancy, despite the fact that they eat rice and soybean products several times a day. This is complemented by the fact that they typically eat lots of fish and vegetables, are very active, and drink lots of green tea, all of which likely contribute to their high health status.

The Mediterranean Diet—based on dietary practices in Greece, Italy, and other countries surrounding the Mediterranean Sea—is rich in vegetables and fish but also includes grains and beans. This is echoed by the Blue Zones studies (mentioned in Chapter 4) of long-lived populations whose traditional diets are high in vegetables and fruits but also include various grains and beans. Humans have been eating grains and beans consistently for at least 10,000 years, and most cultures have built up some tolerance to these foods.

Real Food

Putting all my observations together, I came to the conclusion that the health potential of any particular food is defined by how close that food is to its natural origins. **Whole foods**, made of intact cells—a stalk of celery, mushrooms, zucchini squash, a pear, a filet of salmon—have the highest potential to provide the optimal ratios of nutrients that our cells need to function optimally.

Vegetables should be a central feature of any healthy diet. This is supported by the fact that a high-vegetable diet is the common denominator of the Mediterranean Diet, the Paleo Diet, the Vegan Diet, and the traditional diets in the Blue Zones. I feel better, have more energy, think more clearly, and sleep better when vegetables dominate my diet. And I don't feel deprived because these are foods I enjoy. Michael Pollan captured it so well and succinctly in his book

In Defense of Food with his three guiding rules: "Eat food. Not too much. Mostly plants."

The fresher the food, the more nourishing it is. **Fresh whole foods retain the vital energy of the living source.** Vital energy, however, fades with time. There's only a narrow window in which you can capture the full vitality of fresh whole foods. Fortunately, we live in a time when fresh whole foods are more available than ever before in the history of humankind. The foods with the highest potential to nourish your cells are found at farmer's markets, fruit and vegetable stands, seafood markets, the produce and freezer aisles in grocery stores and—if you are willing to do a little gardening—even in your own backyard.

While fresh food is ideal, it is not always practical or available. Luckily, there are ways to preserve the vitality of fresh foods. Refrigeration and freezing are best. Drying offers an acceptable way of preserving grains, beans, and fruits. Fermentation would seem like a process of decay instead of preservation, but the microbes present offer a whole different level of vital energy. Beans and tomatoes preserve well in a can, but most other vegetables do not. Meat is best fresh or frozen, though oily fish, such as tuna, salmon, sardines, and anchovies preserve well in a can. The more that food is pulverized, packaged, and polluted with chemicals, the less vital energy and nutrition is left to properly sustain your cells.

Even with the availability of healthy food, however, it's all too tempting to reach for carb-loaded, processed food products. It has to do with our ancient tendency toward gorging. Because high-calorie foods were rare in the ancient world, our brain is programmed to prompt us to eat them whenever we see them. It's an urge that most of us struggle with every day. Admittedly, avoiding all processed food products is challenging, but the guidelines I've provided below can help you resist the urge.

To make life simpler, I've developed four guiding principles for balancing the need to nourish my cells with the need to satisfy my taste buds at the same time. I try to live by these principles every day of my life.

1. **Choose fresh whole foods whenever practical.**

2. **Eat more vegetables than anything else.**

3. **Limit pro-inflammatory foods—chiefly sugar, corn, wheat, and red meat—as much as you can.**

4. **Fill the leftover void with fresh whole fruits, beans, nuts, healthier whole grains, such as rice and oats, and healthy protein sources, such as poultry and fish.**

Making the Transition to a Healthy Diet

A healthy diet should be a lifestyle, not a trend. It's important to lay down some basic dietary ground rules and stay with them. Pick something that isn't too restrictive, so that you will be more likely to stick with the plan. My four dietary principles will fit a lot of healthful diet plans.

Start by ratcheting down your consumption of carbohydrates (starches and sugars). This tends to be tough for everyone (myself included), but if you value your health, these foods should be minimized. The list includes cookies, cakes, pasta, breakfast cereals, crackers, snack bars, fruit juices and products sweetened with fruit juices, and sugar-loaded beverages. There's just no room in a healthful diet for these types of food products. If life demands a crunch every now and then, look for crackers made from nut flours or high-protein flour. These still contain carbs, but not as much as most crackers.

Antidiabetic Properties of Herbs

When it comes to controlling carbohydrates and the damage done to your cells, herbal phytochemicals are your best friend. In a study[100] published in 2019, researchers cataloged hundreds of different commonly used herbs that have been found to provide antidiabetic properties by a variety of mechanisms.

Limit products made with wheat and corn flour. Loaded with carbohydrates and calories, but sparse in nutrients, consumption of wheat and corn flours should be kept to a minimum. Wheat and corn promote inflammation in the body. Many people are gluten sensitive and feel much better when gluten grains (wheat, barley, rye) are avoided or minimized. Even though corn has no gluten, it is high in carbohydrate calories and promotes inflammation in the body.

Rice tends to be the best tolerated of all grains. It's hypoallergenic and doesn't disrupt gut flora like many other grains. Quinoa and oats are also well tolerated. All grains, however, are high in carbohydrates and shouldn't make up a significant portion of your diet.

Bread is a problem no matter how you slice it. This is true whether it is regular or gluten-free, white or whole wheat, sprouted grain or thin-sliced. Save it for special occasions or eating out, but don't routinely keep bread at home. For sandwiches, try lettuce leaves in place of bread.

Sugar is sugar. Organic cane sugar, high-fructose corn syrup, honey, agave, maple syrup and rice syrup all contain sugars (just as in table sugar) and do the same harm if used excessively. In addition to

---

100   Salehi B, Ata A, V Anil Kumar N, et al. Antidiabetic Potential of Medicinal Plants and Their Active Components. *Biomolecules*. 2019;9(10):551.

controlling the amounts you add to foods and drinks yourself, be aware of the sugars found in processed food products and beverages.

When you need that sweet taste but want to avoid the calories, try stevia and monk fruit extract, which are natural sugar substitutes. Erythritol and xylitol are good, too, but they both tend to give people gas when eaten in large amounts.

Artificial sweeteners have been associated with a host of issues.

- *Saccharin* has been around the longest. It has a strong aftertaste and carries a lingering concern associated with cancer studies in laboratory animals. It's probably best avoided entirely.

- *Aspartame* consists of two amino acids, aspartic acid, and phenylalanine. Many diet soft drinks and a host of other products contain aspartame. Excessive aspartic acid and phenylalanine could cause imbalances in serotonin and other neurotransmitters, which may contribute to depression and other neurological symptoms. Through the years, a possible aspartame link to cancer has remained controversial, but a new 2021 study raises the question again.[101]

- *Sucralose* is the newest arrival on the artificial sweetener scene. Sucralose is derived from cane sugar, but three of the oxygen atoms in the sucrose molecule are then replaced with chlorine atoms. This creates a stronger chemical bond that is not broken down by enzymes in the human body. Of the three artificial sweeteners described here, sucralose is likely the safest, but it has been associated with weight gain, possible increased risk of diabetes, inflammatory bowel disease, and increased inflammation in the body (just as with table sugar).

---

101 Landrigan PJ, Straif K. Aspartame and cancer - new evidence for causation. *Environ Health*. 2021;20(1):42.

How much is too much carbohydrate? If you're counting carbohydrate grams, 300 grams per day should be your absolute limit, 200 grams is comfortable for most people, and 100 grams if you want to lose weight. (For reference, one-half cup of cooked rice contains about 22 grams of carbohydrate.) How much carbohydrate you can tolerate depends on your activity level: the more active you are, the more carbs you'll burn.

Fruits should be on your list of healthful foods. Fruits are loaded with fiber and nutrients, but should be eaten fresh and kept in much smaller portions than vegetables because of their high carbohydrate content. One banana contains 27 grams of carbohydrate and a medium-sized apple has 25 grams. A cup of blueberries equals 21 grams of carbohydrate. A cup of watermelon contains 11 grams of carbohydrate. Despite the carbs, wild berries are packed with potent antioxidants and protective phytochemicals.

Fill up on vegetables. Vegetables are your best food choice for nourishing your cells. More than half your food each day should be vegetables. This is because vegetables have it all: vitamins, minerals and other essential nutrients for nourishing cells; lower fat content and a modest amount of carbohydrates; beneficial fiber for balancing the microbiome and promoting optimal intestinal motility; and, of course, phytochemicals.

I loosely define vegetables as including **leaves** (such as lettuce and kale), **stalks** (celery, broccoli, fennel), **vegetable-fruits** (zucchini squash, pumpkin, tomatoes, and many others, which are considered fruits, botanically speaking), **roots and tubers** (sweet potatoes are best; limit white potatoes and red potatoes) and the **onion family**, which includes garlic and leeks. Though **mushrooms** are technically fungi, I toss them into the vegetable quota because they provide similar health benefits.

Here's a perk: A high intake of vegetables has been associated with reduced risk of virtually all diseases, including cardiovascular disease, diabetes, and cancer. (Read that sentence again to figure out why vegetarians live longer.) Vegetables have fiber that is essential for normal digestive function and reduces risk of all digestive disorders.

Nonetheless, getting people to consistently eat vegetables is easier said than done. Although vegetables provide ample quantities of essential nutrients for keeping the human body healthy, they aren't loaded with what drive our food cravings the most—namely, carbohydrates and fat. It's a real dilemma. Compared to many modern foods, vegetables seem bland and sometimes downright bitter.

Sugar, Fats, and Feel-Good Dopamine

An article published in *Scientific American* in 2016 noted that calorie-dense foods loaded with sugar and fat stimulate secretion of dopamine in the reward center of the brain.[102] Dopamine is the neurotransmitter associated with feeling happy and content. The more that high-calorie foods become a habit, however, the greater amount of carbohydrates and fats it takes to achieve the same feel-good levels of dopamine. Is it any wonder that a third of the American population is classified as obese?

The key to making vegetables a central part of your life is blending different vegetables with other foods and spices and adding just enough

---

102 Jabr F. How Sugar and Fat Trick the Brain into Wanting More Food. https://www.scientificamerican.com/article/how-sugar-and-fat-trick-the-brain-into-wanting-more-food/. Accessed February 26, 2022.

carbohydrate and fat to make vegetables taste good. Admittedly, a plate of plain steamed broccoli, cabbage, carrots, zucchini, onions, and mushrooms without any seasonings isn't very appetizing. But sauté in sesame oil or grapeseed oil with ginger, garlic, vinegar, lime, cashew or peanut butter, a protein source, such as chicken, coconut milk, and curry powder—served over a small bed of rice—and you have an exceptional *and highly nutritious* meal that meets the vegetable quota!

Top of the Morning Smoothie

I look for every opportunity to add vegetables into my life. Often, my mornings start with a smoothie of frozen wild blueberries, banana, celery, and carrots. Sometimes I add spinach, salad greens, or cucumber to contribute to my vegetable quota. To reinforce the health benefits, I add collagen powder (for joint support), ground flax seeds (for GI regularity), medicinal mushroom powder (from immune-boosting mushrooms such as lion's mane, reishi, or chaga), cat's claw (antimicrobial), and sometimes cocoa powder (rich in antioxidants). Grated ginger is another flavorful addition. You'll need to add a liquid base, such as juice or a type of milk—my current favorite is unsweetened flax milk. If you like, you can add a little sweetness with agave nectar or honey.

Don't overlook vegetables and fruits as significant sources of hydration. By weight, vegetables and fruits are approximately 70% water. Water is slowly released during the digestion process, aiding digestion and providing a constant source of hydration. Vegetables and fruits are also alkalinizing (neutralizes acidity in the body), which aids in reducing the risk of kidney stones and gallbladder stones and supports strong bones.

Fill your phytochemical gap with herbs. Even a healthy diet rich in vegetables doesn't come close to the phytochemical concentrations found in wild plants. Standardized extracts of herbs from the everyday category are the easiest way to compensate for the loss. Herbal phytochemicals protect cells from the damaging effects of glycation, free radicals, toxic substances, and invasive microbes. Herbs also balance hormones disrupted by chronic stress. To gain an extra edge above and beyond a healthy diet alone, taking herbal extracts is a practical choice.

Feed your flora. Another important aspect of vegetables is the fiber they contain. Vegetable fiber not only helps to keep your bowel movements regular but also significantly reduces your risk of colon cancer. Furthermore, when fiber gets to the end of the line—the colon—it feeds your valuable gut flora. In turn, they convert some of that fiber into smaller molecules called short-chain fatty acids, which energize the gut wall.

A common question asked by patients is whether to take a probiotic. In general, unless a person has had an illness requiring antibiotics or picked up an intestinal bug, I don't think taking a probiotic is necessary on a regular basis. A better choice is fermented foods.

Fermented foods. Daily consumption of fermented foods helps to continually seed the intestinal tract with favorable bacteria. Though dairy products such as yogurt and kefir are the most commonly consumed fermented foods in the Western world, fermented vegetables such as sauerkraut (buy it refrigerated, not canned, to gain the benefits of the live bacteria) and kimchi (a fermented savoy cabbage dish from Korea) shouldn't be overlooked, as they are exceptionally good sources of favorable bacteria. Fermented vegetables are also *pre*biotics—foods that provide nourishment for favorable bacteria. In addition to cabbage, some other prebiotic foods include onions, leeks, garlic, chicory, and Jerusalem artichokes.

Make your own food. When someone's grocery cart is loaded down with packages of processed food but no fresh foods, that person's health is, without a doubt, suffering. Though packaged foods might seem cheaper than fresh foods, the hidden costs are higher risk for all chronic illnesses and cancer, along with increased medical bills.

That being said, making all of your food from scratch often isn't practical or necessary. The guiding principle for purchasing prepared foods is this: Can you reasonably prepare that food yourself from fresh ingredients? For example, you probably don't need to go to the trouble of preparing your own mayonnaise, but you should buy a quality product with ingredients on the label that you recognize. If the label has things on it that don't look familiar, it's better to pass it by.

Do a Pantry and Refrigerator Makeover

The reality is that we tend to eat whatever is available. Your refrigerator should be full of fresh foods, especially weighted toward a variety of vegetables and fresh fruit. For snacks, it's a good practice to keep the pantry and fridge clear of high-carb packaged items. And keep healthier items on hand, such as turkey and lettuce roll-ups, celery and hummus, yogurt with blueberries, pecans with dark chocolate chips, or apples and cheese.

Be mindful of your calorie intake. The fact of the matter is that most of us consume more calories than we really need. Calorie demands, of course, vary with daily activity levels. A desk job requires a fraction of the calories necessary for construction work. If your daily calorie demand is on the low side of the spectrum, filling up on calorie-sparse vegetables—celery sticks with hummus or almond butter, salads instead of sandwiches—will reduce your carb cravings.

One strategy for reducing calories is narrowing your eating window to <12 hours a day. Some people call it intermittent fasting. It's great for your digestive system and for preserving your mitochondria. Eating all your food within a short interval of time would seem like an invitation to overeating; however, for most people it has the opposite effect, especially if you stick to the >50% vegetable rule. If you go for more than 12 hours without eating, your stomach will contract down so that when you do eat, you will get full faster.

Eating Less, Living More

Years ago, I knew a gentleman who at age 90 was still active and regularly playing doubles tennis. One time I asked him his secret. I thought he would attribute it to staying physically active, which was obviously part of the answer. He surprised me by stating very emphatically that he thought the one thing that made the most difference was the fact that he only ate one meal a day—at midday—and didn't eat much otherwise. He had followed this diet most of his life.

If you want to give intermittent fasting a try, start the day with tea, coffee, or fresh squeezed vegetable juice and don't snack until noon. Eat a normal lunch and snacks in the afternoon if desired, but try to eat supper before 6 pm (7 pm in the summer). Then, don't eat again until morning. This gives your digestive system a break and, if you're struggling with gut issues, it allows for healing. You will also find that it helps with weight control, as you may enjoy food more but tend to eat less. Another good practice is slowing down, chewing your food, and eating more mindfully.

Balance your diet according to foods that work best for you. Beyond vegetables, your diet should be proportionally divided among other natural food sources. The more diverse your diet, the closer you will come to fulfilling dietary requirements for optimal wellness.

How to divide it up is highly individual—everyone has different food tolerances. Finding what works best for you is often a process of trial and error. Sometimes you have to accept that even though you like a certain food, it may not like you back. You will feel better if you stick with foods that mesh well with your biochemistry. Most everyone has certain foods that they have to work around for one reason or another.

Nuts are great snack foods and can be included in food dishes to add both texture and flavor. Low in carbohydrates, they are good sources of healthful oils, protein, vitamins, and minerals. A handful of nuts, dark chocolate chips, and dried blueberries (preferably unsweetened) tastes much better than any "health" bar on the market. It may be a little less convenient, but creating your own trail mix allows you to personalize it to your taste.

Trail mix, the Ultimate On-the-go Food

Trail mix, the ultimate on-the-go food. There are many commercially available trail mixes, but it's not difficult to make your own. That way, you control the quality of the ingredients you put in it.

Pumpkin seeds (raw or roasted) make a great base for trail mix. Pumpkin seeds contain very healthful fats and are lower in calories than other nuts. Other ingredients might include sunflower seeds, pecans, walnuts, dried coconut, roasted almonds, roasted cashews, roasted pistachios, dried blueberries, dried cherries, dried cranberries, and bittersweet dark chocolate chips.

Beans have a place on the healthy food list. Beans are a good source of protein and complex carbohydrates including fiber. Of all the beans, the most digestible are mung beans and lentils. On the other hand, kidney beans (and some others) are high in compounds called lectins, which some people find irritating to the gut. Most beans do not cause blood sugar spikes, and in fact prevent them. Some exceptions include starchy beans such as lima beans and traditional "baked beans," which have added brown sugar or molasses. It is difficult to comment on refried beans without knowing the recipe involved; the dish is made with mashed pintos or black beans and some form of oil or fat. Some recipes use olive oil, and some call for bacon grease or lard. The sodium load is another issue with refried beans.

You need about 100 grams of "complete" protein each day to replace the turnover of protein in the body. Three ounces of lean meat (about the size of a deck of cards) provides about 30 grams of protein, and one egg provides about 6-8 grams of protein.

A complete protein source is a source that provides all nine amino acids that are defined as "essential". When a nutrient is defined as essential, it means that substance must be obtained from food. There are many amino acids that the body can synthesize internally, but all nine essential amino acids must be obtained from dietary sources for the body to be able to make proteins.

Complete **vegetarian protein sources**, offering all nine of the essential amino acids, include soybeans and fermented soy products such as tofu and tempeh, hemp, buckwheat, quinoa, chia seeds, amaranth, and spirulina. When combined (but not alone), rice and beans provide all essential amino acids and are considered a complete protein source.

Fish, poultry, and eggs are all good sources of animal protein, providing both complete protein and healthful fats. Fish is especially anti-inflammatory. **Beef and pork** tend to have higher concentrations of saturated fat and toxic substances stored in fat. High consumption of red meat promotes inflammation in the body. Therefore, red meat is best eaten only occasionally and in small amounts.

The Dangers of High Meat Diets

Though meat is arguably the best source of complete protein, heavy meat eaters pay a steep price. Beyond the fact that meat, especially red meat, contains high levels of saturated fats that clog arteries, metabolizing lots of extra protein is toxic. When amino acids are metabolized to produce energy, nitrogen is released in the form of ammonia, which is quite toxic to cells and hard on kidneys. High-protein diets are also linked to bone loss, in both men and women. Metabolism of protein generates acid in tissues, which must be immediately neutralized. To compensate, the body pulls calcium carbonate from bones to neutralize the acid and maintain normal blood and tissue pH of 7.4. Finally, high meat consumption stimulates growth of bacteria in the colon that has been associated with colon cancer.

If you choose to eat meat, choose wisely. Most of the meat available at a typical grocery store comes from mass-produced animals that have been fed a grain-based diet. Contrast this with pasture-raised animals that eat a diverse array of wild plants and have significantly higher amounts of phytochemicals concentrated in their meat and milk. You'll also want to look for meat (and dairy) produced without antibiotics, which have been linked to the rise of antibiotic resistance. That certainly builds a case for paying attention to the sources of our meat and dairy products, and for stepping back to appreciate the interconnectedness of food chains.

A few more thoughts about dairy. Dairy products are often touted as health foods, primarily because of calcium content, but the evidence isn't necessarily there to support it. Whole milk is high in both carbohydrates and saturated fat. Many people do not produce adequate levels of the enzyme lactase that is necessary to break down lactose (milk sugar). The undigested lactose is fermented by intestinal bacteria, which causes symptoms of intestinal discomfort, gas and bloating, and loose stools. Some people have sensitivities to casein proteins, which account for 80% of proteins in milk (another milk protein called whey protein, found in many powdered protein supplements, is generally well tolerated).

The bottom line is that if you tolerate dairy and want to use it, look for low-carb, low-fat options. The newest is filtered milk, which has much of the lactose filtered out of it, significantly reducing the carbohydrate content. Filtered milk is available as 2%, which is half the fat of whole milk. An even healthier option is nut milk, such as almond milk, which is low carb, contains healthy fats, and has just as much calcium as cow's milk. Soymilk is a great source of protein and calcium unless soy allergy is an issue.

Cultured yogurt is lower in lactose than milk products and is available in low-fat versions; look for products without added sugar. Hard cheeses (parmesan, Swiss, hard cheddar), are very low in lactose, high in protein, and lower in fat than soft cheeses such as mozzarella.

The healthiest oils for cooking include olive oil, sesame oil, coconut oil, and ghee (clarified butter). Use olive oil only for lower heat cooking, as it has a low smoke point. Grapeseed oil, walnut oil, and avocado oil are good choices for cooking with low heat or in salads. Avoid refined oils, such as soybean, corn, and canola, commonly found in processed food products. Other fats are best obtained from natural food sources—fresh meats, fish/seafood, and whole plant foods such as nuts and avocados. Deep-fried foods are notoriously unhealthy.

Water is the healthiest beverage you can drink. Admittedly, however, plain water is a bit boring. Outside of water, tea of any variety, sweetened with just a bit of sugar, honey, or stevia is the healthiest beverage you can drink (unsweetened is even better). Coffee is fine in moderation because it contains antioxidants. Coconut water is very refreshing after exercise—it's low in sugar and high in beneficial potassium. Soft drinks (diet or regular) and fruit drinks are best avoided completely. Although artificially sweetened diet soft drinks don't contain calories, they have been linked to increased risk of diabetes and heart disease. If you want a healthier alternative to a soft drink, try flavored sparkling water. You can add sweetness with stevia.

Every now and then, you have to indulge. Make a mental list of foods that you eat regularly, but you know are unhealthy. Your list may include things such as bread, cake, ice cream, pastries, pasta, or breakfast cereal. For several months, purge these foods from your diet completely. Once you become comfortable with a healthier diet, you can start allowing yourself occasional indulgences of some of these foods. Examples might include bread when you go out to eat for a special meal, a small amount of pasta once a week, or a snack bar after going for a jog. It's important, however, to avoid falling back into old habits. As my relationship with food changed, I came to appreciate a food's capacity to enhance my health as much as its capacity to satisfy my taste buds.

Nutritional Supplement Support

- **Omega-3** fatty acids are important molecules that our bodies cannot make, and so they must be consumed. The number 3 refers to the position of a certain bond within the molecular chain. "Omega-3s", as they are often called, are a group of especially virtuous unsaturated fats that are found in abundance in oily fish (such as salmon, mackerel, anchovies, and sardines) and krill (small shrimp), as well as in walnuts, pecans, chia seeds, flaxseed, and borage oil.

When you consume omega-3s regularly, they offer extraordinary health benefits. Having healthy blood levels of omega-3s has been closely linked to reduced risk of heart attack. Their anti-inflammatory properties also provide some relief from arthritis and help to prevent it, as well. They also optimize blood lipids and prevent oxidation of cholesterol (which makes cholesterol less atherogenic). Omega-3s also promote brain health and protect cognitive function. Some studies suggest that they may even help with mood stabilization.

For many years, I recommended fish oil to patients as a reasonable and affordable way to get those important omega-3 benefits. However, there's also an alternative, krill oil, that is now commercially available and offers distinct advantages over fish oil. For starters, krill oil causes no fishy burps, reflux, or fishy taste. It is also much easier for the body to absorb omega-3s from krill oil than from fish oil. In fact, it takes 37% less krill oil compared to fish oil to achieve the same omega-3 levels. This is due in part to the fact that krill oil occurs in a form called phospholipids, which are more readily absorbed and used by the body than the triglycerides found in fish oil.

Krill oil's antioxidant power is many times stronger than that of fish oil, thanks mainly to the presence of astaxanthin. Astaxanthin is the chemical that gives shrimp and flamingos their pink color. This potent natural antioxidant promotes optimal heart, joint, brain, eye, and immune function and acts as a natural preservative for the oil. Krill oil also contains choline, a vitamin-like nutrient that supports brain health.

One final reason you might choose krill oil over fish oil is sustainability. Krill is mostly harvested from the waters surrounding Antarctica. Responsible krill harvesters have impeccable traceability and are very active in monitoring krill abundance. Maximal harvest is predicted to only affect 1% of the total Antarctic population of krill. Look for the Marine Stewardship Council (MSC) logo to ensure you are purchasing from a sustainable source.

General suggested dosing ranges are 500-1500 mg of krill oil daily or 1000-3000 mg of fish oil daily. Please note that both fish oil and krill oil are natural blood thinners. Talk with your health care provider before trying these if you are already taking a prescription blood thinner, as a brain hemorrhage could occur with an overdose. If bruising appears, discontinue use or lower the dose.

- **Lutein and zeaxanthin.** Lutein and zeaxanthin are potent antioxidants, called carotenoids, that offer specific protection to the skin and eyes. UV light from the sun penetrates and damages cellular structures within the skin and eyes. This kind of damage can lead to skin cancers, macular degeneration (gradual destruction of the retina of the eye), and cataracts (damage to the lens of the eye). Whether consumed through diet or through supplements, lutein and zeaxanthin build up in the layers of the skin and the retina, absorb some of the UV energy, and thus minimize damage to these sensitive tissues. General daily dosing recommendations are 1-3 mg of lutein combined with 1-3 mg of zeaxanthin. Supplementing with lutein and zeaxanthin within these dose ranges is as safe as eating any natural foods that contain these substances.

- **Pine bark extract.** Bark protects a tree or shrub from many threats, including free radicals, insects, and microbes. Not surprisingly, many tree and shrub barks have remarkable protective properties. One of the most well-studied is maritime pine bark from trees on the coast of France. The phytochemicals in French maritime pine bark have been found to improve the integrity of the entire vascular system by providing potent antioxidants that protect blood vessels, increase blood flow by dilating blood vessels, and reduce thickness of blood (blood thinner). This spectrum of phytochemicals also offers anti-inflammatory properties and support for the immune system (increases natural killer cells). Antioxidant protection extends to eyes and skin.

The Multivitamin Question

I am often asked about the role of vitamin supplements. Do we really need a daily multivitamin and mineral supplement? The answer, really, is individual to a person's needs. In my opinion, people who have good health and eat well are probably just fine without a multivitamin. On the other hand, those who have an increased cellular demand for vitamins will likely benefit from a daily multivitamin supplement. This includes pregnant women, breastfeeding women, surgery patients, burn patients, and people recovering from chronic illness.

It also depends on what vitamins you're talking about. Some people need selected vitamins. For example, supplemental vitamin B-12 is recommended for vegetarians (especially vegans, who don't have a food source of this vitamin); the elderly, who suffer diminished production of a stomach chemical called intrinsic factor that is necessary to absorb B-12; and anyone who takes heartburn medications, because stomach acid normally makes vitamin B-12 more bioavailable (i.e., in a form that is ready to be absorbed).

Vitamin D is another one to monitor. You cannot absorb calcium well if your vitamin D level is low. Moreover, vitamin D is not only an important vitamin, but it's also a hormone that plays a role in regulating many functions in the body, including healthy immune system functions. Our skin makes Vitamin D when exposed to the sun, but our levels tend to dip precipitously during winter. Furthermore, some people do not get much sun exposure in any season. Also, as we age, we lose some capacity to make and activate vitamin D, so supplementing with this important vitamin (in the form of D3) makes sense. Average doses are 1000-2000 IU daily, but people living at northern latitudes may need much higher doses, typically in the range of 5000-10,000 IU daily. Testing your vitamin D level once or twice a year is the best way to gauge your dose. You can do it at your doctor's office, but home test kits for vitamin D are also available.

The conclusion of the medical community is that there isn't enough evidence to support vitamin and mineral supplementation. As recently as 2018, research published in the *Journal of the American College of Cardiology* reviewed data from 179 individual trials and concluded that multivitamin supplements did not help prevent or improve cardiovascular disease.[103] Another study examined data from more than 30,000 people over six years and found that people who took multivitamins had about the same risk of dying as those who didn't take a multivitamin.[104]

You have to consider, however, that all of these studies used synthetic forms of the vitamins. There's a lot of difference between the vitamins in an average multivitamin product and the natural vitamins and minerals found in food. And synthetic versions of vitamins are not always a perfect match for our physiology. For example, vitamin E exists in foods in a variety of different forms in the body, but most vitamin supplements contain only one form of vitamin E, called alpha tocopherol.

---

103 Jenkins DJA, Spence JD, Giovannucci EL, et al. Supplemental vitamins and minerals for CVD prevention and treatment. *J Am Coll Cardiol*. 2018;71(22):2570-2584.

104 Chen F, Du M, Blumberg JB, et al. Association between dietary supplement use, nutrient intake, and mortality among US adults: a cohort study." *Ann Intern Med*. 2019;170(9):604-613.

Another example is B vitamins. Most multivitamin products contain a B vitamin called folic acid. Folic acid is not the natural form of the B vitamin found in the body and 40% of the population cannot utilize it, which can actually be harmful. The natural forms of this B vitamin are folinic acid or methyltetrahydrofolate. Also, minerals in inorganic form, as opposed to natural amino acid chelates found in better quality multivitamin products, are not well absorbed.

So, if you want to take a high-quality multivitamin alongside a good diet, I don't think there is harm in this approach and, for some people, it may be highly beneficial. Just remember that *quality* is the key part of that statement. It's important to pick one with vitamins and minerals in a natural form that the body can easily utilize. A quality multivitamin will typically contain mixed tocopherols (not alpha tocopherol), folinic acid or methyltetrahydrofolate (instead of folic acid), and minerals in an organic form such as amino acid chelates.

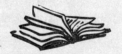

Recommended Reading:

In his 2020 New York Times bestseller *Food Fix*, Mark Hyman, MD details how we can not only save ourselves but also save the planet in the food choices that we make every day. It's an interesting read that shows how much food is interconnected with everything we do and how the food industry contributes to the high rate of chronic illness that has become prevalent in our society.

Chapter Highlights

- Four key principles for a healthy diet:

  ◦ Choose fresh, whole foods whenever practical.

  ◦ Eat more vegetables than anything else.

  ◦ Limit pro-inflammatory foods—chiefly sugar, corn, wheat, and red meat—as much as you can.

  ◦ Include moderate amounts of fresh fruits, nuts, rice, oats, and healthy protein sources such as beans, poultry and fish.

- The protective phytochemicals of herbs help to make up for the phytochemical deficiency in our modern diets and protect cells from the damaging effects of glycation, free radicals, and toxic substances.

12

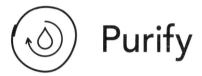 Purify

Nothing makes you more aware of pollution than being near a highway on a cold, still day. Cool air doesn't rise, so if there isn't a breeze, car fumes hang by the roadway like a dense fog.

I happened to be riding my bike on one such day. It was in the middle of the afternoon when traffic was low. Even so, the stench was noticeable. After an hour, my eyes burned and my throat and nasal passages were uncomfortably irritated. I wondered if my liver cells were shifting into overdrive in an attempt to detoxify some of this stuff.

And it's not just the vehicle fumes, of course. When you include coal-burning utilities, industry, and a dizzying array of machines powered by petroleum, you have a significant environmental issue. Beyond those pollution sources, the chemical industry converts petroleum distillates into a nearly infinite variety of compounds used for everything imaginable—from pesticides to plastics.

Fossil fuels—petroleum, natural gas, and coal—are called fossil fuels because they originated from living sources. Coal comes from swamp plants that were trapped within the surface of the earth millions of years ago. Similarly, petroleum and natural gas come from marine organisms—mainly algae and bacteria—that were trapped within the sediments of shallow seas millions of years ago.

If you were able to go back in time and eat the organic matter that would become petroleum and coal, it wouldn't harm you. In fact, it might even be good for you. Millions of years of heat and pressure, however, distorted the organic molecules that make up fossil fuels into configurations that are not compatible with biological life. Coal has the added concern of heavy metals being compressed into it.

In a brief span of a hundred years, the earth's atmosphere has become saturated with hundreds of thousands of unique man-made chemicals that can be sourced to fossil fuels. The European Chemicals Agency has identified 144,000 man-made chemicals in existence, with more being added every day. They're in the soil, the water, the air, and in every living creature. Even animals that live in polar areas with no nearby industries have been found to harbor plastics and other unnatural potential toxicants in their bodies.

Toxic substances migrate up the food chain. It starts with the very smallest creatures in soil and streams, concentrating with each step up the food chain, until toxic substances are most concentrated in the largest creatures on land and the largest fish in the oceans. Being at the top of the food chain, we carry some of the highest concentrations of petrochemical residues and heavy metals of any creature on earth.

You'd be astounded at the long list of toxins that are lurking in your tissues. Though the toxic effects are not usually perceived, you shouldn't discount the potential for toxic substances to weaken your cells and your immune system. Toxic substances disrupt cellular functions, turn on bad genes, and disrupt hormonal pathways in the body. As a society, however, we've been complacent about the harmful effects that man-made toxic substances have on us because these pollution sources are so intimately connected to things that make life comfortable. It's easy to look the other way and ignore the problem.

Chemical toxins aren't the only concern either. The modern world has become a sea of artificial electromagnetic energy and unnatural radiation. We are literally surrounded by our electromagnetic devices: cell phones, computers, copiers, and electric grids. Though all living things emit an electrical field that surrounds them, the energy emitted by artificial electrical devices, power grids, and microwave towers (who knows where we're headed with 5G) is distinctly different from that of living things. Constant exposure to artificial energy fields has the potential to disrupt signaling and cellular energy throughout the body.

If that weren't enough, we're also exposed to unnatural ionizing radiation sources. Ionizing radiation is energy that can damage tissues of biological lifeforms. Natural sources of ionizing radiation include UV rays, x-rays, and gamma rays from the sun and solar system. Every lifeform on earth is exposed, and we have built-in protection—but no one really knows how much we are being affected by additional exposure from routine x-rays for dental and medical concerns and other unnatural sources.

Unfortunately, things aren't likely to change anytime soon. To protect yourself and your family, you must learn to live around it. Fortunately, reducing your exposure isn't as challenging as you might think. Toxic substances can only enter the body one of three ways: by ingestion, breathing, and absorption through the skin. You do have choices: you can control what you eat and drink, what you slather on your skin, the air you breathe (to some extent, anyway), indoor lighting, use of electronic devices, and more.

Foods That Help Us Detox

Preventing exposure to toxins is the best strategy, but what about those toxins that we inevitably take in through our diet? (Hey, it's not a perfect world.) At that point, the goal is to neutralize toxins and remove them from the body. Eating fresh vegetables and fruits can help you accomplish this because they provide protective antioxidants, hydration, and fiber that promote normal digestive and liver functions—all of which are essential for natural detoxification. The antioxidants are important for neutralizing free radicals. Once toxic substances are neutralized, dietary fiber from vegetables and fruits binds to those toxins and funnels them out of the body with the feces.

Eat organic foods whenever practical. Foods produced using chemical pesticides, hormones, and antibiotics have obvious health concerns. We pay the costs in the long run in terms of both our health and damage to the environment.

The prices tend to be a bit higher on organic products. If you've won the lottery, you'll want to make *all* of your food choices organic, as assurance that there is some oversight to the farming methods involved. But if you are looking to stretch your food budget a bit, buy organic varieties when you are selecting thin-skinned vegetables and fruits, as any pesticide residues tend to accumulate on the peel. In general, it is less of an issue with thick-skinned vegetables and fruits that will be peeled or that have a thick outer rind.

As the Environmental Working Group (ewg.org) suggests on its website, even if you can't make 100% of your purchases organic, continue to eat fruits and vegetables anyway because the health benefits outweigh the risks. The Environmental Working Group, a nonprofit organization, lists the following in its 2021 Shopper's Guide to Pesticides in Produce:

Dirty Dozen (Buy these organic, if you can): *strawberries, spinach, kale (also collard and mustard greens), nectarines, apples, grapes, cherries, peaches, pears, bell and hot peppers, celery, tomatoes.*

Clean Fifteen (Produce with the least pesticide residue in their recent tests): *avocados, sweet corn, pineapples, onions, papaya, sweet peas (frozen), eggplant, asparagus, broccoli, cabbage, kiwi, cauliflower, mushrooms, honeydew melon, cantaloupe.*

That might leave you with questions about produce that isn't on either list. For example, what about America's favorite fruit, bananas? They have a peel, so you'd think they would make that Clean Fifteen list. But bananas are very susceptible to fungi and are routinely sprayed with fungicides. While only low levels of fungicide are usually detectable in the edible part of a banana, it did not make it to their Clean Fifteen, at least for 2021.

The ultimate solution is to start a home garden where you choose not to use pesticides. You will, however, draw a crowd of hungry bugs to your buffet. And you'll have to be both vigilant and willing to settle for a few holes in your collard greens and maybe a less-than-perfect tomato. Gardening is rewarding, but it's a fair amount of work. If home gardening is not for you, then hedge your bets by diversifying the sources of your foods. Check out local farmers' markets. And if you have a choice of grocery stores in your area, rotate among them when shopping for produce because they likely source from different suppliers.

Buying meat? Be cognizant that any chemical contaminants in the animal feed is stored and concentrated in the animal's fatty tissues. The largest animals—cows, pigs, and even large fish, such as tuna and swordfish—have the highest concentrations of toxic substances in tissues. So, if meat is part of your regular diet, you should go small and look for "grass-fed" and organic, whenever practical. If you eat fish, stay with smaller fish and limit consumption of large fish such as tuna and swordfish. Salmon tend to be low to moderate in their load of toxic substances and heavy metals, with wild-caught generally lower than farm-raised.

Water

One option for ensuring clean water is installing a filter for your drinking water. You can accomplish much with a modern water-filtering system. Under-the-kitchen-sink systems are available as well as whole-house systems. Reverse osmosis systems remove the most contaminants, but be aware that they also remove most minerals, including calcium and magnesium.

Another option is purchasing filtered spring water or alkalized water. Many health food stores have this available to fill your own containers, preferably in glass or bisphenol-A (BPA)-free plastic containers.

Avoid drinking from plastic bottles whenever practical. Many types of plastic bottles emit hormonally active chemical compounds. These substances have been linked to hormonally active cancers including breast and prostate cancer. It's hard to avoid plastic completely, but minimizing it is a good practice. Try to buy beverages in glass containers or BPA-free plastics whenever possible. Carry or store water in glass or stainless steel containers.

Air

Ventilate spaces where you live and work. Changing the filters on your HVAC system is important for reducing the concentration of dust and allergens in the air. If you are sensitive, you may want to take the added step of having a freestanding HEPA air-filtering system, especially in rooms where you sleep. Freestanding HEPA filtration units can be purchased at any home improvement center.

In regard to flooring, wood flooring is preferred over carpet because carpet fiber holds dust and other allergens. Wood floors are also easier to clean. If you really want carpet, search for non-toxic fiber and backing, and be sure to request low-VOC (volatile organic compounds) foam padding. Most modern interior paints and building materials are now fairly low in volatile chemicals, but if you repaint, be sure to use low-VOC paints.

Prevent mold. Mold produces toxins that are highly disruptive to our immune system functions. Mold thrives in warm, damp places—the tightly sealed modern construction, used for homes and buildings, holds in moisture that promotes the growth of mold. The industrial HVAC systems used in offices and apartment buildings are also notorious for growing mold. As a result, sick building syndrome is common and seldomly recognized. Basements, crawl spaces, attics, and bathrooms are among the many problem areas. The best way to prevent mold is by keeping the interior of the house dry. Ventilate bathrooms and kitchens well. Install dehumidifiers in the crawl space and basement. Promptly replace wet carpet (including padding), floorboards, insulation, and drywall in any water-damaged areas. You will probably need to do some research to find experienced professionals to do this work.

Use safe cleaning products. Regarding cleaners, you have probably noted the array of products available. An inexpensive but surprisingly versatile choice is plain white vinegar. You can dilute it to clean windows and other surfaces. Never mix vinegar and chlorine bleach because toxic and potentially fatal chlorine gas is released. Avoid using cleaners containing synthetic chemicals to which you may develop chemical sensitivity. The Environmental Working Group (ewg.org) posts guidelines for safe cleaners and other household chemicals.

Visit natural outdoor areas as often as possible. There is nothing more revitalizing than spending time in nature. Documented benefits of being outdoors include increased alertness, improvement in mood, reduced allergies, and increased immune function. In a landmark 2008 study, researchers in Japan documented the health benefits of walking in a pine forest, commonly called "forest bathing".[105] They found that spending time in a pine forest increased natural killer cells, boosted immune functions, reduced anxiety and depression, and improved the sense of well-being of their study participants. The effect was attributed, in part, to compounds called phytoncides, which are airborne phytochemicals that many plants naturally emit to deter pathogens and insects. Pine forests, of any variety, are especially rich sources of phytoncides.

In a later study, the same researchers were able to reproduce those results in an artificial controlled setting.[106] Volunteer medical students kept in hotel rooms were exposed to an aerosol of the cypress phytoncides for three days. The cypress aerosol mimicked the level found in the forest air. Participants experienced the same level of increased natural killer cells, boosted immune functions, reduced anxiety and depression, and improved sense of well-being as the subjects in the forest-bathing study.

The positive experience of nature goes beyond the air. Artificial sounds and lights are very disruptive to brain functions. So, a walk in the woods helps to rebalance our brains and reduce stress.

Bring nature indoors. There's little doubt that natural environments are better for us than artificial environments, but can artificial environments be made more like natural environments? One of the most obvious ways that you can bring nature inside is to bring plants inside—and the more the better. Plants are nature's purifiers. They pull many pollutants from the air while also generating those beneficial phytoncides.

---

105 Li Q, Morimoto K, Kobayashi M, et al. A forest bathing trip increases human natural killer activity and expression of anti-cancer proteins in female subjects. *J Biol Regul Homeost Agents.* 2008;22(1):45-55.
106 Li Q, Kobayashi M, Wakayama Y. Effect of phytoncide from trees on human natural killer cell function. *Int J Immunopathol Pharmacol.* 2009;22(4):951-959.

Essential oils. If plants aren't an option, or you want to go one step further, essential oils contain phytoncides and other beneficial volatile phytochemical compounds. An essential oil diffuser emits an aerosol of the oils into a room. Good choices include tea tree oil, frankincense, and essential oils from coniferous trees.

Skin

Be wary of exposing skin to irritating or potentially toxic chemicals. Purchase disposable gloves and store them everywhere you might use them—kitchen, bathroom, laundry area, garage or workbench, and vehicle.

When shopping, read the labels on skin care products and select ones derived from natural sources. Antiperspirant/deodorant products not containing aluminum are preferred. Creams, lotions, and other topically applied substances are often overlooked as a source of toxins and allergens. The Environmental Working Group regularly posts lists of safe skin care products.

Sunlight—the Good, the Bad, and the Ugly

Being in sunshine warms your body as well as your soul. And sun exposure is the best way to naturally make vitamin D (often called the "sunshine vitamin"), essential for calcium absorption, maintaining healthy bones, optimal immune system functioning, and more.

The sun, however, is a potent force. We all know that a full day in the sun—even with sunscreen and protective clothing—can be quite draining. Ultraviolet (UV) light from the sun is a major source of damaging radiation to our skin and eyes and its "collagen crunching" abilities contribute to wrinkling. Radiation from the sun does damage as it strikes molecules in tissues of the skin and eyes, generating free radicals. Antioxidants such as lutein, zeaxanthin, phytochemicals found in pine bark extract, and resveratrol absorb excess energy and neutralize free radicals, minimizing the damage to our cells. This protects our valuable collagen and thereby reduces wrinkle formation.

Clothing and sunglasses offer the best protection against sun exposure. Some protection can also be gained by regularly eating certain yellow-orange vegetables, which are loaded with chemical compounds called carotenoids. Carotenoids build up in the skin and in the retina of the eyes, helping to counteract some of the damaging effects of sun exposure. Eating or juicing two carrots a day is a good practice.

Though using sunscreen is a good idea, many sunscreens contain chemical compounds that can become carcinogenic when exposed to UV light. Use sunscreens that are free of potentially carcinogenic chemicals. As mentioned previously, the Environmental Working Group (ewg. org) maintains a list of sunscreens that are free of potentially harmful chemical compounds.

Moreover, sunscreens block UV light, which means that they limit our skin's ability to produce vitamin D for us. About 15-30 minutes of sun exposure without sunscreen, several days a week, is enough to generate daily requirements of vitamin D. Even so, having your vitamin D levels checked and supplementing as indicated makes sense.

Other Toxic Threats

Limit alcohol. There's no way around it: alcohol and the metabolites of alcohol are highly toxic to living cells, especially liver cells. This is partially balanced by the fact that alcohol has some anxiety-relieving properties, but only with low to moderate consumption (no more than 1-2 glasses of wine or beer per day). In addition, red wine contains resveratrol, the previously mentioned phytochemical found in grapes known to have strong health benefits. Beer also contains favorable yeast that can provide health benefits. The bigger picture, though, is that alcohol is one of the most addictive substances on earth and stopping at a single alcoholic beverage is a real challenge for many people. If for you, one drink leads to another and then another, it may be best to avoid alcohol completely.

If you smoke, stop. Smoking adds yet another source of heavy metals, especially cadmium, organic toxins, and electron-deficient positive ions, along with a host of other toxic chemicals. Cigarette smoke is a notorious "collagen cruncher" that will age skin rapidly and prematurely.

Cook in stainless steel or ceramic pans. Stainless steel and ceramic are the most inert cooking surfaces. Ceramic is silicon dioxide, the same compound found in glass and sand. Nonstick ceramic pans are typically aluminum with a thin, ultrasmooth layer of ceramic applied to the surface. Although they don't last as long as some other nonstick surfaces, they don't shred into potentially toxic particles. Overall, ceramics are fairly durable and are a good option if you don't love scrubbing pans.

Be mindful of your medicines. Most drugs are therapeutically dosed toxicants. Though there is a place for drug therapy, the potential toxicity of drugs should be respected. Use drugs only in the lowest doses necessary. If you follow all the recommendations in this book, your need for drug therapy will be greatly reduced and possibly eliminated.

Check for radon. Some damaging radiation comes from the earth. Most of it fits into the category of background radiation, which we are designed to tolerate. However, one type that all homeowners should be aware of is radon gas. This radioactive gas is emitted from the soil in some locations. The gas collects in basements and crawl spaces and can be a threat. Testing kits are commercially available and protecting yourself is a matter of ventilating the space and installing a simple barrier. If you live in an area where radon gas is a problem, testing your home would be wise. Testing kits are available in many hardware stores and some drugstores. A simple internet search for "radon gas high-risk areas" is worthwhile to learn more about your general vicinity.

Protect Your Energy

Although the jury is still out on how much the artificial energy field from devices such as cell phones, laptops, computers, and computer screens disrupt cellular processes,[107,108] putting as much distance between you and electronic devices as is practical makes sense. Some proactive steps you can take include not keeping your cell phone constantly on your person and taking breaks from computers whenever possible.

Artificial lighting can also be disruptive. In the evenings, try to break away from your computer and cell phone screens, as reducing your exposure to the blue light from these devices will help you sleep better. You will notice a difference! Also, try to get outdoors daily in open natural spaces away from devices, excessive noise, and artificial lighting.

Find a quiet place. When you can't control the noise around you, earplugs are a simple solution. And noise-canceling headphones are well worth the investment if you travel on airplanes or work in or near construction zones or high-traffic areas. Find solace in natural areas that are free of artificial noise pollution as often as is practical.

---

107 Kim JH, Lee JK, Kim HG, Kim KB, Kim HR. Possible effects of radiofrequency electromagnetic field exposure on central nerve system. *Biomol Ther (Seoul)*. 2019;27(3):265-275.

108 Kıvrak EG, Yurt KK, Kaplan AA, Alkan I, Altun G. Effects of electromagnetic fields exposure on the antioxidant defense system. *J Microsc Ultrastruct*. 2017;5(4):167-176.

How Detoxification Happens

Fortunately, the body does have the ability to eliminate toxins via a very sophisticated detoxification system. Detoxification never stops. The body is continually processing toxic substances every minute of every day.

Detoxification starts at the cellular level. Plasma, the liquid that passes from the bloodstream into spaces around cells, flushes away toxic substances and metabolic wastes that have been purged by cells. Increased blood flow from physical activity or a sauna enhances the removal of toxic substances from cells. The cells of your body absolutely depend on periodic sustained surges of blood flow to purge the buildup of waste products and toxic substances.

Toxic substances and metabolic waste that have been purged from cells are delivered to the liver, where they are neutralized and converted into water-soluble substances. From there, they are either delivered to the kidneys or secreted in bile into the intestinal tract for removal from the body. Remember that vegetable fiber is crucial for binding toxic substances in the gut and whisking them out of the body, keeping them from being reabsorbed.

Vegetables provide other detox-related functions, too. Leafy greens are your best source of l-methylfolate and other "methyl donors" that are necessary for the detoxification process. Cruciferous vegetables, including cabbage, cauliflower, collards, Bok choy, Brussels sprouts, kale and especially broccoli, enhance the liver's ability to neutralize hormonally active toxic substances. These same vegetables also influence the way the liver metabolizes estrogens in the body, which may reduce the risk of breast cancer and other estrogen-related cancers.

Toxic substances get backed up when the load of toxins coming into the body exceeds the capacity of the liver to neutralize and process them. If you feel well, it's a good indication that you haven't exceeded your body's capacity to purge toxic substances. On the other hand, if you feel "toxic" or you are experiencing symptoms of chronic illness, it's likely that toxic substances are getting backed up in your tissues. While a ten-day detox may help you feel better temporarily, this is a long-standing issue that needs to be addressed.

In youth, the body has a high capacity to process toxic substances because liver functions are at peak performance. As aging occurs, however, the liver's processing ability declines as the liver loses functional liver cells. Poor health habits compound the problem.

To stay ahead of toxic accumulation, detoxification support needs to be a lifelong habit. In other words, consistently following healthy dietary practices, minimizing exposure to toxic substances, exercising regularly, taking steps to keep stress under control, and protecting your liver with herbal supplements.

Detoxification Support

Herbs are your insurance policy. Herbs from the everyday category provide potent antioxidants and a host of other beneficial phytochemicals that protect cells in tissues and organs throughout the body from the damaging effects of toxic substances and unnatural radiation. They also neutralize toxic substances at the cellular level and balance hormone systems in the body that have been disrupted by hormonally active toxic substances.

Certain herbs, such as milk thistle, are especially important for protecting liver cells. In our toxic world, the liver takes a real beating. The detoxification process generates free radicals that over time cause damage to the cells of the liver. As we age, this affects not only our ability to detoxify but other liver functions as well, such as managing cholesterol and blood sugar levels. This makes protecting your liver as you age a high priority. One of the best ways to do that is herbal phytochemicals.

- **Milk thistle (*Silybum marianum*).** Native to southern Europe and North Africa, milk thistle has been used for thousands of years for the treatment of jaundice and other liver conditions. Silymarin, the primary active component of milk thistle, offers potent antioxidant protection for liver cells and increases bile flow. Very importantly, milk thistle has been found to stimulate the formation of new liver cells. It is the most widely researched of all hepatoprotective (liver-protective) herbs and is well known for its low toxicity (see the complete profile on milk thistle in Chapter 9).

- **Chlorella (*Chlorella* spp.).** Chlorella is a fresh-water algae known for its detoxifying properties. Chlorella contains many health-enhancing substances, but chlorophyll may be the most important for removing toxins. Chlorophyll holds onto and pulls toxic substances away from cells, which expedites their removal. It is primarily effective for removal of organic toxins (less so for heavy metals). Chlorella is also nutrient-dense with high concentrations of vitamins, minerals, amino acids, and antioxidants. Taking chlorella is especially important while overcoming any type of chronic illness.

  Suggested dosing: 3-10 grams per day. Chlorella can be obtained as a powder or small tablets. A typical dose for daily maintenance is 10-15 tablets, one to two times daily. The dose can be increased to enhance detoxification.

  Potential side effects and precautions: Chlorella is generally well tolerated. Intestinal side effects, such as bloating and loose stools can occur, but are more common at higher doses. Note, having green stool is normal.

- **Glutathione, NAC, alpha lipoic acid.** Limiting free-radical damage is essential for life. Cells are armed with protective antioxidants, but the ability to generate these important compounds declines with age and chronic illness. Glutathione is the primary antioxidant that protects cellular function. It also plays an essential role in the detoxification process. Natural sources of glutathione include asparagus, spinach, avocados, squash, garlic, and melons. This protection can be augmented by glutathione supplements, which also provide detoxification support and antiviral properties. Alpha lipoic acid and N-acetyl cysteine (NAC) help to recharge glutathione that has been oxidized by free radicals, restoring its functions.

Suggested dosing: Glutathione 500-1000 mg, one to two times daily. NAC 500-1000 mg, one to two times daily. Alpha lipoic acid 50-300 mg, one to two times daily. Dosing can vary depending on the supplement taken.

Potential side effects and precautions: Generally well tolerated. Alpha lipoic acid can cause reflux at higher doses.

Chapter Highlights

- Toxic substances can only enter the body by three pathways: ingestion, breathing, or through the skin.

- Reducing exposure to toxic substances involves eating organic foods (when possible), drinking beverages made from filtered water, and taking steps to keep air clean where you live and work.

- The capacity for detoxification declines through life because of the loss of liver cells.

- Taking milk thistle, an herb with liver-protective properties, is one of the best ways to protect liver function.

- Additionally, herbs protect the cells of the body from the damaging effects of toxic substances and unnatural sources of radiation.

13

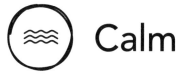 Calm

Our ancient ancestors didn't know stress in the same way that you and I might know stress. Every day was the same: rise with the sun, forage all day, and then sleep after sunset. Their primary concern in life was finding enough to eat, which wasn't something that could be scheduled. It was just life.

Their primary emotional stress was confrontation with an acute threat such as a tiger or another hostile human. And that couldn't be anticipated—it simply happened.

Being chased by a tiger elicits the classic fight-or-flight reaction. Resources of the body are immediately refocused on dealing with the imminent danger at hand. Vision becomes acute, mental functions sharpen, reflexes quicken, and heart rate increases to pump more oxygen and glucose to contracting muscles.

Functions that aren't essential for dealing with the threat, such as digestive system functions and immune system functions, are placed on hold until the threat has passed. With the tiger gone, all systems would return to normal, and the daily grind of foraging for food could be resumed.

In our modern world, however, the "tiger" never goes away.

The perception of an acute threat is gnawingly present for most waking hours. It comes with schedules, deadlines, appointments, financial obligations, interrelations with other people, and a long list of other ever-pressing concerns. If that wasn't enough, we have all of the world's stress coming at us through television, radio, cell phones, and over the internet almost continually. Just thinking about it all is enough to make your pulse quicken.

Curiously, we seem to be drawn to it. When stress doesn't find us, we often seek it out. Conflict, or even the perception of conflict, stimulates adrenaline, the hormone associated with the fight-or-flight response. Adrenaline makes us feel alive. It pumps us up. The fight-or-flight response also taps you into your dopamine (reward) and serotonin (pleasure) centers in the brain.

Historically, humans have satisfied the need for a periodic adrenaline fix through activities that were physical, such as adventure, hunting, or sports. All too often today, people get it from television, computer, and cell phone screens—which doesn't require any physical effort at all.

The impact on cells is devastating. It's like revving your car engine with the brakes pressed all the way to the floor—sooner or later, the motor is going to burn out (in this case, the mitochondria inside your cells). Adrenaline energizes cells, but if the mobilized energy isn't used, then it becomes destructive, causing cells to burn out faster.

Adrenaline stimulates the heart to beat harder and faster, but without physical activity, all it does is increase blood pressure to unhealthy levels. Adrenaline also mobilizes glucose stores to provide energy for the fight-or-flight response, but without the fight or flight, it just raises blood sugar levels and promotes glycation of tissues.

Right behind the wave of adrenaline comes a surge of cortisol, a steroid hormone designed to direct the resources of the body to where they are needed for the given circumstances. When life is calm and balanced, cortisol secretion follows a gentle circadian rhythm that balances all functions in the body. In the evening, a natural dip in your cortisol levels initiates a tide of calming hormones that surge into your brain and induce sleep. In the morning, around 5 a.m., there is normally a boost of cortisol that leads to a surge of stimulating hormones that wake you up and get you going.

During stress, adrenaline and cortisol work seamlessly together to keep you going by shifting resources away from everyday concerns (such as sleep, digesting food, and repairing cells) toward handling some imminent conflict. The body is designed to do this intermittently, but when the perception of threat never goes away, keeping the body poised in high alert is quite destructive; cells never have an opportunity to recover, and the body starts breaking down.

The HPA Axis

It's not actually your adrenal glands that are the problem. It's how your brain perceives the world around you. Your brain constantly monitors what's going on outside the body and modifies the activity of cells in the body to match. It does so by acting through a major hormone network called the hypothalamic-pituitary-adrenal axis (HPA axis for short).

Central in the HPA axis is the hypothalamus, a walnut-sized structure at the base of the brain. You can think of the hypothalamus as the thermostat of your body. When your brain senses change outside the body, it regulates what's happening inside the body by turning different parameters of the thermostat up or down. Through the hypothalamus, the brain can regulate functions throughout the body—**metabolism and energy, mood and emotions, hunger, digestion, reproductive functions, pain perception, and immune system functions**.

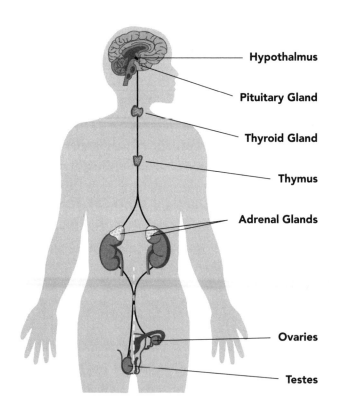

Hypothalmus

Pituitary Gland

Thyroid Gland

Thymus

Adrenal Glands

Ovaries

Testes

To make change happen, the hypothalamus routes messages through the pituitary gland to the adrenal glands, thyroid gland, reproductive glands (testes, ovaries), and autonomic nervous system. The hypothalamus also stimulates growth hormone production and is a source of endorphins, the "feel-good" molecules that relieve depression and are important for optimal immune system function and the suppression of pain.

When the brain is chronically overstimulated, neural pathways associated with the stress response become dominant. In other words, if pushing the stress button is a routine part of life, the brain becomes more reactive to stress. It becomes a vicious cycle that disrupts the balance of the HPA axis and everything it regulates. Once established, any kind of stress or unnatural stimulation plays into the cycle: artificial lighting, computer screens, excessive noise, medications, chronic illness, surgery, and even normal life changes such as menopause.

What happens when the balance within the HPA axis is chronically disturbed? Lots of things, including digestive problems, low energy, low pain tolerance, stress intolerance, elevated blood sugar, chronic sleep disturbances, weight gain, temperature fluctuations (including hot flashes in menopause), inhibited sexual energy, and suppressed immune function.

One of the most pronounced effects of chronic mental stress is the disruption of sleep. If the brain continues to be excessively stimulated into the evening hours with artificial lighting, computer screens, and leftover stress from the day, then cortisol secretion is sustained into the night. The tide of hormones that initiate sleep is impeded, and sleep becomes dysfunctional.

Cellular wellness is simply not possible without adequate sleep. Sleep is when the cells of the body have downtime to recover from working all day, the immune system is functioning at a peak level, and the brain stores memories and purges the buildup of toxic metabolic waste. Without at least 7-9 hours of good sleep every night, including at least 4 hours of deep sleep, all systems of the body suffer, and the incidence of disease increases.

Restoring Balance

Not all stress is bad for you. Just the right amount of stress is actually motivating, especially if it gets you off the couch and gets you moving. It's unrelenting stress that disrupts the HPA axis. Eliminating all harmful stress is often not practical, but you can learn to live around it. It's a matter of putting things in proper perspective.

How tense are you? It's natural to brace against stress, whether that's walking out into the cold or having an intense discussion with someone. We brace against stress by reflexively tightening up the muscles of the back, neck, and shoulders and breathing in a rapid, shallow fashion. When stress is chronic, back, neck, and shoulder pain, as well as tension headaches, can result from built-up muscle tension. Periodically doing a simple tension assessment can help you stay more relaxed.

Tension Assessment

- **Is your breathing shallow and quick or deep and slow?** Shallow and quick breaths in the upper chest are a sign of building tension.

- **How tense are the muscles of the shoulders and neck?** Tension of neck and shoulder muscles is a sure sign of a tense state.

- **Are your hands cold and clammy, even when the temperature is warm?** Adrenaline causes constriction of peripheral blood vessels. A relaxed state is associated with warm feet and hands.

Learn to recognize the feeling of your body bracing against stress. Consciously relaxing your shoulders, maintaining an upright posture, and calming your breathing automatically neutralizes the stress response. This simple exercise is amazingly effective. Get in the habit of doing it several times a day. By evening, you will have less built-up tension.

Set priorities. Everybody keeps a to-do list, but having more on your list than you can actually accomplish causes stress. Try limiting your list to three priorities. Only those things should enter your conscious mind. Keep chipping away at each item until it's solved. Once a task or problem is solved or completed, a new one can go on your list. All items on your list should be actionable. If it's not something within your power to change, it doesn't go on the list.

Cultivate positivity. Try to put a positive spin on completing tasks. Does completing the task make your life or someone else's life better? Or does completing the tasks free up your time in a way that allows you to focus on things that enhance your life? Can you make a stressful task more enjoyable by adding upbeat music or asking other people to help? Address any feelings of anger, frustration, or fear so that they do not consume your life and rob your health.

Allow yourself to have simple problems to solve. Life is full of difficult problems with complex solutions. Anxiety occurs when you're confronted with a problem that doesn't have an easy solution or doesn't appear to be solvable. As long as that problem is at the top of your concerns, your brain will focus on it. And it will continue to eat at you. One way to take a break is temporarily exchanging that problem for a solvable problem. After you've had a break (and a good night's sleep), you can come back to the more difficult problem with a fresh mind. Often that, in itself, will open up solutions that you didn't see before.

The solvable problem you're using for escape needs to be something that requires enough of your attention to occupy your mind and give you an escape from more frustrating problems. Examples include crossword puzzles, jigsaw puzzles, landscaping in your yard, and hobbies of various sources. Also, sometimes a bigger problem can be broken down into smaller parts and solved at intervals that generate less anxiety.

To offset the mental stress of writing this book, I took on an alternate problem that was decidedly physical—I built a 14-foot skiff. As a solvable problem with no particular deadline, building the boat provided balance to my life. Each day, I could work for an hour or two and see visible progress toward a well-defined goal. It was exactly the kind of distraction I needed to clear my brain to make this book happen.

Take a break from stress. Intentionally (but temporarily) disconnect yourself from life's priorities. In fact, this should happen several times a day. There are many ways to do this: meditate, take a nap, go for a walk, enjoy a hobby, do some yoga, qigong, or other exercise.

One of the quickest ways to neutralize pent-up stress or anxiety is to do something physical. Taking a walk is often the simplest option. While you're walking, focus on everything around you—flowers, people, trees, buildings, sky—anything except what's going on inside your brain. While you're walking, stress hormones will normalize and you'll get a boost of endorphins. Your whole outlook on life will be improved!

Get out in nature. Research has repeatedly shown that nature—be it a secluded hiking trail, wide-open space, or urban green area—is an effective antidote to stress and its harmful side effects on your health. There are several likely explanations, including that nature helps give our brains a much-needed "break" from the influx of information it otherwise must deal with in the course of our regular day.

We humans evolved from living in natural environments. Simply put, living amongst and in a more natural setting is embedded in our DNA, and as such, it's comforting. So the more time you can spend outdoors, surrounded by greenery or water or mountains, the more likely you are to be able to relax and recharge.

Give meditation a try. Your thoughts are powerful. When you start thinking about a future potential negative event, such as a confrontation with a spouse or boss, you start living that experience in the present. Your body starts reacting as though it was happening—pulse quickens, your stomach starts to churn, and you become anxious—even though that experience may never actually happen.

Fortunately, there is a way to short-circuit those stressful thoughts. It involves letting go of negative thoughts and focusing on positive thoughts. If you imagine a positive experience, then your body will respond as though you were actually having that experience. That's what meditation is all about—becoming detached from negative thoughts by focusing on positive thoughts. Meditation will make you more resilient as it resets the HPA axis and brings adrenaline and cortisol levels back to baseline.

Granted, meditation takes a bit of practice, but it isn't as difficult as you might imagine. All you need is a quiet place, earphones that help block noise, and possibly an audio device such as a smartphone. There are plenty of guided meditations that will talk you through the process. Try various ones to find what works best for you. There are many different ways to go about meditation, but the common themes with all forms of meditation are calming thoughts and a positive focus.

Turn down the volume a notch. Literally. When you feel stressed, listen to some relaxing music. Sometimes just pure quiet is best. Turn off the news and filter your media. When you over-consume alarming news, you're more likely to perceive a greater "threat," which then activates and, more importantly, sustains your body's fight-or-flight response for a longer period of time. So, as much as possible, seek out balanced and less sensational new sources, consume news with a more critical eye, and try to limit your exposure throughout the day. That doesn't mean burying your head in the sand, rather it's about making smarter choices about where, how, and especially how much you take in news and other information.

Tips for Smartly Filtering Your Information:

- Turn off news alerts on your phone, and instead set aside time once or twice a day to update yourself.

- Avoid constantly checking social media or spending long periods passively scrolling through the endless links.

- When you can, leave your phone at home, or use the "do not disturb" settings.

- As you're consuming news or other info, especially if it stirs up anger, anxiety, or other strong, negative emotions, ask yourself how you might take action or what you can do — or if you're getting riled up over something you have little control over.

- If you find that stress is becoming debilitating or severely impacting your mental or physical health, consider taking a news or social media holiday and focusing on your personal wellness and healthy coping strategies.

Make sleep a priority. Give your cells the break they need—aim for at least 8 hours of sleep every night. The key to a good night's sleep is a calm day. Artificial lighting, computer screens, and noise pollution irritate the nervous system and prohibit restful sleep. Try to make a habit of turning down the lights, cutting off the TV, computer, and cell phone, and listening to easy, restful music for at least an hour before you turn in for bed. You will be rewarded by better sleep at night and a productive day the next day. If sleep disturbances are a chronic frustration, occasional use of calming herbs can be beneficial.

Herbs That Promote Calm

The phytochemicals in certain herbs support a state of calm in the mind and body through a variety of mechanisms. At the cellular level, potent antioxidants counter free radicals and cellular stress factors. Calming herbs also help to balance hormone systems that have been disrupted by stress. The herbs allow cells and tissues to communicate more effectively, which allows everything in the body to run more smoothly and is especially important for optimizing our immune system.

- **Ashwagandha (*Withania somnifera*).** Native to India and Africa, ashwagandha is derived from the root of a plant distantly related to tomatoes and potatoes. Ashwagandha is a calming adaptogen that is particularly useful in balancing the HPA axis in the brain (the control center for hormone regulation). By restoring balance in this important pathway, ashwagandha improves stress resistance, allows for improved sleep, reduces brain fog and fatigue, and eases the transition through menopause, especially hot flashes. These properties also are useful for weight loss and controlling carbohydrate craving. In addition, ashwagandha offers anti-inflammatory, antioxidant, anti-mutagen and immune-enhancing properties. It is also known to normalize low thyroid function.

Benefits of ashwagandha:

o   Supports stress management

o   Encourages mental focus

o   Promotes homeostasis (hormonal balance in the body)

o   Antioxidant and immune-supporting properties

o   Helps balance the HPA axis

o   Supports memory and cognitive function

o   Generally regarded as a calming adaptogen

o   Supports normal thyroid function

Suggested dosing: 100-300 mg, one to two times daily for a powdered extract or 2-3 mL, one to three times daily for tinctures. Look for products standardized to at least 10% withanolides for maximum potency. Ashwagandha pairs well with L-theanine and other calming herbs for counteracting chronic mental stress.

Potential side effects and precautions: Ashwagandha has an excellent safety profile and is well tolerated by most people. Ashwagandha contains iron so it may help with iron deficiencies, but should be avoided for those with hemochromatosis or other conditions with elevated iron. Ashwagandha also stimulates low thyroid function. Please consult a knowledgeable health care provider before using ashwagandha if you have a thyroid condition or are taking thyroid medication.

- **L-theanine.** L-theanine is a unique amino acid found only in green tea and certain mushrooms. Considering half the population of the world drinks green tea daily, an awful lot of L-theanine is consumed every day. This makes L-theanine second only to caffeine as the most consumed medicinal substance on earth. L-theanine crosses into the brain and competes with excitatory neurotransmitters in such a way as to induce calmness and improve mental focus. L-theanine has a wonderful calming effect with little potential for side effects. At the same time, it improves focus and concentration. Consumption of L-theanine is also associated with a positive mood. It counters the negative effects of caffeine and stress-induced adrenaline secretion. It does not cause sedation during the day, making it ideal for daytime use, but it does promote natural sleep at night.

  Suggested dosing: 100-200 mg can be taken up to three times a day.

  Potential side effects and precautions: L-theanine is very safe and has a low potential for side effects. (General precautions for natural substances with the potential for causing sedation can be found at the end of Chapter 9.)

- **Passionflower (*Passiflora incarnata*).** In its native Amazon, the woody vine of passionflower climbs into the rainforest canopy. Local inhabitants enjoy the fruit, but it was traditionally used for relieving pain, calming nervous energy, and promoting sleep. The name originates from when Spanish missionaries first saw the large white flowers with pink centers, and they thought it resembled the crucifixion of Christ. Passionflower is now grown worldwide, and the beneficial properties of passionflower have been well documented in clinical studies.

For someone suffering from nervous tension and poor sleep, passionflower can be a real lifesaver. Passionflower has been long revered for its characteristic sedative properties. It has a reputation for restoring restful sleep without causing a next-day hangover. It also offers muscle-relaxing and pain-relieving qualities.

Suggested dosing: 150-300 mg of 10:1 passionflower extract, one to three times daily as needed or at bedtime to promote restful sleep.

Potential side effects and precautions: Rare. Passionflower is on the FDA's GRAS (Generally Recognized As Safe) list. That being said, there are theoretical concerns that passionflower may potentiate the effects of prescription sedatives and anti-anxiety medications, so caution is advised if using them together. Avoid use with older type antidepressants such as MAO inhibitors. (General precautions for natural substances with the potential for causing sedation can be found at the end of Chapter 9.)

- **Lemon balm (*Melissa officinalis*).** Lemon balm is a hardy herbaceous plant in the mint family that's relatively easy to grow, delightfully aromatic, and has been used medicinally for millennia. Its small white flowers bloom and fill with nectar in late summer, attracting bees, hence the name *melissa* is Greek for honey bee. The use of lemon balm dates back at least as far as Hippocrates around 400 BCE and was used by the ancient physicians Dioscórides and Galen.

This multipurpose herb is a gentle, yet effective ally for a variety of mental, emotional, and digestive ailments. Its relaxing and grounding qualities make it well suited for clearing the mind and relaxing the body for quality sleep and digestion.

Unwinding periodically throughout the day is a crucial step in preparing for sound sleep. Lemon balm is thought to naturally increase a neurotransmitter called GABA, which helps turn down the dial on incoming stimuli.

Ongoing research also suggests that lemon balm may provide some benefit for cognitive degenerative conditions because it gently boosts cholinergic activity (necessary for brain functions), which may help compensate for the loss of functioning neurons.

Lemon balm also calms the digestive tract. It is rich in aromatic oils that stimulate the digestive system and promote the smooth flow of food through the GI tract. This in turn helps reduce GI inflammation, indigestion, and gas. Furthermore, lemon balm is also *antispasmodic,* which means it reduces intestinal spasms and discomfort.

Suggested dosing: 200-600 mg of lemon balm extract, one to three times daily to promote a natural feeling of calm.

Potential side effects and precautions: Lemon balm has a very good safety profile and long history of safe use. At high doses, lemon balm may interfere with thyroid hormone medications. (General precautions for natural substances with the potential for causing sedation can be found at the end of Chapter 9.)

Chapter Highlights

- In the modern world, the "tiger" never goes away—stress is continually present throughout the day.

- The body is designed to tolerate chronic mental stress intermittently, but when the perception of the threat never goes away, cells do not have an opportunity to recover, and the body starts breaking down.

- Be aware of how tension builds in your body and take steps early to diffuse it.

- Allow plenty of time for adequate sleep.

- Take balancing herbs, such as ashwagandha, passionflower, and lemon balm, to tone down the impact of stress.

14

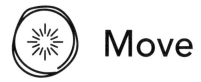 Move

Humans are designed to move, and for the vast majority of the past 200,000 years, humans have been in perpetual motion. Most of that movement has not been running, leaping, or lifting heavy things, but instead lower intensity, constant movement—walking, picking up objects, digging roots, skinning animals, preparing food, and, later, farming.

This kind of movement is so essential that wellness is not possible without it. When you tally up the reasons you should be more physically active in this way, the consequences of *not* doing so become quite apparent.

Physical activity increases heart rate. The heart pumps harder to move more blood and carry more oxygen to active muscle fibers. Blood vessels automatically dilate, allowing increased plasma flow to all cells. Improved blood flow normalizes blood pressure and optimizes cardiovascular function. Moving blood flushes the spaces around your cells, which reduces congestion and buildup of toxic substances. This not only allows your cells to breathe, but it also reduces buildup of plaque in your arteries.

On a deeper level, regular exercise re-energizes mitochondria, the powerhouses of cells. Oxidants such as nitrous oxide (NO), one of the free radicals generated by exercise, cause dilation of blood vessels, which increases blood flow in all parts of the body, especially the heart. The increased oxidative free radicals generated by exercise, however, turn on genes that make protective antioxidants and reduce inflammation in the body.

Active muscles require glucose and fat for energy, and vigorous physical activity mobilizes glucose and fat stores in the body. This has the effect of normalizing blood sugar, an important factor in decreasing the incidence of insulin resistance and diabetes. And if losing weight is your goal, making a commitment to exercise makes you more likely to lose those pounds *and keep them off.*

In fact, using muscles activates genes that support maintenance of muscle mass. Being physically active also supports healthy bones by a number of different mechanisms. The old saying "use it or lose it" definitely applies—the price of not being physically active is muscle atrophy and loss of bone mass.

Physical activity is the endpoint of our natural fight-or-flight response. Exercise normalizes the adrenaline and cortisol levels elevated by feeling stressed. Indeed, exercise is one of the best ways to diffuse the stress that has become so pervasive in modern life. That alone should motivate you to move more!

By stimulating blood flow, normalizing blood sugar levels, and balancing stress hormones, physical activity improves brain functions. It clears out the mental cobwebs and enhances cognition, memory, and mood. If you want to enhance your mental productivity, one of the best ways to do it is by getting up and moving around.

A good night's sleep always comes easier after a physically active day. Normalizing adrenaline and normalizing cortisol allows the tide of neurotransmitters needed to induce sleep to flow more naturally. Physical activity during the day is also associated with the buildup of a substance called adenosine, an important factor for promoting restful sleep.

Regular exercise boosts immune system functions. It triggers the release of anti-inflammatory cytokines (chemical messengers) from muscles and helps modulate metabolic signals related to immune function. Exercise helps flush toxins, viruses, and other garbage from the body. When cells are healthy and the immune system is functioning optimally, your cells are less vulnerable to invasion by microbes.

The Endorphin Connection

With the benefits of physical activity being so obvious, you would think that people would be stepping all over each other trying to get out and run around the block. Initiating movement, however, comes with the disincentive of discomfort. It's because the simple act of contracting muscles and moving ligaments across bones generates friction that causes damage and pain. If it weren't for our natural pain-fighting chemicals called endorphins, movement wouldn't be comfortable; even the slightest movement would hurt too much.

Regular physical activity stimulates secretion of endorphins—it's one of the greatest benefits of exercise. Endorphins (opioid polypeptides) are chemical compounds produced by the hypothalamus and pituitary gland. These "feel-good" chemicals elevate mood and allow us to go about our normal daily activities without significant discomfort. As a bonus, endorphins boost immune system functions, including natural killer cells. The name *natural killer* comes from the fact that these cells have the job of taking out abnormal cells that could turn into cancer and cells that have been infected with microbes.

Endorphins not only limit the pain of movement, but also stimulate the stem cells necessary to generate new tissue and allow healing. Physical movement is a continual balance of damage and repair. The more regularly you exercise, the more endorphins are generated internally, and the better you feel—naturally. Regular movement is the best antidepressant on the planet!

Making Physical Activity a Priority

When looking for the best ways to move, look to the past. Our ancient foraging ancestors didn't do what they wanted to, they did what they had to. They were probably active throughout the day. The main thing they had to do was collect food, which involved a lot of low-intensity movement—walking, stopping to gather food, digging roots, and occasionally sprinting after wild game. Mimicking this type of activity is the most natural form of exercise you can do.

In other words, being physically active doesn't have to be defined as a sport. Walking the dog, raking the yard, picking berries, and gardening are good examples of physical activities that are in line with natural forms of movement. Kayaking, swimming, rowing, biking, and hiking over hills take the intensity up a notch. Lifting light weights and running short distances are good for muscle toning (after you're warmed up, of course). For wellness, however, consistency is more important than intensity.

Warm up slowly. If your body isn't accustomed to regular physical activity, start slowly with activities that feel comfortable and safe. Walking is a good place to start. Try to do just a little more each day.

It takes about 20 minutes to warm up (the uncomfortable part). After the body is warmed up, wonderful things happen. Blood vessels dilate and blood flow increases to all parts of the body, and endorphins start flowing. It doesn't take intense exercise to gain all the benefits, only consistency—and the more you do, the better you'll feel!

Exercise moderately as long as it feels good. Make sure you cool down adequately. If physical exertion results in a next-day hangover (pain and increased fatigue), allow time to recover, and back down on the level of intensity.

Respect your limits. Being physically active has a downside—any degree of movement causes microscopic damage to skeletal muscles, heart muscle, ligaments, bones, and support structures of the body. This damage must be continually repaired. If you repeatedly exceed your body's ability to repair damage, it will set you back. Not surprisingly, performance athletes are plagued by chronic injury. Seeing a top athlete in any competitive sport beyond the age of 40 is rare because competitive athleticism is very hard on the body.

Accept that being physically active is a balance of continual damage and repair. If you are training for a higher level of fitness, allow for adequate rest and recovery. Learn your limits and gradually increase activity as the healing process allows. Follow the 70% rule: do not exceed 70% of your full capacity. Staying within your limits will prevent injury.

Chronic inflammation can be a significant impediment to being active. If tissues are inflamed—from heavy exertion or from a chronic illness—it's even more important not to overdo it. A high-vegetable diet and comprehensive herbal therapy both help to curb inflammation.

Another common roadblock to exercise is excessive body weight because this is commonly associated with back, joint, and foot problems, which obviously reduce the incentive to exercise. It takes real perseverance. It will initially involve some discomfort, but if you persist, your stamina will gradually improve, your discomfort will lessen, your muscle tone will increase, you will shed some pounds, and a larger variety of activities will become possible.

Get outside. No matter where you live, seek out natural places when you can. Whenever weather allows, do something active outside. It's great for your vitamin D level and your mood! Rake your yard. Pull some weeds. If you have the option, ride a bike to get groceries.

Find an activity that fits you. Embracing an athletic activity can be very rewarding. Low-intensity activities such as biking, hiking, golf, pickleball, or kayaking can be continued well into later years. If youth allows, tennis, soccer, basketball, and similar ball sports can be very fulfilling, but the higher potential for injury must be respected.

Consider a yoga class. Yoga is perfect for maintaining a healthy body. Nearly anyone—at any level of fitness and stamina—can participate at some level. Classes are widely available in most communities. Yoga stretches muscles and ligaments and improves posture. It also encourages blood flow to areas of the body where flow can be restricted, such as the spine. Yoga is also a great way to generate those mood-elevating endorphins!

Give qigong a try. For indoor movement that can be done anywhere, anytime, and by anyone, qigong is an excellent choice. Qigong is an ancient Chinese art of movement that follows consistent natural movements. It's so simple, you can even do it beside your desk at work. It can be easily learned from videos, but classes are gradually becoming more available. Tai chi is a complex form of qigong.

Movement gets your brain juices flowing. Stuck on a mental problem that you can't figure out? Get up and move around or go for a walk. The solution will come to you. Moving clears your brain and moves toward creative right-brained thinking. If you have a desk job, set a timer and take movement breaks regularly throughout the day. You will be more productive and gain greater satisfaction from your job.

Keeping Your Structure Strong

Your entire body is held together by a protein called collagen. It's the most abundant protein in the body. Collagen is made up of three strains of specialized elongated proteins twisted together like twine. Collagen fibers come together to form the tendons and ligaments that provide support for the entire skeleton. Cartilage in joints is made of collagen. For added support, collagen is present throughout muscles. Collagen also provides a matrix for bones and teeth to form.

Collagen, along with another protein called elastin, provides support for skin that covers the entire body. Wrinkling is a direct result of the compromise of these important support structures. Collagen also provides support in blood vessels, eyes, intestines, and really anything in the body that needs to be supported. In other words, collagen holds all of your cells in place.

When collagen strands are broken, the collagen structure collapses. I call things that break collagen strands "collagen crunchers". Collagen crunchers are not only the enemies of collagen, but they are also the primary forces that cause aging.

Keeping your collagen strong is important as you go through life. There are many enemies of healthy collagen, however. By now, you should have a pretty good idea of what those factors might be—and how you can protect yourself.

The Primary Collagen Crunchers

- **Sunlight.** Ultraviolet (UV), infrared, and visible light from the sun are potent collagen crunchers of skin. Sunblock protects against UV, but not infrared and visible light, which are the primary causes of skin wrinkling. The best way to optimize skin protection is through the high consumption of natural antioxidants, which build up in skin layers and provide protection. Lutein and zeaxanthin (carrots, yellow vegetables, kale) and anthocyanins (blueberries, red cabbage, purple potatoes) should be dietary staples. These antioxidants also protect collagen in blood vessels and other parts of the body.

- **Free radicals.** Free radicals associated with inflammation and from toxic substances are a threat to collagen everywhere in the body. Minimizing the forces that promote inflammation and chronic illness, plus reducing your exposure to toxic substances (smoking is a terrible collagen cruncher) is the answer here. The antioxidants previously mentioned and phytochemicals from daily herbs also help minimize collagen damage.

- **Glycation.** The protein-sticking effect of glucose from excessive consumption of starches and sugar is one of the most notorious collagen crunchers. If you value your collagen, you need to ratchet down your carbohydrate consumption. Certain foods are especially good for collagen. Kale and other deep green leafy vegetables, fermented soy (tofu), cucumbers, fish such as salmon, eggs, celery, and olives are a few foods that stand out as being beneficial for protecting collagen in the body.

- **Physical stress.** Extreme physical activity causes excessive wear and tear on joints and ligaments. Follow the 70% rule (as previously mentioned) for not overtaxing your structural collagen. The practice of yoga helps maintain healthy ligaments, good posture, and skeletal support.

- **Stress and poor sleep.** Being stressed and not sleeping inhibits the ability of cells to repair damaged collagen. You need 8 hours of sleep every night to keep your structure strong.

- **Microbes.** Many bacteria use collagen as a nutrient source and generate inflammation as they break down collagen. Yes, you likely have some microbes buried in your tissues right now. In general, herbs provide antimicrobial protection for your collagen. If your immune system has been compromised or you have arthritis symptoms, the addition of any of the antimicrobial herbs can be a collagen saver.

Supplements to Support an Active Lifestyle

- **Hydrolyzed collagen.** Though taking collagen as a supplement shouldn't be considered a replacement for protecting the collagen you already have in your body, it can provide extra benefits. The body can readily make collagen, but it needs the right raw materials. Collagen is made of very specific amino acids. It's especially rich in an amino acid called hydroxyproline. While you can get all of the amino acids necessary for making collagen from any protein sources, collagen is the best source. In ancient times, humans got a lot more dietary collagen than we do today. Although they ate meat, they also gnawed the cartilage off of bones and ate other collagen-rich parts of hunted animals.

  There are a number of different ways of getting supplemental collagen, including bone broth (stewing fresh chicken or beef bones), eating gelatin, and hydrolyzed collagen powder. Any will work, but hydrolyzed collagen powder is possibly the easiest. Hydrolyzed means that the collagen is broken down so that it can be easily absorbed and used by the body. It is an animal product, typically from poultry (chicken) or bovine (cow) sources. For bovine sources, look for grass-fed and pasture-raised. A typical daily dose is 20 grams. The powder doesn't have a strong taste and can be added to smoothies or milk-based drinks, such as coffee or hot chocolate.

- **Cannabidiol (CBD) oil.** CBD oil can help with a lot of things. It normalizes the response to pain, improves stress resistance, improves resilience and stamina, promotes natural sleep, and enhances the sense of well-being. It also does wonderful things for the immune system, both fine-tuning the system for better function and reducing inflammation in the body. All in all, it can be a great friend to have around when life gets to be too much.

CBD, short for cannabidiol, is the primary chemically active component of hemp. Hemp is a variety of *Cannabis sativa*, the same plant also known as marijuana. While hemp and marijuana plants look the same, they are distinguished by their unique chemical composition. Marijuana contains varying levels of the infamous euphoria-inducing substance, THC, whereas hemp contains mostly CBD with only trace amounts of THC. In fact, to be legally defined as hemp, the plant extracts must contain <0.3% THC.

CBD and THC act very differently in the body. Both of these substances act on the endocannabinoid system in the body. The endocannabinoid system is a complex regulatory system in the body that influences mood, sleep, stress reaction, memory, pain responses, metabolism, immune functions, and reproductive functions.

THC binds to endocannabinoid receptors very tightly, so an exaggerated response occurs that causes euphoria—in other words, you get high. It also suppresses or downregulates natural chemical messengers of the endocannabinoid system (called endocannabinoids), which promotes dependence and habituation, a serious drawback to marijuana use.

CBD binds to endocannabinoid receptors very weakly, having the effect of increasing natural endocannabinoids instead of suppressing them. This evokes a normal response—you feel better, but without experiencing euphoria, drug-like effects, or any risk of habituation. In addition, CBD affects serotonin receptors in the body, positively affecting mood and gastrointestinal function, and it naturally increases endorphins, the feel-good chemicals that we naturally produce to suppress pain.

It's not just the CBD in hemp that provides benefits. Extracts of the whole hemp plant, known as CBD oil, provides a range of other cannabinoids and terpenes, chemicals that are also found in essential oils. Natural terpenes provide a spectrum of benefits that includes suppressing threatening microbes, boosting immune system functions, reducing anxiety and depression, and even healing the esophagus lining that's been damaged by acid reflux. Terpenes are broadly anti-inflammatory, something that all of us can benefit from.

Benefits of CBD:

○ Anti-inflammatory

○ Decreased pain

○ Enhanced sense of well-being

○ Increased calm

- ○ Improved sleep

- ○ Reduced stress (thanks to CBD's adaptogenic properties)

Suggested dosing: **The average dose range is 10-80 mg of CBD, one to three times per day, though much higher doses of 100-500 mg are generally well tolerated.** Some people will notice benefits at the lower end of the dose range, but most people will need 30-60 mg to notice any effects. As with any medicinal herb, start at a low dose and gradually build up to a higher dose as you get used to the effects of the substance.

Potential side effects and precautions: Reported side effects of hemp oil with CBD are generally mild and uncommon and can include tiredness, loose stools, and slight changes in appetite and weight (either increased or decreased). Both hemp oil with CBD (hemp flower-bud extracts) and purified CBD (CBD isolate) have been shown in both animal and human clinical trials to be remarkably safe and well tolerated. The risk of habituation with the chronic use of CBD oil is zero. It will not cause euphoria at any dose. (General precautions for natural substances with the potential for causing sedation can be found at the end of Chapter 9.)

- For additional joint, muscle, and bone support, see recommendations in Part Four, in Chapter 18 (Bone Health) and Chapter 22 (Joint Health).

Chapter Highlights

- Get moving! Physical activity increases blood flow, which optimizes the removal of toxic substances and metabolic waste from cells.

- Regular physical activity increases endorphins, stimulates immune system functions, and balances stress hormones.

- Sugars and starches are collagen "crunchers"; other factors that cause collagen collapse include prolonged sun exposure, free radicals, physical wear and tear, poor sleep, and microbes.

- We are not consuming the same amount of collagen as our ancestors, so collagen supplementation can be helpful.

- Antioxidants and herbal phytochemicals help to minimize collagen damage.

- If your immune system has been compromised or you have arthritis symptoms, supplementation using an antimicrobial herb can be a collagen saver.

15

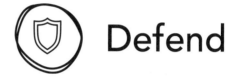 Defend

There's always something circulating around out there waiting for an opportunity to invade your body. Currently, over 2,000 pathogens have been identified, and that's just the ones we know about. Over 200 different viruses can cause a common cold.[109] Though most of them are not life threatening, they can still make you sick—especially if you're vulnerable.

No matter the threat, healthy cells and a strong immune system increase your resistance to infections. Which means, of course, keeping yourself at peak resilience by consistently eating a healthful diet, minimizing exposure to toxic substances, keeping your stress down, and staying active. Beyond following a healthy lifestyle, the

---

109 Wein H. Understanding the Common Cold Virus. National Institutes of Health. April 13, 2009. https://www.nih.gov/news-events/nih-research-matters/understanding-common-cold-virus. Accessed February 28, 2022.

everyday herbs give you a basic level of protection from microbes that stays with you all the time.

Resistance and exposure are two different things, however. Just being healthy doesn't protect you from actually catching something. The best way to avoid being sick at all is minimizing your chances of exposure. The COVID-19 pandemic has taken modern society to a whole new level of awareness and vigilance. We need to keep that up, even after COVID-19 subsides. With 7.8 billion people on the earth who are more mobile than ever (with 40% of them not having enough water to consistently wash their hands), there will always be new threats.

- **Wash your hands** or use hand sanitizers after being in public places and exposed to other people. The active ingredient in most hand sanitizers is plain old alcohol, which is toxic to microbes, but not toxic to you. The fact that handwashing is one of the most effective and least expensive ways of minimizing spread of many types of infectious diseases has been proven time and time again.

- **Avoid heavily crowded public places** as much as practical. When you can't avoid the crowd, wear a mask. A randomized trial conducted by researchers from Yale University, Stanford Medical School, the University of California, Berkeley, and the nonprofit Innovations for Poverty Action carried out among more than 340,000 adults living in 600 rural communities in Bangladesh defined that use of face masks significantly reduced the incidence of COVID-19 in a real-world setting. If a mask can reduce your risk of COVID-19, it can help protect you from other airborne microbes.[110]

---

110 Abaluck J, Kwong L, Styczynski A, et al. The Impact of Community Masking on COVID-19: A Cluster-Randomized Trial in Bangladesh. Innovations for Poverty Action. September 1, 2021. https://www.poverty-action.org/publication/impact-community-masking-covid-19-cluster-randomized-trial-bangladesh. Accessed February 27, 2022.

That being said, wearing a mask is uncomfortable and not always necessary. It's most valuable in tightly crowded places, such as inside airplanes or subways at rush hour. It is also most important during pandemics, such as COVID-19 or influenza, and during months of the year when viruses are at peak spread. Developing a habit of having a mask in your pocket or purse handy could save you a week or two of misery.

- **Stay home when you're sick.** Please. If you have to go out, wear a mask to protect others.

- **Vaccinate against the big threats.** The more threatening a microbe is, the more important vaccination becomes. It also tends to be true that the more threatening a pathogen is, the more effective the vaccine. Vaccines are very effective against highly threatening infections, such as smallpox or polio. All vaccines carry risks of adverse reactions, however, so that risk must be weighed against the degree of protection offered by the vaccine. Vaccines take time to develop for new threats (average is 1-2 years), and few vaccines are 100% effective (average effectiveness for the flu vaccine is 40-60% in the adult population ages 18-64). COVID-19 proved that reaching the threshold of herd immunity worldwide for a pandemic is challenging.

- **Protect against biting insects.** Who hasn't been bitten by a mosquito, tick, flea, or some type of biting insect? Every new bite, however, is an opportunity for microbes to enter your bloodstream. Reducing risk is a matter of maintaining vigilance, wearing protective clothing, and using chemical deterrents when your exposure is elevated, such as a hike in thick woods or possibly even working in the garden in a high-risk area for ticks. Products containing natural essential oils can be quite effective for deterring insect pests, but aren't nearly as toxic as synthetic chemicals, such as DEET.

- **Protect during sexual contact.** It's not just syphilis and gonorrhea that you need to worry about—many microbes (that aren't routinely tested for) take advantage of intimate human contact to spread to new hosts. Condoms can go a long way in minimizing exposure to these microbes.

- **Minimize risk during travel.** Keep in mind: foreign places have microbes that are foreign to you!

  ○ **Food.** When traveling in general, but especially in developing nations or on a cruise ship, following some simple rules can prevent a gastrointestinal nightmare.

    ■ Eat only foods that have been freshly prepared. Avoid foods that have been sitting out.

    ■ Eat only cooked foods. Avoid salads or fruits that have been peeled.

    ■ Fruits that you peel yourself are okay.

    ■ Drink only bottled or filtered water.

  ○ **Public transportation.** When traveling by planes, trains, buses, or any crowded public transportation, wear a mask and wash your hands when you get off.

- **Take care of your teeth and gums.** Oral health is an important component of overall health. Gengival microbes shed into the bloodstream from diseased gums and teeth are commonly found in association with atherosclerotic plaques, diseased heart valves, dementia, and other chronic illnesses. Good oral hygiene includes regular brushing and flossing, along with having your teeth cleaned by a dental hygienist twice a year.

Natural toothpastes containing essential oils, such neem or tea tree can help reduce buildup of bad bacteria.

- And finally, as emphasized throughout this entire book: **take herbs!** Herbs are your secret weapon against microbes. None of us live in a bubble, and some exposure to microbes is inevitable as you go through life. A core regimen of daily herbs can offer good protection against a wide range of different microbial threats. However, if and when you come into contact with a new microbial threat, you'll want to boost your defenses with stronger herbs that contain antimicrobial properties.

The Herbal Advantage

Though antibiotics and antivirals are important when acute infections occur, antibiotics only work for bacteria, and antivirals are specific for certain viruses. Too often, you don't know what you've got. For example, during the COVID-19 pandemic, less than 25% of symptomatic individuals who were tested for the virus were actually found to be positive for SARS-CoV-2. It means that there are a lot of other viruses out there that can cause the same symptoms. And that's just respiratory infections.

The good news is that herbs cover a lot of bases, and they're always there for you. The antimicrobial properties of many herbs are well documented by scientific studies. I believe that herbs are the most reliable option we have for protecting against threatening microbes, especially when there aren't any other options. In addition, herbs offer some clear advantages over drugs:

- The protection provided by herbs is due to the actions of dozens of phytochemicals with a broad-spectrum antimicrobial activity against a wide range of microbes, including bacteria, viruses, protozoa, and yeast (as opposed to one chemical found in antibiotics or antivirals). Because herbal phytochemicals inhibit growth of microbes by a variety of mechanisms, bacterial resistance doesn't occur like it does with antibiotics.

- Unlike antibiotics, herbs typically do not disrupt normal flora in the gut. In fact, herbs suppress pathogens in the gut, which allows normal flora to flourish. This is especially beneficial for infections with foodborne pathogens.

- Most herbs have very low potential for toxicity and therefore do not add stress to the body, which helps to promote recovery.

- Japanese knotweed, Chinese skullcap, andrographis, ginger, and garlic are just a few examples of herbs that have been found to have robust activity against a range of respiratory viruses, including influenza and SARS-CoV-2. Unlike antiviral drugs, which only inhibit specific viruses by one mechanism, herbs inhibit different viruses by a variety of mechanisms. And the coverage provided by these herbs isn't limited to viruses: each of these herbs also has antibacterial, antiprotozoal, antifungal, and antiparasitic properties.

Protocol for Acute Infections

- **Hydrate.** Warm fluids such as hot tea are particularly beneficial. Try ginger tea with honey if nausea is a concern. Reduce your overall intake of food to allow resources of the body to be shifted toward healing. Chicken noodle soup is actually an excellent choice for colds and flu.

Fresh Ginger Tea Recipe

Ginger tea is my go-to for colds, flu, or intestinal bugs, but it can be enjoyed anytime. Fresh ginger is a potent antiviral. It contains nearly a dozen antiviral compounds, including some that seem to be especially effective against common cold-causing viruses. This spicy plant is also well known for easing nausea associated with an upset stomach.

Recipe for homemade ginger tea:

1. **Wash 1 large piece of ginger root** and chop into small pieces.

2. **Heat 1-2 quarts of water** (preferably filtered spring water) in a large pot and add the ginger.

3. **Simmer for 5-10 minutes**. When cooled, pour through a strainer into another container to remove the ginger..

4. Sweeten as desired and enjoy hot or cold.

- **Get plenty of rest.** Take time off of work if possible, or at least follow an abbreviated work schedule. Put projects on hold until you feel better. Avoid strenuous exercise or activity in general until you feel better.

- **Boost with vitamins and minerals, in particular:**

  ○ **Vitamin C** – when cells are stressed by infection, they use up a lot of vitamin C. Vitamin C has been shown to reduce the severity and duration of a viral illness, but you have to take enough. Take 500-1000 mg every few hours up to 4000 mg per day with the onset of a viral illness and continue until symptoms subside. Use buffered vitamin C (EsterC) to prevent stomach upset.

  ○ **Zinc** – essential for normal immune function. Take 20-40 mg daily until you're well.

  ○ **Vitamin D** – also essential for normal immune function. Adequate supplementation is essential, especially during winter when sun exposure is limited. Have your vitamin D levels checked at the beginning of cold and flu season.

- **Load up on antimicrobial herbs.** There are a variety of herbs known to shorten the length and severity of mild acute infections, such as colds and flu. My favorites include andrographis, ginger, garlic (stabilized allicin extract), Japanese knotweed, and Chinese skullcap. Echinacea and elderberry are also effective and widely recommended choices, but are strong immune stimulants (whereas the others mentioned are immunomodulators).

  ○ **Andrographis.** One of my favorite antiviral herbs for colds and flu (see complete profile in Chapter 10).

  ○ **Garlic.** Antiviral and general antimicrobial properties are among the many benefits of garlic that have been documented by scientific studies (see complete profile in Chapter 10).

  ○ **Japanese knotweed.** A systemic antimicrobial herb often used to treat any type of infection (see complete profile in Chapter 10).

- **Chinese skullcap.** A potent antimicrobial used traditionally to treat respiratory infections (see complete profile in Chapter 10).

- **Ginger tea.** Ginger is a potent anti-inflammatory with antiviral properties. Ginger tea is especially good for reducing nausea and settling an upset stomach. See the previously mentioned recipe.

- **Elderberry.** Commonly found as a syrup or elixir, juice from berries of the black elderberry tree (*Sambucus nigra*) offers immune-stimulating and anti-influenza properties. Elderberry syrup is a good choice for children because it has a pleasant taste and is well tolerated. It should be used with caution in severe COVID-19 infections, however, because it can overstimulate the immune system. It shouldn't be used for more than two weeks.

- **Mullein.** Traditional treatment for bronchitis. It reduces inflammation and is an expectorant. It also soothes inflamed mucous membranes.

- **Echinacea.** Immune stimulant. Some studies show a reduction in severity of common cold symptoms when Echinacea is taken when symptoms first start. There are several types of Echinacea, and not all studies show benefit. It is a great antiviral, but also has antibacterial properties. Echinacea is an immune stimulant and therefore should only be used for durations of fewer than 2 weeks. It also should be avoided with severe respiratory illness and in individuals with ragweed allergies.

My Personal Defense Protocol

From the very first moment that I feel like I'm coming down with something—the first hint of a scratchy throat or nasal stuffiness—I take 1000 mg of buffered vitamin C and double doses of herbs including andrographis, garlic extract, Japanese knotweed, reishi, and Chinese skullcap. I repeat the doses of vitamin C every several hours up to a total of about 4000 mg a day and repeat the herb doses one or two more times each day until the symptoms are gone. I also take a vitamin supplement with zinc and selenium. My perception is that the length and severity of viral illnesses in the decade or so that I've been using this protocol is dramatically reduced as compared to the years prior to using herbs. I just don't suffer like I used to.

- When to see a health care provider:

    ○ Persistent fever higher than 101 degrees

    ○ Persistent sore throat

    ○ Severe or debilitating symptoms, such as shortness of breath or inability to stand

    ○ Prolonged symptoms — symptoms persist and do not improve for greater than a week

    ○ Dehydration — inability to drink, severe vomiting, or severe diarrhea

Chapter Highlights

- Microbes are always looking for an opportunity to invade your body.

- Keeping your immune system strong is essential for staying well.

- Take steps to reduce potential exposure to new infections whenever possible.

- Take everyday herbs to increase your general resistance to microbial threats and have antimicrobial herbs on hand for use when common viral symptoms arise.

Part Four

Problem Solving

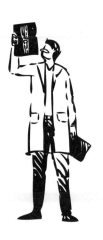

If you follow the concepts laid down in the book thus far—namely, a diet rich in fresh vegetables, a healthy lifestyle, and a regimen of daily herbs—your potential for wellness will be greatly enhanced. Even so, most people have at least one problem area that needs extra attention.

This part of the book applies the concepts of cellular wellness to common health issues. While this information shouldn't be considered a replacement for any medical therapy you may be receiving, cultivating an environment inside your body that allows stressed cells in your body to heal often results in reduced need for medical therapies and a higher level of wellness.

16

Andropause

Andropause, the male loss of reproductive function associated with aging, is often paralleled to menopause in women. However, they are not the same. The decline in estrogen production associated with menopause is specifically caused by loss of eggs in the ovaries. All women have a set supply of eggs in their ovaries that lasts until midlife. When the ovaries run out of eggs, estrogen levels decline sharply, along with reproductive function. Typically, this happens fairly abruptly over the course of a few years.

In comparison, testosterone is produced in men by cells in the testes. Though testicular cells are subject to gradual loss of function associated with aging, they are designed to last until the end of life. This means that the natural decline in testosterone production is very gradual. Testicular function should be able to maintain adequate testosterone levels until the end of life.

That being said, there seems to be an epidemic of middle-aged men with low testosterone levels. Even men in their thirties and forties are being found to have low testosterone. That's not natural. It's a sign that testicular cells are being unnaturally stressed. When testicular cells are stressed, they can't do their jobs, and testosterone levels go down. Beyond decreased libido, symptoms of low testosterone include fatigue, muscular atrophy, loss of bone mass, and increased atherosclerosis.

If your testicular cells are unnaturally stressed, you can bet other cells in your body are stressed too. Low testosterone is a telltale indication of poor health in general.

Possible contributing factors to low testosterone:

- **Refined carbohydrates:** Our entire food supply is now saturated with processed carbohydrates. The habit of a bowl of cereal with cow's milk for breakfast, a burger and bun with fries for lunch, and pasta for dinner leads to chronic elevation in insulin secretion from the pancreas. Elevated insulin occurs long before diabetes sets in. Elevated insulin and central obesity (excess weight around the midsection) have been linked to low testosterone levels.[111]

- **Hormones in meat:** Whether hormones used in the beef, pork, and dairy industry affect testosterone levels is unknown, but high dietary consumption of red meat is associated with increased risk of many chronic illnesses. If you're a meat and potatoes kind of guy (or girl), it may be contributing to poor health and possibly even low testosterone levels. Vegetables are a better choice for your health and your testosterone levels. Certain vegetables, such as celery and cruciferous vegetables, may actually have a positive influence on your testosterone levels. When you do eat meat, insist on grass-fed, hormone-free meat and dairy.

---

111 Rao PM, Kelly DM, Jones TH. Testosterone and insulin resistance in the metabolic syndrome and T2DM in men. *Nat Rev Endocrinol.* 2013;9(8):479-493.

- **Xenoestrogens:** There are thousands of man-made chemicals present in the environment that were not here a hundred years ago, and many of them have estrogen-like activity. Eating organic food is one of the best ways to avoid them.

- **Estrogens in your water:** Estrogens, from women taking pharmaceuticals containing synthetic estrogens, are showing up in municipal water supplies. The best protection is installing a reverse-osmosis filtering system in your drinking water or buying filtered water.

- **Stress:** If you are constantly running from the tiger, or more commonly known as being stressed out, your reproductive ability is likely to suffer. Chronic stress raises cortisol levels, which suppresses central hormone pathways. This also suppresses reproductive hormone secretion, including testosterone.

- **Beer:** Believe it or not, the hops in most types of beer have estrogen-like properties and can adversely affect testosterone production. Just another reason to avoid having a beer gut!

Erectile dysfunction (ED) also has ties to low testosterone. However, it's more specifically linked to plaque formation (atherosclerosis) in the blood vessels supplying the erectile tissues of the penis. All of the same factors that contribute to loss of reproductive function and low testosterone also contribute to ED.

Solutions for Low Testosterone

One solution is testosterone replacement. All it takes is a simple lab test to confirm low testosterone at the doctor's office, and an injection of testosterone solves the problem. There's a catch, however. Within a couple of weeks, the injection wears off. Regular injections are required every 2-4 weeks. Testosterone patches are another option, but the patch must be worn continually.

The newest option for testosterone replacement is the testosterone pellet. The pellet is inserted during a simple office procedure. It releases testosterone continually for a period of about 4-6 months, after which time, another pellet must be inserted. There's also a pellet option for menopausal women that releases estrogen and a lower level of testosterone. Hormone pellets have become extremely popular for managing both andropausal and menopausal symptoms. The biggest disadvantage of the pellets, however, is the necessity of repeat insertions and cost. Pellet insertions can run anywhere from $350-$650 and aren't always covered by insurance.

Alternatively, using herbs and lifestyle modifications to support normal testosterone secretion by testicular cells can be just as effective as testosterone replacement and less costly. It's in keeping with the idea that if you take care of your cells, they'll take care of you. Low testosterone, especially in younger men, is often associated with poor health habits and poor health in general. Good health habits and daily herbs preserve cellular functions throughout the body, including testosterone secretion by testicular cells.

Two of the herbs on the everyday list, rhodiola and shilajit, are recognized for supporting sexual vigor, but there are others. Herbs categorized as energizing adaptogens are specifically recognized for their ability to restore vital energy, promote sexual vigor, and support healthy bone and muscle mass.

Energizing Adaptogens

Energizing adaptogens are herbs that energize the body without having drug-like effects. By counteracting stress factors, stimulating healing, and protecting cells and mitochondria in the body, energizing adaptogens leave you with more energy to work with. This allows you to feel energized and function better, even when you are stressed.

The effect is very different from caffeine, which stimulates the body by mimicking adrenaline. Caffeine drives the body harder and actually robs energy from your body. In contrast, the enhancements made possible by adaptogens are real. They leave you feeling normal— possibly a better and more invigorated version of normal, but still normal—not artificially pumped up.

Like other adaptogenic herbs, energizing adaptogens balance the HPA axis, but in a way that positively influences anabolic hormones, including testosterone. Anabolic hormones build muscles, support bone mass, and improve physical performance. These same hormones can restore normal sexual vitality affected by aging.

All of these features make energizing adaptogens particularly attractive to athletes. Energizing adaptogens are widely used by performance athletes, and many studies have documented benefits for performance and recovery. If performance athleticism is your goal, energizing adaptogens are your best asset for staying in the game.

Even though there are a number of energizing adaptogens, the following are a list of my favorites, especially for promoting sexual vigor.

- **Eurycoma (*Eurycoma longifolia*).** Also known as *tongkat ali* and *longjack*, Eurycoma is an invigorating adaptogen native to Southeast Asia. In 2021, a 6-month duration, double-blind study found that Eurycoma extracts of 200 mg improved erectile dysfunction and raised testosterone levels in a group of male volunteers.[112] Though Eurycoma is best known for invigorating sexual performance

---

112 Leitão AE, Vieira MCS, Pelegrini A, da Silva EL, Guimarães ACA. A 6-month, double-blind, placebo-controlled, randomized trial to evaluate the effect of Eurycoma longifolia (Tongkat Ali) and concurrent training on erectile function and testosterone levels in androgen deficiency of aging males (ADAM). *Maturitas*. 2021;145:78-85.

for men and women, improving strength and muscle mass, and increasing bone mass, traditional uses have also included increasing general vitality with aging, reducing anxiety, improving stress tolerance, fighting infections, relieving constipation, ameliorating diabetes, improving energy, reducing glandular swelling, and as a general health tonic. Because Eurycoma is quite bitter, it is best taken as a standardized powdered extract in capsules.

Suggested dosing: The average dose found in most supplements containing Eurycoma is 200-400 mg per day.

Potential for side effects and precautions: Eurycoma is reported as well tolerated in all studies. Side effects are mild and few. There was no evidence of toxic effects to the liver or kidney function in any studies. In animal studies, there were no adverse effects noted in pregnancies. The lethal dose of Eurycoma, as determined by rat studies, is 3000 mg/kg. For an average 160-lb human, that's 210,000 mg per day.

- **Epimedium (*Epimedium grandiflorum*).** In the Western world, Epimedium is primarily known for its libido-enhancing properties. However, in native China, Epimedium is a highly revered herb that has been used for a variety of purposes for at least 2,000 years. In traditional Chinese medicine, Epimedium was used to restore vitality and strengthen the body. Vital support provided by this energizing adaptogen includes supporting muscle and bone mass, strengthening the heart and cardiovascular system, promoting joint health, restoring energy, supporting optimal immune functions, and slowing the aging process. Studies on animal models have also confirmed Epimedium's ability to enhance testosterone levels.

Suggested dosing: An average dose in supplements is 250-500 mg of a standardized extract.

Potential for side effects and precautions: Epimedium is generally well tolerated, but has been known to cause nausea at higher dose ranges. There are no reports of significant side effects or toxicity. There have not been studies to evaluate the effect on liver function and kidney function in humans or effect on pregnancy in humans. However, there is no history of adverse reports.

- **Ashwagandha (*Withania somnifera*).** Although ashwagandha, a mildly energizing adaptogen, is best known for balancing the HPA axis and promoting calm under stress, it has also been found to increase testosterone levels in men. A 2019 randomized, placebo-controlled study using 240 mg of standardized ashwagandha extract raised testosterone levels in male volunteers by 11%.[113] A complete profile on ashwagandha can be found in Chapter 13.

- **Pine pollen.** Though not an adaptogen, pine pollen is a source of natural testosterone. Pollen comes from the male part of the plant, and not surprisingly, it contains phytochemical compounds with androgenic activity. The pollen from scotch pine, among other pine trees, contains natural testosterone, along with a range of other compounds that have androgenic (male) activity. Pine pollen has been used in traditional Chinese medicine and Ayurvedic medicine of India to restore male vigor for over a thousand years.

  Potential for side effects and precautions: Because of the strong androgenic actions of pine pollen, it is in the yellow cautionary zone on the herbal spectrum. Therefore pine pollen is best used under the guidance of a certified herbalist.

---

113 Lopresti AL, Smith SJ, Malvi H, Kodgule R. An investigation into the stress-relieving and pharmacological actions of an ashwagandha (Withania somnifera) extract: A randomized, double-blind, placebo-controlled study. *Medicine (Baltimore)*. 2019;98(37):e17186.

Chapter Highlights

- Andropause refers to the gradual but steady decline of testosterone production in men.

- Accelerated decline in testosterone levels has been linked to excessive carbohydrate consumption, xenoestrogens, and chronic mental stress.

- Testosterone replacement is one potential solution, but it is costly and doesn't mimic natural testosterone production.

- Carb control and regular exercise, along with energizing adaptogens such as eurycoma, epimedium, and ashwagandha, can help restore natural testosterone production.

17

Blood Sugar Control

Metabolic disorders such as obesity, insulin resistance, and Type 2 diabetes were rare before the middle of the twentieth century. The reason was simple: the availability of dietary carbohydrates in the food supply was sparse as compared to today. The only way to become obese, insulin resistant, and diabetic is consistently consuming excessive dietary carbohydrates. It was only after the industrial-scale production of grains, chiefly wheat and corn, began to saturate the food supply with refined carbohydrates (starches and sugar) that this was possible.

Once it began happening, however, the rate of these disorders began a steady climb. Today, the rate of obesity in the U.S. population is now over 35%, with insulin resistance not far behind. The incidence of type 2 diabetes is the highest it's ever been in the history of humankind.

Carbohydrates include starches and sugars. Starches, such as potatoes or bread, are made up of long chains of the simple sugar, glucose, linked together. Table sugar and high-fructose corn syrup are equal parts of glucose and fructose. Fructose is also referred to as fruit sugar, because fruits contain mostly fructose.

When you eat a pastry, slice of bread, or a bowl of sugary cereal with sliced banana, the starches and sugars are immediately broken down into the simple sugars, glucose and fructose, and then absorbed. Glucose enters the bloodstream directly, but fructose is mostly converted into glucose or fat by the liver. Glucose and glucose converted from fructose, flow directly into the bloodstream to be used to generate energy in muscle and brain cells.

The fact that glucose molecules are loaded with energy also makes the molecules highly reactive. As such, glucose molecules have a noxious habit of sticking to proteins in the body. This is the "protein-sticking" effect mentioned in Chapter 2, called glycation. Glycation accelerates aging and contributes to immune dysfunction, atherosclerosis, arthritis, eye damage, and every known illness, including cancer.

Because of glycation, blood sugar levels must be tightly controlled to prevent damage to blood vessels and other tissues. That's the job of insulin, a hormone secreted by cells in the pancreas in response to rising blood sugar levels. Insulin works like a key opening a lock on a door—it allows cells of your body to take up glucose, thus lowering blood glucose levels back to a normal level.

If overconsumption of carbohydrates is a habit, cells become resistant to the effects of insulin, such that higher and higher levels of insulin are required to hold blood glucose to tolerable levels. This condition, called insulin resistance, has become remarkably common in all age groups, including children.

Elevated insulin has been linked to immune system dysfunction. Elevations in insulin and a related hormone called IGF-1 promote cell growth and may play a role in cancer. Chronically elevated insulin levels not only throw a monkey wrench into the glucose-regulating system, but also have a negative influence on all of the hormone systems of the body. This cascade of dysfunction impacts the adrenal hormones, testosterone levels, and even the way the brain functions.

Insulin resistance drives an increased appetite for carbohydrates, creating a self-sustaining cycle of dysfunctional eating habits and carbohydrate craving. Ironically, insulin resistance is often associated with episodes of low energy because glucose stored in the body is less available if insulin levels remain high. This phenomenon, referred to as hypoglycemia (low blood sugar), translates into an insatiable hunger, craving for carbohydrates, and exercise intolerance. In addition, elevated insulin blocks fat removal from fat stores, driving the incidence of obesity.

Interestingly, it's this fat, the fat converted from excess carbohydrates in the liver, that's the source of the type of LDL cholesterol your doctor is worried about. The fat generated from excess carbs is transported through the bloodstream by way of particles called lipoproteins. To keep the particles stable, the liver adds in cholesterol. After the transport is made and the fat is deposited in fat cells, the leftover lipoprotein particle contains only residual fat, protein, and cholesterol. That particle, now called LDL cholesterol, continues to circulate in the blood and can become embedded in arterial plaques, contributing to the process of atherosclerosis. (For more information on preventing atherosclerosis, see Chapter 20, Cardiovascular System Health.)

If carbohydrate overconsumption continues unchecked, blood sugar levels start to rise, along with accelerated glycation of proteins. Eventually, the ability of the body to maintain normal blood sugar levels is exceeded, signaling the onset of type 2 diabetes.

Excessive blood levels of glucose are especially hard on nervous tissue and blood vessels. The eyes and the feet are the first to suffer. Loss of vision is of grave concern, and diabetic neuropathy of the feet results in debilitating symptoms of chronic tingling, burning, loss of sensation, pain, and eventual ulceration. The heart, kidneys, and brain also suffer damage with diabetes.

The symptoms of insulin resistance may be subtle. And unless you have your blood glucose levels checked regularly, you may not realize that you are on a slippery slope toward type 2 diabetes. Symptoms of insulin resistance progressing to type 2 diabetes may include fatigue, lack of energy, more thirst than usual, more frequent urination, weight gain (especially in abdominal fat), lightheadedness, inability to concentrate, general irritability, mild headache, and frequent craving for carbohydrates. Fortunately, most of these symptoms can be prevented and even reversed with dietary modifications and improved health habits.

Solutions

The solution seems straightforward: curb the carbs. But in a world saturated with dietary carbohydrates, that's often easier said than done! The problem is that we are hardwired to seek and eat carbohydrates because generating energy from glucose, specifically, is so efficient. Our cells, however, are designed to run lean; we just don't need the amounts of carbohydrates found in most of the foods we tend to eat.

It requires some willpower, but you can learn to live on fewer carbs and still enjoy food. One key is to simply not eat *refined* carbohydrates. One of the easiest ways to do that is by cutting out products made with flour—not just wheat flour, but any flour. This pertains to bread, pastries, cookies, pasta, grain bars (even the ones that are cleverly marketed to make you think they are "health foods"), and anything else made from flour. And yes, it also includes these same products made from gluten-free flour.

Sweetened beverages (with refined sugar, high-fructose corn syrup, and/or fruit sugar) are also major contributors to a typical daily diet. Yes, we're referring to soft drinks, fruit drinks, coffee drinks/lattes, and the like. Carb counts for these products can range from 35-60 grams of carbohydrates in one serving! And, by the way, sugar is sugar! Don't be deceived by food labels that tout "natural sugars"; these are all equally destructive in the body. This includes organic cane sugar, brown sugar, maple syrup, agave nectar, honey, molasses, high-fructose corn syrup, beet sugar, and others.

As recommended in Chapter 11 (Nourish), keep your carb count below 300 grams of carbohydrate a day when eating an average 2000-calorie diet, but less than 200 grams per day is more ideal.

Often by midlife, irreversible changes have occurred such that the ability of the pancreas to produce insulin has been permanently compromised. Even with strict dietary modification and exercise, glucose levels may remain elevated. In this case, supplements and medications may be necessary to normalize blood glucose levels.

Testing and Monitoring

Diabetic or not, it's worth checking your blood glucose concentration periodically to see if things are changing. The time of day matters; our blood glucose tends to be lowest in the morning, right when we wake up and before we've had breakfast. Checking your blood sugar first thing in the morning gives you a benchmark, which is called a fasting blood sugar. Then, after you eat a meal, blood sugar levels will climb for a couple of hours afterward, peak, and then go down.

The two primary indicators for monitoring glucose metabolism include blood glucose measurements and hemoglobin A1c. Both of these measurements can be done without stepping foot in a doctor's office.

Blood glucose. Measuring blood glucose requires a test kit, which includes a blood glucose monitoring device, test strips, and a lancet device to draw blood. Test kits cost around $30 and can be obtained from any pharmacy or through the internet without a prescription.

Blood glucose testing is simple and requires only a single drop of blood. Follow the kit directions. The standard for testing is obtaining fasting blood glucose (generally referred to as fasting blood sugar or FBS) in the morning before you eat anything and then 2 hours after any meal. The latter is known as postprandial blood sugar.

Ideally, you want to see a fasting blood sugar below 90 mg/dL. A fasting value of 100-125 is considered prediabetic, and overt diabetes is suspected with a value over 126. If you've drawn the blood sample after a meal (remember to wait 2 hours after the meal because that is when much of the food will have been digested and glucose will have been absorbed into the bloodstream). Ideally, your postprandial blood glucose reading should be less than 120 mg/dL. (It should not be over 140.) If you measure your blood sugar level after different meals, you will quickly begin to notice how your blood glucose varies with different foods. What happens after you eat eggs? Oatmeal? Donuts?

If you are monitoring your own blood glucose, keep a record of what time of day the blood sugar was checked and if it was a fasting blood sugar or a postprandial value. And if your goals are not achievable with diet modifications alone, you should consider the addition of supplements or medical therapy directed by your health care provider.

Hemoglobin A1c (HbA1c). Hb A1c is a very valuable test because it gives you a "big picture" of what your blood sugar levels have been over the past 3 months. Hemoglobin is the protein that carries oxygen in your bloodstream. A drop of blood is used to determine how much of your hemoglobin has glucose stuck to it. You'll recall that this protein-sticking effect is called glycation, which tends to happen more when there is excess glucose in the bloodstream. By measuring the percentage of hemoglobin bound with glucose, this test can, by association, indicate the load of blood glucose over the past 3 months. The higher the average blood glucose level, the higher the rate of glycation. Furthermore, the amount of "sugar coating" of our hemoglobin indirectly implies the relative rate of glycation and damage occurring *throughout the body.*

The range of normal is 3%-5.7%. Ideal is less than 5.3%. A level of 5.7%-6.4% indicates prediabetes, and a level greater than 6.5% indicates diabetes. People with poorly controlled diabetes may have a value greater than 8%, but with effort, that can be brought down to 6% or below. A concerning trend in America is HbA1c test results indicating prediabetes in about 35% of the population. Hb A1c home test kits can be obtained through any pharmacy or the internet without a prescription for $30-$50.

Complete lipid (cholesterol) profile. Your health care provider may recommend this because elevated blood glucose and insulin resistance are risk factors for abnormal blood cholesterol levels and atherosclerosis.

Regular eye exams. Digital imaging of the retina offers noninvasive screening for progression of hypertension, diabetes, and atherosclerosis. This type of computerized screening is another tool to look for vascular changes, as the blood vessels of the eye are a window to the entire vascular system.

Sugar Substitutes

Here are some natural sugar substitutes that I believe to be safe to consume. Use them sparingly.

- **Stevia.** An extract of leaves of a plant native to South America. The sweetening capability of the plant comes from several molecules of glucose fused together in a way that cannot be broken down by the human body, so it does not elevate blood sugar level. It has been used by humans for over a thousand years. The only "side effects" noted so far are that it lowers blood sugar and also lowers blood pressure.

- **Monk fruit.** Native to Southeast Asia, this fruit is so named because it was first eaten by monks centuries ago. Don't look for it on the produce aisle, though; it is usually sold as a powdered sweetener. And how sweet it is: monk fruit is about 250 times sweeter than table sugar! So, a little goes a long way. It has been deemed "generally recognized as safe" by the U.S. FDA for just about everyone, including children and pregnant women. Look carefully at the package label because monk fruit is often blended with erythritol (see next paragraph), which gives some people gas.

- **Sugar alcohols (xylitol and erythritol).** Sugar alcohols are found naturally in berries, plums, peaches, mushrooms, corn husks, and certain fermented foods. They are as sweet as sucrose, but only carry 1/3 of the calories. There is no aftertaste. Xylitol and erythritol are absorbed more slowly than glucose and have less impact on insulin levels, thus they are safe for diabetics. One interesting feature of xylitol is that it appears to prevent tooth decay and reduce plaque, which is why you will often find it in sugar-free chewing gum. Although sugar alcohols are not a significant calorie source for you, they are broken down in the gut by bacteria, which can give you gas and/or diarrhea.

Herbal and Other Supplements

There are many herbal and other natural substances that have antidiabetic properties, either by lowering absorption of glucose, normalizing insulin, or affecting uptake of glucose by cells. Several of the everyday herbs, including rhodiola, gotu kola, and shilajit have a positive effect on blood glucose levels. If you're struggling with insulin resistance and your blood glucose and HbA1c levels are starting to rise, but you haven't crossed the line into being defined as a diabetic, these supplements can help you get it back under control.

All of the following herbs and supplements are generally well tolerated. Though they normalize blood glucose, they typically don't promote episodes of hypoglycemia, unless they are combined with antidiabetic medications. Herbs with blood glucose–lowering properties can accentuate the blood glucose–lowering effect of any antidiabetic medications. Therefore, tell your doctor before starting any of these supplements if you have been prescribed medications to lower blood glucose. For dosing, follow the recommendations for the product you purchase. The following ingredients can often be found combined in a single supplement.

- **Bitter melon (*Momordica charantia*).** This is from a cucumber-like fruit used in Chinese and Indian cooking. Extracts have been found to lower blood glucose levels by a variety of mechanisms. Numerous studies have documented bitter melon's ability to normalize blood glucose levels and promote favorable HbA1c levels. Bitter melon extracts have also been found to inhibit synthesis of triglycerides. Additional benefits of bitter melon extracts include anticancer properties for oral and pancreatic cancer. Bitter melon extracts are generally well tolerated.

- **Banaba (*Lagerstroemia speciosa*).** Extracts made from the leaves of the banaba tree have been shown to be able to lower fasting blood glucose levels and improve blood glucose levels in general. The primary blood glucose-lowering ability of banaba appears to come from increasing sensitivity of cells to insulin.

- **Gymnema (*Gymnema sylvestre*).** Gymnema extracts provide a wide range of health benefits, including blood glucose control. Numerous studies have documented gymnema's ability to normalize blood glucose levels, improve blood lipids, and promote weight loss. Gymnema appears to act primarily by increasing insulin secretion and insulin sensitivity. Other documented benefits of taking gymnema include anti-allergenic, antistress, and anticancer properties. It also promotes healing of stomach ulcers.

- **Fenugreek extract (*Trigonella foenum-graecum*).** Fenugreek extracts lower blood glucose levels by slowing glucose absorption and increasing secretion of insulin. Additional benefits of fenugreek extracts include anticancer, anti-inflammatory, and antimicrobial properties. Fenugreek extracts also promote healing of stomach ulcers.

- **Cinnamon (*Cinnamomum verum*).** Induces very mild increase in insulin release. Cinnamon supplements contain the spice cinnamon in powder form. Cinnamon sugar, of course, neutralizes the blood glucose–lowering actions of taking cinnamon.

- **Garlic.** Stabilizes blood glucose and improves circulation. Has a favorable effect on cholesterol.

- **Chromium picolinate.** The mineral, chromium, plays an important role in the normal function of insulin. It also increases affinity for insulin in tissues. Before taking a chromium supplement, review the amount of chromium present in any other supplements being taken, such as a multivitamin. Total daily dose should not exceed 600 micrograms (mcg).

- **Vinegar.** Two tablespoons of apple cider vinegar before meals tends to improve digestion and also helps lower blood glucose levels, according to the American Diabetes Association. The vinegar may be diluted in a glass of water.

Pharmaceutical Therapies

- **Glucophage (metformin).** Improves the sensitivity of tissues to the effects of insulin. This drug is most commonly used in treatment of type 2 diabetes, but has also been found to be useful in individuals with insulin resistance. The drug decreases absorption of glucose and increases sensitivity of tissues to insulin. Improving sensitivity of tissues to insulin helps break the cycle of carbohydrate craving. Though inexpensive if covered by insurance as compared to herbs, metformin is associated with side effects including loose stools and fatigue. It also doesn't offer the wide range of additional benefits provided by herbs. Metformin is available by prescription only. Metformin use tends to cause a deficiency in vitamin B-12, so daily supplements of B-12 are recommended.

- **Insulin.** This is the gold standard for treatment of type 1 diabetes as well as type 2 diabetes that is not controlled by other measures. When diet, supplements, and insulin-sensitizing drugs do not adequately control diabetes, insulin is indicated and can actually help conserve remaining beta-cell function in type 2 diabetics. Available only by prescription. If you are using insulin, do not start herbal therapy without consulting a health care provider and closely monitoring your blood glucose levels. This is because many herbs have the same effects as the insulin and, when that effect is compounded, your blood sugar level may crash. However, careful and gradual addition of certain herbal supplements may ultimately allow the amount of needed insulin to be reduced.

Other Considerations

Regular, moderate exercise is an essential component for managing insulin resistance and type 2 diabetes. Ideally, you should exercise for at least 30 minutes per day. (Yes, walking counts!) Many people are able to achieve glucose normalization and weight-management goals through exercise alone or in combination with dietary changes.

Reducing your stress is also important. Remember that stress can cause our hormones to be "out of whack". This factor can affect hormones that regulate hunger, satiety (sense of fullness after you eat), digestion, the insulin response, and fat storage.

Recommended Reading:

Dr. Bernstein's Diabetes Solution: The Complete Guide to Achieving Normal Blood Sugars by Richard Bernstein, M.D. should be considered an essential read for anyone with type 1 or type 2 diabetes.

Chapter Highlights

- The modern epidemics of obesity, insulin resistance, and type 2 diabetes are almost exclusively related to excessive carbohydrate consumption.

- The solution is straightforward: reduce total carbohydrate intake.

- Certain herbs, including bitter melon, banaba, gymnema, fenugreek, and cinnamon, have been shown to normalize insulin and blood glucose levels.

18

Bone Health

Although we don't tend to think about it, our skeleton is very much alive. Each bone is constantly being remodeled for maximal strength. As with everything else that happens in the body, this attribute is made possible by living cells. Cells called osteoblasts and osteoclasts break down a bit of bone tissue daily and reconstruct it to compensate for wear and tear. Because of this ability, bones can heal after being injured or broken.

Of course, bone cells age like all cells in the body. As bone cells decline in functional capacity and number, bone density gradually declines. Though bone loss occurs in both sexes, women start with about 20% lower bone density than men and tend to lose bone mass at higher rates. This loss occurs most significantly at menopause, with the potential for loss of up to 20% of bone mass in the first 5-7 years after menopause.

When bones reach a point of decline where they become porous and brittle, it's defined as osteoporosis. Though osteoporosis is most prevalent in postmenopausal women, there are other risk factors that may predispose anyone to weaker bones; chief among them is a diet high in meat, wheat, and corn but low in other vegetables. Other risk factors include White race, sedentary lifestyle, soft drink consumption, chronic use of stomach acid blockers, alcohol abuse, smoking, heredity, and corticosteroid use.

The danger associated with osteoporosis is increased risk of fracture with poor bone healing after fracture. The most commonly affected bones include the spine, hips, and wrists. Vertebral fractures in the spine can lead to symptoms of back pain, compromised posture and mobility, and nerve compression. Hip and spine fractures lead to hospitalization, surgery, immobility, and increased risk of death. Elderly individuals are at increased risk for falls, compounding the risk for fracture.

The Calcium Conundrum

The best way—the natural way—to maintain strong bones is through a diet high in vegetables and fruits, along with moderate, daily weight-bearing exercise. Most people know that there is calcium in bones, but there's some dynamic chemistry involved. And if you are looking for bone health, it isn't simply a matter of popping calcium pills. Yes, calcium is important for bone hardness, but just consuming a calcium supplement doesn't necessarily mean that it ever reaches or stays in your bones.

The pH Factor

The density of bones is closely related to body pH (acid-base balance). Chemical reactions in the body occur optimally when our blood and tissues are maintained at a slightly alkaline pH of 7.4. This is so important that the body maintains complex buffering systems to ensure this specific pH.

The metabolism of certain foods—namely meats, dairy products, and grain products—generates acids. If meat, dairy, and grain are a person's dietary norm, the body must constantly neutralize this acid to maintain a stable pH. Though some acid can be removed by way of the lungs and kidneys, the body also depends on alkalizing minerals from other food sources—primarily fruits and vegetables—to neutralize acidity. If alkalizing foods are not consumed regularly, the body must pull minerals such as calcium phosphate and calcium carbonate from bones to maintain a stable pH in the blood and tissues.

After calcium is leached from bones to neutralize acid, it may even be deposited in other parts of the body. Regularly consuming foods that generate metabolic acid may also be a factor in the formation of kidney stones and bone spurs.

Step up your consumption of vegetables and fruits to help prevent or slow accelerated bone loss!

The Milk Myth

Milk is high in calcium, but whether milk has a positive long-term effect on bone density is still widely open for debate. For many years, Americans have dutifully strolled along the dairy aisle, certain that milk is good for our bones; yet, the evidence is contradictory. Some studies show benefits and others don't. Though small studies haven't provided definitive answers, population studies are hard to ignore. The United States and Europe have the highest rates of milk consumption in the world, but also have the highest rates of osteoporosis in the world. On the other hand, China has the lowest consumption of dairy products of any country on earth, yet it has the lowest rates of osteoporosis of any culture. The message is that we have to look beyond milk alone if we want to maintain healthy bone mass.

Keeping Bones Healthy for Life

The best overall strategy for addressing bone loss is prevention. Peak bone mass occurs by age thirty. Poor health habits in general contribute to low peak bone mass. Children who do not receive adequate nutrition are at greater risk of developing problems associated with bone loss later in life. Adequate dietary calcium is best obtained from fresh vegetables (especially leafy greens) and nuts (especially almonds). Weight-bearing exercise such as walking is also essential for maintaining healthy bones throughout life.

Loss of bone mass isn't just about calcium, however. Poor health habits cause cellular stress and accelerate the loss of cells associated with aging. A decline in functional bone cells is a significant contributor to accelerated bone loss. In combination with good health practices, taking herbs protects cells throughout the body, including bone cells.

If you've spent your life leaching calcium from your bones, putting it back may not be easy, but you can start slowing the loss right now by changing your dietary and lifestyle habits!

- **More than half of your diet should be metabolically alkalizing.** Alkalizing foods (foods that neutralize acid) that promote healthy bones include most vegetables and fruits, pumpkin seeds, flax seeds, coconut oil, olive oil, sesame seeds, almonds, avocado, lima beans, white beans, lentils, tofu, sea salt, and alkalized water. Alkaline grains include buckwheat, quinoa, and spelt.

- **Minimize or avoid metabolically acidic foods that rob bones of calcium.** This list includes soft drinks, refined sugar, grain products (especially those made with wheat and corn), dairy products, meat, many types of beans, refined oils, and artificial sweeteners (especially aspartame).

- **Consume calcium-rich foods.** Good sources of dietary calcium include nuts (especially almonds), beans (especially soy, chickpeas, lentils, and mung beans), figs, kelp, collards, broccoli, kale, okra, chocolate (!), fish (especially sardines and salmon), and scallops. Dairy products including yogurt and hard cheeses such as cheddar, Swiss, and parmesan are acceptable sources of calcium but should not outweigh other sources.

- **Take about 2 tablespoons of apple cider vinegar in 6-8 oz of water with meals.** This may seem counterintuitive because you've just read that you should minimize consumption of metabolically acidic foods. However, the acetic acid in vinegar actually promotes absorption of calcium and helps keep calcium in bones. Stomach acid is necessary for the absorption of calcium. This is why drugs that block stomach acid (commonly used for heartburn) have been linked to increased risk of osteoporosis. The acetic acid in vinegar is a weak acid. In the stomach, acetic acid aids digestion, but when acetic acid reaches the small intestine, it is neutralized and absorbed into the bloodstream as acetate, an alkalizing buffer that protects calcium in bones!

- **Stay physically active.** Weight-bearing exercise is essential for the maintenance of optimal bone mass. Set a goal of at least three miles of walking per day, or 10,000 steps. Make it a lifestyle habit.

- **The estrogen connection.** In women, the onset of menopause with declining estrogen levels is associated with a rapid decrease in bone mineral density. Postmenopausal estrogen replacement reduces this decline, but the benefits of therapy must be balanced by possible increased risks of breast cancer, stroke, and heart attack. The associated risks are highly dependent on the type and dose of hormonal therapy used and the individual's risk profile. Micro doses of estrogen have been found to have a favorable influence on bones without increasing risk of other illnesses.

- **Vibrational therapy.** The problem of bone loss in astronauts subjected to the weightless environment of space appears to be relieved by exposure to vibration. Studies using subtle vibrations in animal models with rats, turkeys, and lambs have also shown profound effects on artificially induced bone loss. Oscillating platforms have been available for use in exercise and weight loss for some time. Vibrational platforms appear to be safe, but precautions should be followed to guard against exercise-related injuries and any other precautions advised by the manufacturer.

- **Yoga.** The regular practice of yoga improves structural integrity of the skeletal system and increases bone density by providing gentle stress on bones.

- **Qigong.** Qigong is an ancient Chinese practice of meditation in movement. The movements of qigong are designed to stretch muscles and ligaments, restore health, and energize the body. Clinical studies in China have demonstrated the reduction in bone loss markers with regular practice of qigong.

Supplement Support

- **Vitamin D.** Vitamin D has many roles within the human body with one of the most important being promoting bone formation, mineralization, and the regulation of the calcium/phosphorus ratio. Vitamin D is manufactured in the skin with exposure to sunlight. With a higher proportion of the population working indoors and using sunscreen during sun exposure (sunscreen blocks 95% of vitamin D production), vitamin D deficiency is common. Supplementation should be considered for individuals at high risk for bone loss or with limited sun exposure; this is best guided by a lab test that measures vitamin D levels in the blood. The average dosage of vitamin D is 400-1000 IU daily for most adults and 1000-2000 IU or more daily for postmenopausal women. In winter time in northern latitudes, however, many individuals need upwards of 10,000 IU daily. Supplemental vitamin D should say on the label that it is in the form D3.

- **Calcium supplementation should be considered in individuals at risk for bone loss.** There are several forms of calcium supplements available. Calcium carbonate is the least expensive but is not ideal for supplementation. Of the less expensive calcium supplements, calcium citrate (and/or calcium malate) is the best tolerated and absorbed. In addition, calcium citrate and calcium malate are known to decrease the risk of kidney stones.

    Calcium in the form of microcrystalline hydroxyapatite (MCHC) provides the most benefit for preserving and restoring bone health. MCHC is a standardized extraction of natural whole bone providing optimal ratios of calcium, phosphorus, trace minerals, collagen, bone amino acids, organic factors, and growth factors in a bioavailable form. Clinical studies have shown significant reduction of bone loss markers with use of this supplement. MCHC is well tolerated and has an excellent safety profile.

As mentioned, calcium is best absorbed within an acidic stomach environment; therefore, calcium supplements should be taken with food. Calcium should always be taken with vitamin D and magnesium for adequate absorption and incorporation into bone.

Avoid overzealous calcium supplementation. Studies suggest that supplementing with calcium may increase calcium deposits in atherosclerotic plaques associated with "hardening of the arteries".

- **Magnesium.** Magnesium is the second most important mineral for bone health and should be included in any bone health supplement. At least half the population over 40 lacks adequate dietary magnesium, which is contained in leafy greens, whole grains, lentils, almonds, and yogurt, among other foods.

Herbs for Bone Support

Certain energizing adaptogenic herbs help to balance the hypothalamus and pituitary glands in a way that positively influences anabolic hormones. These are the hormones that build muscles, support bone mass, and improve physical performance. (They also increase libido, just so you know!) These herbs are known to have a positive effect on bone mass in both men and women. Note that these herbs are normalizing—meaning they do not promote excessive testosterone in men or women.

- **Eurycoma (*Eurycoma longifolia*).** Also known as *tongkat ali* and *longjack*, Eurycoma is an invigorating adaptogen native to Southeast Asia. Eurycoma improves strength and muscle mass and promotes increased bone mass. Because Eurycoma is quite bitter, it is best taken as a standardized powdered extract in capsules. (See Chapter 16 for a complete profile.)

- **Epimedium (*Epimedium grandiflorum*).** In the Western world, Epimedium is primarily known for its libido-enhancing properties. But, in its native China, Epimedium is a highly revered herb that has been used for a variety of purposes for at least 2,000 years. In traditional Chinese medicine, Epimedium was used to restore vitality and strengthen the body. Vital support provided by this energizing adaptogen includes supporting muscle and bone mass, strengthening the heart and cardiovascular system, promoting joint health, restoring energy, supporting optimal immune functions, and slowing the aging process. Epimedium is also used to ease the normal symptoms of menopause. (See Chapter 16 for a complete profile.)

Screening for Osteoporosis

Bone loss is silent, and symptoms in the form of fracture only show up in later stages of disease. Screening for early evidence of bone loss, especially in postmenopausal women, can reduce the need for toxic medical therapies necessary to manage advanced osteoporosis.

- **Risk assessment.** Your risk of osteoporosis can be determined with the use of a tool developed by the World Health Organization. This useful questionnaire is available online through the International Osteoporosis Foundation at www.iofbonehealth.org. The International Osteoporosis Foundation is also a good source of current information about osteoporosis screening tests.

- **Dual-energy x-ray absorptiometry (DXA).** This is the gold standard in measuring bone loss for defining osteoporosis.

Bone densitometry is a simple, low-intensity, x-ray test that is now widely available. Bone mineral density is interpreted by comparing the individual tested with the peak bone density of an average, healthy, twenty-year-old of the same sex.

- **Vitamin D levels.** As discussed earlier, vitamin D is critical to absorbing calcium, yet many people unknowingly have a vitamin D deficiency. The best guide to supplementation is getting your blood vitamin D level checked. (Home test kits are available.)

- **Testing for other causes of bone loss.** Basic testing should include a complete blood count and blood chemistries, liver function, serum (blood) calcium levels, c-reactive protein, and complete thyroid function. If serum calcium levels are high, parathyroid function should be measured to rule out a problem with the parathyroid glands (which normally regulate your calcium levels). Testing for reproductive hormone function (including FSH, estradiol, DHEAS, and testosterone) is sometimes indicated for menopausal women.

Chapter Highlights

- Restructuring of bones to maintain bone mass and strength is an ongoing cellular process throughout life.

- The loss of bone cells occurs as part of the natural aging process, but it is accelerated by poor health habits.

- In women, bone loss is accelerated after menopause and is associated with declining estrogen levels.

- A diet high in vegetables and other calcium-rich foods and regular exercise are the best ways to curb bone loss associated with aging.

- The androgenic effect of energizing adaptogens supports normal bone and muscle mass in men and women.

19

Brain and Nervous System Health

The brain is the primary processing center for the entire body. It constantly monitors the environment outside the body with the five senses and, through the nervous and endocrine systems (hormones), continually adjusts what's happening inside the body to match.

In other words, our brain enables us to navigate the world in which we live. For most of human existence, that's mostly been about finding something to eat, competing with other creatures and humans for something to eat, avoiding being eaten by some other creature (sometimes even other humans), and creating offspring to provide food when age or disability made acquiring food impractical or impossible.

No doubt, life today is quite a bit more complicated than ever before, but we have the processing power to keep up. Brain processing is performed by cells called neurons, the biological equivalent of a semiconductor in a computer. The brain contains about a 100 billion neurons, but each neuron has as many as a thousand connections. This gives the human brain a capacity for 100 trillion connections. In computer terms, it's the equivalent of a storage capacity of *2.5 million gigabytes* and a processing speed of *one billion-billion calculations per second*. The largest computer on earth doesn't come anywhere close to matching that kind of speed or capacity.

To function properly, neurons require a support staff made up of a variety of other cells. *Neurons* are surrounded by *astrocytes*, which hold neurons in place and help to enable nerve impulses. *Oligodendrocytes* insulate nerve fibers from each other by wrapping a fatty substance, called myelin, around nerve fibers like the plastic coating on a copper wire. Without the myelin coat, nerve impulses short out. *Microglia* are the immune cells of the nervous system. They not only protect nerve cells from microbes, but are also the garbage collectors of the brain. Microglia clean up debris and remove dysfunctional and dying cells to keep the neuron network running smoothly.

All that cellular activity uses a lot of energy. Though the brain accounts for only 2% of body mass, at rest, it consumes 20% of the body's energy. Using all that energy generates a lot of metabolic waste. To clear waste, the brain depends on the *glymphatic drainage system*, sometimes referred to as the sewage system of the brain.

The glymphatic system channels cerebrospinal fluid throughout the brain to flush away the buildup of debris and waste generated by cells. If this essential flow becomes compromised, then brain cells suffer. Though glymphatic drainage is always happening, it happens most intensely during sleep. This means that a good night's sleep is essential for having a "clear head" in the morning.

Enemies of Brain Cells

Like anywhere else in the body, the health of the brain is a function of the cells that make up the brain. Though all cells in the body are sensitive to the same stress factors, certain stress factors are especially disabling to brain cells. Because neurons have the lowest capacity to regenerate of *any cells in the body*, the impact of stress factors on brain cells is greater than any cells in the body.

- **Glycation.** If excessive carbohydrate consumption is a regular habit, expect to get by with reduced processing power. The protein-sticking effect of glycation inhibits not only the functions of neurons, but also the different cells that support neurons.

- **Toxic substances.** Many toxic substances, including many pharmaceuticals, disrupt transmission of nerve impulses and slow mental functions.

- **Stress and poor sleep.** Chronic stress not only stresses cells in the brain directly, but it also affects sleep. Adequate sleep is essential for normal brain function, especially with aging. Sleep is when the brain is reshuffling files and memories are stored. It is also when the glymphatic system is working most efficiently to clear debris and toxic metabolic wastes. Without sleep, cognitive function suffers and aging of brain cells is accelerated.

- **Trauma.** Concussions kill brain cells directly, but also disrupt blood flow to brain cells. Because the capacity for neurons to regenerate is limited, lost functions must be rerouted to other areas of the brain. Severe or multiple concussions set the stage for other chronic illnesses and cognitive dysfunction with aging.

- **Microbes.** The brain studies mentioned in Chapter 3 strongly suggest that having a brain microbiome composed of hundreds of different species of bacteria and other microbes is a normal state. They arrive there from the skin, gut, and outside the body. This is a very new finding; much is still unknown. Even so, microbes have to eat, and if they're present in the brain, *their primary source of food is brain cells.*

The Aging Brain

After age 50, your brain loses about 2%-3% of its total mass for every decade that you're alive. This accounts for loss of functional cells in both grey matter and white matter associated with the normal aging process. The brain, however, is remarkably plastic, meaning it's constantly rerouting and reworking neural pathways to compensate for any loss. Therefore, it's possible to maintain normal cognitive functions right up to the end of your life.

When brain cell loss is accelerated by stress factors such as glycation, toxic substances, radiation, chronic stress, poor sleep, or head injury, however, the brain's ability to compensate is exceeded, and cognitive functions suffer. Increased cellular die-off puts strain on the aging immune system, compromising the immune system's ability to keep the microbes of the brain microbiome in check. More aggressive bacteria gain the upper hand as brain cells weakened by stress become vulnerable to invasion. As an overtaxed immune system shifts from anti-inflammatory to a defensive proinflammatory state, inflammation becomes a chronic destructive process, and cognitive functions decline even further.

Of course, there are a variety of ways that cognitive decline associated with aging can occur. What type depends on genetics, how different stress factors come together, and which microbes a person picks up through life. One of the most feared forms of cognitive decline is

Alzheimer's dementia. With Alzheimer's, a person gradually loses all long-term memory and becomes a shell of their former self.

The conventional medical approach to treating Alzheimer's provides yet another example of flawed logic supported by nearsighted science. One of the key features of Alzheimer's is the buildup of a proteinaceous substance called *amyloid-beta*. Research for treating Alzheimer's is focused primarily on creating drugs that eliminate amyloid-beta. The mistake is assuming that amyloid-beta is the root of the problem.

No doubt, amyloid-beta buildup is toxic to cells, but no one stopped to ask why the amyloid-beta was there in the first place.

Brain cells produce amyloid-beta for a reason. The functions of amyloid-beta include protecting cells from invading microbes, repairing leaks in the blood-brain barrier, promoting cellular recovery from injury, and regulating synaptic function.[114] Production of amyloid-beta goes up when brain cells are stressed and returns to normal upon recovery. Accumulation of amyloid-beta is a clear sign of unrelenting stress. Though excessive accumulation of amyloid-beta is toxic to cells, single-minded therapy of artificially targeting amyloid-beta strips away brain cells' primary defense mechanism and leaves them even more vulnerable to stress.

Is it any wonder that drugs targeting amyloid-beta have such a poor track record? And yet, the pharmaceutical industry continues to push these drugs on an unsuspecting public, all the while suppressing scientific evidence of natural therapies that address the underlying causes of cellular stress. The latest is a drug called Aduhelm (generic name aducanumab). Despite evidence of marginal short-term benefit, a high rate of side effects and adverse reactions, and the unanimous opinion of the science board of advisors to the FDA against approval

114 Brothers HM, Gosztyla ML, Robinson SR. The physiological roles of amyloid-β peptide hint at new ways to treat Alzheimer's disease. *Front Aging Neurosci.* 2018;10:118.

of the drug, the FDA, bending to pressure from the pharmaceutical industry, went ahead and approved it.

Causes Versus Manifestations of Illness

One common practice used by medical scientists is mislabeling *manifestations* as *causes* of illness. Manifestations of illness result *from* underlying causes. Symptoms are manifestations of illness. Inflammation is a *manifestation* of illness (not a cause, as it is often mislabeled). Similarly, misfolded proteins associated with dementia are a *manifestation* of the illness, not a cause. Buildup of amyloid-beta is a *manifestation* of the illness, not cause. Underlying factors (glycation, toxic substances, microbes, etc.) cause the inflammation, misfolded proteins, amyloid-beta buildup, and therefore, the symptoms.

Not only is this type of mislabeling bad science, it also leads to erroneous therapies. Instead of treating or addressing underlying causes, this type of science leads to drug therapies that treat the manifestation of the illness, which *never* results in wellness. This may be the point. It's where the money is. Big pharma invests mostly in finding *patentable* chemicals that temporarily block manifestations of illness, but don't address underlying causes, so the chronic illness never resolves.

The solution for any type of accelerated cognitive decline is the same as any other chronic illness: reduce the factors that promote cellular stress and, simultaneously, protect cells from stress to create an internal environment that allows cells to recover. Possibly, there is a place for drugs to acutely reduce the toxic effects of accumulated amyloid-beta, but pursuing that as a singular therapy is nothing short of narrow-minded.

How to Protect Your Brain

Brain and nerve cells don't regenerate if injured. In other worlds, you don't make new brain cells—you've got what you've got. Fortunately, the brain can rewire itself, a feature called *neuroplasticity*. Everything you've learned in your life—how to talk, how to walk or ride a bike, a new profession—set down fixed nerve pathways so that you don't have to relearn those skills every time you want to use them. If those pathways are damaged or lost, sometimes it's possible to relearn those skills by laying down new neural pathways in other parts of the brain. This keeps your brain engaged in staying alive.

The pathway to wellness is also the pathway to brain health. All aspects of staying healthy are important for brain health, but there are key areas that are especially important.

- **Cut back on carbs.** Glycation is a primary enemy of brain health.

- **Keep your brain active.** Learn new things. Develop new skills at every opportunity. Challenge yourself.

- **Get plenty of sleep.** Sleep is essential to clear buildup of amyloid-beta from the brain.

- **Stay physically active.** Physical activity increases blood flow, which helps flush toxic waste from brain tissue.

- **Take herbs every day.** The standard regimen of daily herbs provides exceptional support for brain health, but there are certain herbs that provide support for specific brain functions.

Brain Support Supplements

Though all of the herbal supplements mentioned in this book support cellular health, and therefore support brain health, certain herbs are known for being particularly beneficial for some aspects of brain health.

- **Cat's Claw** (*Uncaria tomentosa*). The phytochemistry of cat's claw has been specifically defined to have value for supporting the immune system and an ideal balance of microbes in the body. Traditional use of cat's claw included supporting cognitive function with aging. A 2019 study found that cat's claw reduced brain plaques and tangles—commonly associated with memory problems and cognitive decline, especially in Alzheimer's disease—through specialized anti-inflammatory and antioxidant properties.[115] Another study from 2014 found that alkaloids from cat's claw increase the neurologic growth factor BDNF and moderate other neurological changes associated with stroke.[116] (See complete profile on cat's claw in Chapter 10.)

- **Bacopa** (*Bacopa monnieri*). Native to India, bacopa has been used for thousands of years for treating sleep disturbances and anxiety. It specifically calms an overactive nervous system. Overactive is the key word—if the nervous system is not revved up, sedation is not especially pronounced. It helps people sleep better and stay calmer, but does not have drug-like effects.

  Benefits to the nervous system go well beyond calming properties. Bacopa has been mostly studied in modern times for enhancing cognitive function (improved brain function). Use of bacopa

---

115 Snow AD, Castillo GM, Nguyen BP, et al. The Amazon rain forest plant Uncaria tomentosa (cat's claw) and its specific proanthocyanidin constituents are potent inhibitors and reducers of both brain plaques and tangles. *Sci Rep.* 2019;9(1):561.

116 Huang H, Zhong R, Xia Z, Song J, Feng L. Neuroprotective effects of rhynchophylline against ischemic brain injury via regulation of the Akt/mTOR and TLRs signaling pathways. *Molecules.* 2014;19(8):11196-11210.

has demonstrated enhanced cognitive function in children with attention deficit disorder (ADD), college students during exam time, and elderly dementia patients in controlled studies.

Beneficial properties:

∘ Rebalances nervous system function in the face of stress

∘ Calms overactive nerve function

∘ Improves sleep

∘ Enhances cognitive function

Suggested dosing: 200-400 mg standardized to at least 20% bacosides.

Potential side effects and precautions: It is well tolerated with rare side effects. Some individuals notice more sedation than others. Sedation can be either decreased or enhanced by combining bacopa with other herbs.

- **Lion's Mane** (*Hericium erinaceus*). Beyond its long history of being used as a food (it tastes similar to crab or lobster meat), when lion's mane mushroom is extracted and prepared as a supplement, **it supports a variety of cognitive and immune-boosting qualities.**

  Lion's mane has a long history of use (1,000+ years) in traditional Chinese medicine (TCM). Traditional use includes digestive issues, insomnia, and fortifying the central nervous system.

  Numerous animal studies and several high-quality human studies support the traditional use of lion's mane mushroom for improvement of memory, mental clarity, and focus.

In one small double-blind, placebo-controlled study of Japanese men and women aged 50 to 80 who had been diagnosed with mild cognitive impairment, **participants showed marked improvement in cognitive function after taking lion's mane during a 16-week period.**[117] The study also found that participants' cognitive performance scores dropped back to pretreatment levels within 4 weeks of discontinuing lion's mane, indicating the need for ongoing use for optimal benefits.

Lion's mane **provides nourishment for the brain, crossing the blood-brain barrier to directly support brain cells.** Compounds called erinacines and hericenones are two major constituents of lion's mane that are known to cross the blood-brain barrier and stimulate nerve growth factor (NGF).[118]

NGF is a natural peptide produced in the body that's essential to the growth, maintenance, and survival of nerve cells. **NGF helps create new brain cells, strengthen old ones, and promote brain plasticity, which is important to brain development and repair.** Lack of NGF is considered a contributing cause of certain neurological problems such as Alzheimer's and dementia.

Lion's mane contains polysaccharides called beta-glucans, which have been shown to support immune health and overall wellness, as well as healthy cell growth and turnover. As is common with nearly all herbs and fungi, lion's mane appears to have some **mild antimicrobial qualities** that may contribute to its ability to support a healthy microbiome and promote gut health.

---

117 Mori K, Inatomi S, Ouchi K, Azumi Y, Tuchida T. Improving effects of the mushroom Yamabushitake (Hericium erinaceus) on mild cognitive impairment: a double-blind placebo-controlled clinical trial. *Phytother Res.* 2009;23(3):367-372.

118 Mori K, Obara Y, Hirota M, et al. Nerve growth factor-inducing activity of Hericium erinaceus in 1321N1 human astrocytoma cells. *Biol Pharm Bull.* 2008;31(9):1727-1732.

Suggested dosing: Depending on the product quality and concentration, general dosing ranges are between 250 mg and 500 mg, one to two times daily.

Potential side effects and precautions: This mushroom has a very good safety profile. Avoid use if you are allergic to mushrooms.

- **Ashwagandha** (*Withania somnifera*). Well known for counteracting the negative effects of stress and balancing mood, but also studied for supporting optimal cognitive function. Like other herbs in the formula, it also provides robust support of normal immune system functions. (See complete profile in Chapter 13).

- **Ginkgo** (*Ginkgo biloba*). Ginkgo is one of the oldest living trees on earth, dating back 225 million years. The trees can live up to a thousand years. Fortunately, the bioactive substances in ginkgo come from the leaves, so the tree is unharmed by use of this herb. Current and traditional use includes enhancing blood flow and protecting brain and nerve functions.

Well over a hundred scientific studies have been done on ginkgo, with at least a third involving human participants. Of these, the majority showed potential benefit for preventing cognitive decline in the elderly, tinnitus (ringing in the ears), hearing loss, depression associated with cognitive decline, and peripheral vascular disease (venous insufficiency).

Suggested dosing: 100-500 mg, one to two times daily.

Potential side effects and precautions: Occasional side effects include upset stomach, headache, allergic skin reactions, and pounding heartbeat. Ginkgo is a stimulating herb that should be avoided in higher dose ranges (500-1000 mg per day), especially in individuals with anxiety, insomnia, or hypertension. Lower doses of 100-150 mg daily are generally well tolerated. Potential drug interactions with higher dose ranges include MAO inhibitors, anticoagulants, diuretics, anticonvulsants, and antidepressants.

Chapter Highlights

- The brain uses a lot of energy and generates a lot of metabolic waste.

- Brain cells rely on the glymphatic system to continually clear metabolic waste.

- Poor health habits compromise glymphatic drainage, weaken brain cells, and increase vulnerability to invasive microbes.

- Amyloid beta is a marker for stressed brain cells.

- Good health habits and supporting herbs keep brain cells healthy and promote optimal cognitive function.

20

Cardiovascular System Health

The cardiovascular system is the lifeline for all cells in the body. When the cardiovascular system is compromised, all cells in the body suffer. Illness involving the cardiovascular system can include problems with the pump (heart), problems with the pipes (blood vessels), or both (which is most typical). As with all diseases, some people are more prone to have cardiovascular disease than others, but the fact remains that *cardiovascular disease is the #1 killer in America.*

The most common cardiovascular condition is plaque formation in major arteries. We all start with clean arteries when we're born, but, with time, the walls of arteries develop waxy deposits called arterial plaques that build up inside blood vessels. There are two main problems stemming from plaque buildup: it slowly but surely inhibits blood flow (like a slow-draining, partially clogged pipe), and pieces of plaque may break loose and end up in a smaller blood vessel, where they suddenly plug it and cut off blood flow. That is what happens in some heart attacks and strokes.

Everyone eventually forms some degree of arterial plaque, but the rate varies from person to person. The process of plaque formation and arterial damage is technically called atherosclerosis (commonly called "hardening of the arteries"). Atherosclerosis is closely tied to blood viscosity (thickness). Blood is a complex mixture of red blood cells, white blood cells, proteins, fats (triglycerides), cholesterol-containing lipoprotein particles, dissolved nutrients, immune factors, platelets, and coagulation factors. It flows more like a thin milkshake than like water.

Blood viscosity is of concern because when blood is thick, it creates friction as it is pushed through the arteries—especially where arteries twist and turn, such as the tortuous arteries of the heart and brain. Over time, friction erodes delicate blood vessel walls, causing damage that would be similar to a rug burn on your skin.

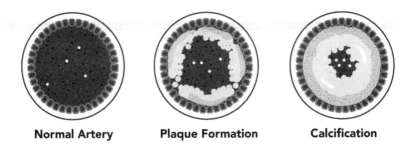

Normal Artery   **Plaque Formation**   **Calcification**

The body seals the wound with clotting factors, including fibrin and platelets, much like it would seal an abrasion on the skin. Other things carried in blood—fat, cholesterol, white blood cells, and even bacteria—stick to that site, making it thicker and more gooey. With time, calcium becomes deposited in the plaque (calcification), causing the classic hardening of arteries.

As plaque builds up in the vascular system, blood vessels become stiffer, and blood flow is further restricted. This increases back pressure in the heart, and blood pressure steadily rises. As pressure builds, heart muscle cells become stressed from having to work harder to pump blood through the system. Chronic emotional or mental stress exacerbates blood pressure issues. Chronically elevated blood pressure (**hypertension**) not only damages the heart, but also the vascular system itself. When the vascular system breaks down, all cells in the body suffer.

Plaque formation happens fastest in arteries where rate of flow is brisk, such as the coronary arteries, carotid arteries, aorta, and large arteries of the legs, but it happens to arteries throughout the body. Coronary arteries (the ones supplying the heart) and carotid arteries (those supplying the brain) are the vessels most affected by plaque formation. As plaque builds up, flow is restricted to these vital organs. Reduced flow to heart muscle can cause symptoms of chest pain (angina), shortness of breath, exercise intolerance, and heart irregularities. Reduced flow to the brain results in cognitive dysfunction. Complete blockage of a coronary or carotid artery from a piece of loose plaque or a blood clot lodged in a narrowed vessel can result in a heart attack or stroke.

Atherosclerosis also commonly affects the aorta (the large artery coming out of the heart) and the large arteries supplying the legs. In the aorta, buildup of plaque weakens the wall of the vessel, causing it to balloon into an aneurysm, which can rupture and cause instant death. Plaque buildup in leg vessels causes weakness and chronic pain.

Factors That Drive Atherosclerosis

Obviously, any factors that thicken the blood increase the likelihood of plaque formation. Although there are genetic factors that influence blood viscosity, a person's diet and lifestyle play significant roles in reducing the risk of cardiovascular disease. Despite the fact that some people have a greater genetic risk of developing cardiovascular illness, dying a premature death from cardiovascular illness is largely avoidable.

Diet

A diet dominated by grain, meat, and dairy is highly linked to increased risk of cardiovascular illness primarily because these foods increase blood viscosity and promote inflammation. Fat obviously doesn't dissolve in water. This is especially true of saturated fat from red meat. The more saturated fat you eat—bacon, hamburger, butter, cream—the thicker your blood is. The thicker your blood, the faster plaque builds up.

But dietary fat isn't the only factor; excess consumption of starch and sugar indirectly increases blood viscosity. Any consumed starch and sugar that aren't immediately used for energy are converted into fat by the liver. Some of it is transported as free-floating fats, called triglycerides, in the bloodstream, but much of it is transported as specialized particles called lipoproteins. The liver loads the newly minted fat into lipoproteins. It also incorporates cholesterol to stabilize the particle. Some of this cholesterol comes from your diet, but your liver actually makes most of it (75% of cholesterol is synthesized by the liver).

Eating too much starch and sugar loads the bloodstream with lipoprotein particles, which increase blood viscosity. That's not the only issue, however. Once the fat has been delivered to fat cells for storage, the leftover particle containing residual fat and cholesterol is left floating in the bloodstream. This particle, called low-density lipoprotein (referred to as LDL), is the one your doctor is worried about.

The buildup of LDL particles in the bloodstream not only increases viscosity but also accelerates plaque formation in other ways. LDL particles can become "oxidized" by free radicals in the bloodstream. Common sources of free radicals include fried foods, refined oils found in many processed food products, and toxic substances from sources such as smoking cigarettes or auto fumes at rush hour. Oxidized LDL particles increase damage to blood vessel walls when they become embedded in plaques.

Fortunately, all is not lost, as a scavenger particle called high-density lipoprotein (HDL, for short) picks up vagrant LDL cholesterol and returns it to the liver. HDL particles are the "good guys"—and your risk of atherosclerosis is partially defined by the ratio of HDL particles to LDL particles. The higher the level of HDL, as compared to LDL, the better.

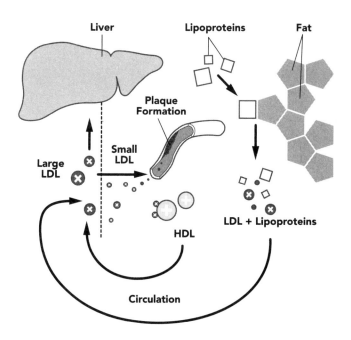

Toxic Substances

Cigarette smoking has long been linked to accelerated plaque formation. However, general exposure to low levels of other toxic substances is an invisible threat to almost everyone. Many toxins contain free radicals that oxidize LDL particles and damage the cells lining the vascular system directly, which accelerate plaque formation.

Most toxic substances are ultimately neutralized in the liver. Chronic exposure to toxic substances destroys liver cells, which are gradually replaced with fat cells. Loss of liver cells affects the liver's ability to manage cholesterol, which means that the liver gradually loses the ability to clean up those leftover LDL particles. As this occurs, LDL blood levels gradually rise over time.

Most people are exposed to some toxins almost daily—vehicle fumes, cleaners, mold, smoke, paints, plastics, pesticides, and other noxious chemicals. Each time, some liver cells are destroyed. As we age, the cumulative damage becomes more obvious as our liver can no longer tightly manage cholesterol. This means that protecting liver function as you age is vital! Herbs such as milk thistle are the best way to do that.

Sedentary Lifestyle

Physical activity dilates blood vessels, which enhances blood flow and reduces plaque formation. Being sedentary does the exact opposite. Inactivity allows blood flow to become stagnant. Stagnant blood flow accelerates accumulation of fat, LDL particles, and other substances in plaque. Vessels become more constricted as plaque accumulates. As blood flow becomes increasingly compromised, cells suffer.

Chronic Stress

Stress activates the fight-or-flight response, which in the ancient past, would have been intermittent (conflict with another human or a confrontation with a lion) and almost always associated with vigorous physical activity. Adrenaline, the hormone associated with the fight-or-flight response, causes the heart to beat faster to increase blood flow to active muscles.

In our modern times, however, activation of the stress response is often chronic and not associated with physical activity. Heart rate is increased, but without physical activity, dilation of blood vessels doesn't occur. Much worse, *blood vessels become constricted*. Increased heart rate with constricted blood vessels increases blood pressure. Increased blood pressure increases friction and accelerates damage to vessels. It also increases back pressure on the heart, which ultimately damages the heart muscle.

Another interesting aspect of the stress response is that it increases the potential for blood to clot. This makes sense when you think about it. The normal stress response would have been associated with confrontation, which could involve lacerations to skin and bleeding. Increased clotting could save a person's life in a confrontation with a lion, but it isn't such a good thing with a confrontation with an angry boss.

Microbes

Microbes of every variety use the vascular system as a transit system. Bacteria and viruses are constantly trickling across barriers into the bloodstream from our gums and teeth, sinuses, intestinal tract, and skin. The flow of microbes across barriers is accelerated with infected teeth (possibly including root canal–treated teeth) and gum disease (gingivitis), sinus infections, dysbiosis (disruption of the balance of bacteria in the gut), and skin diseases. Some microbes latch onto heart valves and become embedded in arterial plaques. Various microbes—cytomegalovirus and Borrelia, the bacteria associated with Lyme disease, just to name a couple—can invade and damage heart muscle directly, causing heart failure.

Sex

Before age 50, men have a greater risk of dying of cardiovascular disease than women. It's possible because in the ancient past, men were more apt to become slashed or injured during confrontations than women. So, men tend to have higher concentrations of red blood cells (therefore higher viscosity) and increased potential for blood clotting. For women, estrogen provides a protective effect. The hormone estrogen positively affects cholesterol levels and has a protective effect on blood vessels. After menopause, however, women lose this advantage, and the risk of cardiovascular disease rises to equal that of men.

Genetics

Though some people have a greater genetic risk of developing cardiovascular illness, dying a premature death from cardiovascular illness is largely avoidable. Yes, genetics is a factor, but it's less than you might expect: the incidence of the inherited form of high cholesterol, called familial hypercholesterolemia, is only 1 in 500 (0.2% of the population). Even people with familial hypercholesterolemia, with proper medical therapy, coupled with natural supplements as well as dietary and lifestyle modifications, can live a normal lifespan and not die prematurely of cardiovascular illness. No matter what your family history, you can outrun your genes by adhering to a healthful lifestyle and adopting herbs to help protect your cells.

Heart-Friendly Solutions

The place to start is with regular checkups at your doctor's office. Cardiovascular disease is a silent killer—you don't know that you have a problem until something terrible happens. Regular blood pressure and cholesterol checks are important for defining risk. If your blood pressure and cholesterol are elevated enough to increase your risk of cardiovascular disease, medications may be indicated. But don't stop there.

A comprehensive approach to cardiovascular health starts with a heart-healthy diet rich in vegetables and low in starches, sugar, dairy, and meat (red meat especially). Regular exercise and stress reduction are also an integral part of heart health. Ideally, a 3-mile walk (or equivalent) should be a heart-strengthening part of your day. Regular physical activity increases blood flow and normalizes stress hormones at the same time. Taking care of your liver by reducing exposure to toxic substances is also more important than you might realize. And, all adults can benefit by taking selected supplements that gently reduce blood viscosity while also reducing oxidative stress (free radicals) and protecting the liver.

If LDL isn't lowered to acceptable levels, you may need medications, but a heart-friendly lifestyle and supplements may allow you to stay at minimal dosages. This is important because the statin drugs commonly used to lower cholesterol have side effects of muscle pain (which reduces your incentive to exercise) and can cause liver damage (which causes your cholesterol to go up).

Lowering cholesterol isn't the only way to lower risk. Lowering blood viscosity is just as important. Reducing saturated fat associated with consuming red meat and dairy is one step in the right direction. Men, especially, tend to have high red blood cell volume (indicated by elevated hematocrit) and can benefit from regularly donating blood. Regularly donating blood is associated with reduced risk of cardiovascular disease.

Heart-Friendly Supplements

All of the everyday herbs protect the heart and vascular system. However, if you develop any type of cardiovascular issue, whether that is hypertension or evidence of plaque formation, the following supplements can add extra protection and benefits.

- **Hawthorn (*Crataegus* spp.).** Hawthorn does a lot of things for the heart. It helps the heart work more efficiently, with a reduction in irregular heartbeats and improved coronary artery blood flow. It normalizes blood pressure in hypertensive individuals (without affecting blood pressure in individuals without hypertension). Hawthorn has been found to improve exercise tolerance, cause a modest reduction in blood cholesterol, and reduce vascular inflammation. Its anti-inflammatory properties have also proven useful for digestive issues, connective tissue ailments, kidney problems, and anxiety (providing a calming effect on the nervous system).

  Benefits of Hawthorn:

  - All-around cardiovascular tonic

  - Anti-inflammatory

  - Calms stress and nervous tension

  - Supports healthy blood lipid profiles

  - Promotes connective tissue health by stabilizing collagen

Suggested dosing: 500-600 mg, one to two times daily for a powdered extract or 3-5 mL, two to four times daily for tinctures.

Potential side effects and precautions: Generally well tolerated by most people.

- **Garlic.** Wonderful for cardiovascular health! Garlic reduces serum cholesterol and triglyceride levels and has a positive effect on HDL cholesterol. Importantly, garlic also acts as an antioxidant to help prevent oxidation of fats in the bloodstream; this reduces plaque formation in arteries. Garlic also offers antimicrobial properties. (See complete profile in Chapter 10.)

- **Pine bark extract.** The phytochemicals in pine bark extract have been found to improve the integrity of the entire vascular system by providing potent antioxidants that protect blood vessels, increasing blood flow by dilating blood vessels, and acting as a mild blood thinner. This antioxidant protection extends to eyes and skin. Additionally, pine bark extract offers anti-inflammatory properties and immune system support. (See complete profile in Chapter 11.)

- **Japanese knotweed.** This herb is an excellent source of *resveratrol*, the age-defying, life-enhancing chemical compound also found in grapes and red wine. Japanese knotweed contains high concentrations of *trans*-resveratrol, the active form of the compound most useful to the human body.

  Resveratrol offers significant cardiovascular benefits including support of optimal heart function, enhanced blood flow from dilation of blood vessels, enhanced integrity of blood vessels, and reduced blood viscosity (thickness). It is also a potent antioxidant with anti-inflammatory properties, and it offers protection to the nervous system, immune system, and liver.

Japanese knotweed also offers antimicrobial properties. (See complete profile in Chapter 10.)

- **Milk thistle.** *Silymarin,* the primary active component of milk thistle, offers potent antioxidant protection for liver cells. It also increases natural antioxidants found in liver cells. Milk thistle has been found to induce regeneration of liver cells. It is the most widely researched of all hepatoprotective (liver-protective) herbs and is well known for low toxicity and high safety. (See complete profile in Chapter 9.)

- **Omega-3 fatty acids.** Often called "omega-3s", these health-enhancing substances are particularly abundant in certain fish such as salmon as well as in walnuts, flaxseed, and krill oil. Omega-3s reduce inflammation, protect against damage from free radicals, reduce platelet aggregation, and also reduce blood viscosity (acts as a mild blood thinner). An advantage of krill oil is that its omega-3s are in a form that is more easily absorbed and used. Krill oil also contains a potent antioxidant called astaxanthin. (See complete profile in Chapter 11.)

- **Nattokinase/serrapeptidase.** Nattokinase, an enzyme found in a fermented soy food called natto (popular in Japan) breaks down fibrin, a key component of arterial plaque. The fact that the rate of cardiovascular disease in Japan is one of the lowest in the world may be partially due to consumption of natto (along with high fish and vegetable consumption, as well as an active lifestyle). Serrapeptidase, another enzyme produced by bacterial fermentation, has similar properties.

- **Red yeast rice.** This is a yeast that grows on rice that happens to produce substances that block the formation of cholesterol in the human body. Interestingly, one of those chemical substances, monacolin K, was the source of the first statin drug, lovastatin. While red yeast rice isn't as potent as statin drugs, it is associated with a lower incidence of muscle pain and other side effects. Because of its drug-like effects, however, red rice yeast is in the yellow cautionary herbal zone and should only be used under the guidance of a certified herbalist or knowledgeable health care provider.

At Your Doctor's Office

Routine screening tests are available to assess risk factors for cardiovascular illness. Sometimes persistent elevation in blood pressure, cholesterol, triglycerides, or blood glucose requires medical intervention. But, the good news is that dietary and lifestyle modifications with supplement support often restore normal parameters and reduce the need for medical therapy. Symptoms such as chest pain, irregular heartbeat, and shortness of breath should be evaluated by cardiologists.

- **Blood pressure.** Traditional blood pressure assessment is a direct measure of the integrity of the cardiovascular system. It is also an indirect measure of the degree of hardening of the arteries and of stress. The average normal blood pressure is 120/80, but it varies with age. Hypertension is defined as resting blood pressure consistently greater than 140/90. Although having regular blood pressure checks at a doctor's office is a good practice, you can check it yourself. You can get your own sphygmomanometer (blood pressure device) and measure your blood pressure frequently at home, where you are more relaxed. Keep a record and show it to your health care provider.

- **Hit the scales.** It's no secret that excess weight is associated with a higher risk of cardiovascular disease. If you are overweight, shedding a few pounds may significantly reduce your risk.

- **Blood cholesterol levels.** (Lab test involves a simple blood draw). LDL cholesterol is most closely associated with elevated cardiovascular risk and should ideally have a value below 130. LDL cholesterol is the long-standing blood marker for cardiovascular risk because drugs approved for lowering cardiovascular risk are almost exclusively directed at lowering cholesterol. A normal HDL value should be above 40, but the higher the better; values above 60 are more ideal for HDL. Your risk of atherosclerosis is best evaluated by looking at the ratio between LDL and HDL. Ideally, the LDL/HDL ratio should be less than 4.5 (aim for 3.5).

- **Triglycerides.** These are free-floating fats in the bloodstream. High concentrations of triglycerides increase viscosity of blood, especially if composed mostly of saturated fat. Obviously, a high-fat diet can produce elevated triglycerides in the blood. However, for most people, elevated triglycerides are actually a reflection of high carbohydrate consumption.

- **C-reactive protein (CRP).** An important marker for cardiovascular inflammation. Elevated levels are commonly associated with the presence of disease-causing stress factors including oxidative stress (free radicals), toxins, oxidized fats (predominantly dietary) and microbes. Elevated CRP indicates the increased likelihood of oxidized LDL particles; a value over 10 predicts at least a two-fold increased risk of heart attack.

- **Blood viscosity.** It is possible to measure blood viscosity, but it isn't routinely used to measure the risk of atherosclerosis because drug therapies don't directly lower blood viscosity. Instead, blood viscosity is assessed indirectly by hematocrit level, triglyceride level, and blood cholesterol measurements.

- **Hematocrit.** Though blood cells are designed to flow easily without getting stuck, they're still solid and therefore make a significant contribution to blood thickness. The greater the concentration of red blood cells (RBCs), the greater the blood viscosity. The concentration of RBCs in blood can be measured by a test called a hematocrit that is typically part of a routine blood test called a complete blood count (CBC). A hematocrit less than 48.6% in men and less than 44.9% in women is considered normal, but closer to 40% is more ideal.

- **Essential fatty acid analysis.** Mounting evidence suggests that measurement of omega-3 fatty acids in the blood is an important indicator of atherosclerosis risk, possibly with even more predictability than traditional markers such as HDL and LDL. The ratio of omega-3 to omega-6 fatty acids may also be useful for predicting risk of inflammatory diseases such as arthritis and diabetes. The ideal ratio of omega-6 fatty acids to omega-3 fatty acids should be no more than 6:1.

- **Metabolic markers.** Blood glucose control is essential for managing risk. Fasting blood glucose levels should ideally be maintained at less than 90 mg/dL. Hemoglobin A1c is an *excellent* test for assessing your long-term blood sugar control (over about the last 3 months). Levels should be maintained at less than 5.6 and ideally closer to 5.0. If your level is 6.0 (borderline prediabetic) or higher, you've got work to do! There are home test kits available to measure your hemoglobin A1c.

  Elevated insulin levels indicate the presence of insulin resistance. Complementary lab tests include liver function and thyroid function.

- **Regular eye exams.** Digital imaging of the retina offers noninvasive screening for the progression of hypertension, diabetes, and atherosclerosis. Once standardized, this new type of computerized screening will offer an effective way to determine the presence and progression of disease, as the blood vessels of the eye are a window to the entire vascular system.

- **Coronary calcium scan.** It's a CT scan that measures calcium deposits in coronary vessels. It's an indirect way of assessing the degree of plaque formation in vessels. Coronary calcium scans provide a way for asymptomatic individuals to assess risk.

- **Treadmill EKG.** A diagnostic tool for assessing risk in symptomatic individuals (those with chest pain, exercise intolerance).

Chapter Highlights

- The cardiovascular system is the lifeline for all cells in the body.

- When blood flow is compromised by plaque formation in blood vessels, all cells in the body suffer.

- High blood viscosity is a key factor initiating plaque formation.

- A healthy diet, regular exercise, and natural supplements (including herbs and omega-3 supplements) are great ways to reduce plaque formation.

21

Gastrointestinal Health

We don't tend to think about it this way, but the human body is basically a tube within a tube. It allows us to take in food at one end, extract nutrients and water that our cells need, and expel waste material at the other. As an extension of the outside, it's filled with bacteria and substances that are foreign to our bodies and our immune system.

The wall of the intestinal tract forms a protective barrier that keeps foreign substances and bacteria in food material separated from our tissues. The cells that line the intestinal tract secrete and maintain a mucus layer to protect the lining from bacteria and foreign substances in food material. We also depend on our normal flora—these are the "good guys"—to coat the inside of the large intestine (colon) and prevent threatening bacteria from gaining a foothold.

Problems in the intestinal tract are predominantly related to breakdown of this essential mucus barrier.

Gastrointestinal dysfunction manifests itself in many ways—everything from heartburn and stomach ulcers to gallbladder issues, chronic constipation, diverticulitis, celiac disease, Crohn's disease, and ulcerative colitis.

Most digestive dysfunction can be linked to three primary factors:

- Slow motility
- Bacterial overgrowth
- Eating the wrong foods

Recipe for Digestive Dysfunction

Keeping things moving is essential for normal digestion. When the flow of food material through the tract gets backed up, symptoms occur. The biggest culprit of slow motility is stress—any kind of stress, such as chronic emotional stress or even the stress of being chronically ill. Another major factor is lack of dietary fiber, which can slow transit throughout the intestinal tract.

When motility is slow, things get backed up in the stomach. Reflux esophagitis occurs when the stomach doesn't empty properly because partially digested food material stuck in the stomach sloshes up into the esophagus. Slow motility is associated with low acid secretion. Acid is necessary to break down proteins. When acid secretion is low, that doesn't happen properly.

Stomach acid also reduces the concentration of foreign bacteria and other microbes found in food. Normally, the concentration of bacteria is lower in the stomach than anywhere else along the intestinal tract. When acid is low, potentially harmful bacteria in food are not eliminated. Slow gastric emptying allows partially digested food material to sit in the stomach and gradually erode away at the protective barrier of the stomach lining, which sets the stage for ulcers to occur. Bacteria, such as *H. pylori*, take advantage of the opportunity and invade irritated and inflamed tissues, causing ulcers to form.

Once food material has been churned in the stomach with acid and protein-digesting enzymes, it enters the small intestine. Although stomach acid greatly reduces the bacterial concentration, it doesn't totally eliminate all bacteria from food material entering the small intestine. If intestinal motility is slowed, then bacteria keep growing. Overgrowth of bacteria in the small intestine causes symptoms of bloating, gas, and discomfort, called small intestinal bacterial overgrowth (SIBO).

Slow motility also affects the liver and pancreas. The liver and gallbladder produce bile, which is necessary for digesting fat and removing neutralized toxic substances from the body. When motility is slowed, bile flow is inhibited, which leads to liver congestion and gallbladder disease, such as formation of gallstones. Secretion of digestive enzymes by the pancreas is also inhibited, which compromises digestion.

The dysfunction caused by stress-induced slow motility is often compounded by the foods that people eat. High-carbohydrate foods (starches and sugar) fuel the rapid growth of bacteria. It stimulates overgrowth of a yeast called candida, too. Slow motility concentrates all the calories in one place, and in response, bacterial growth is explosive. Overgrowth of bacteria erodes the mucus barrier protecting the lining of the small intestine. This can lead to "leaky gut" where bacteria and foreign food materials leak into the bloodstream, causing symptoms such as fatigue and achy joints and muscles.

High-starch foods can promote another problem, since grains and certain beans contain substances called lectins. Lectins are irritating by design. From the plant's point of view, they are meant to deter consumption by other creatures by damaging the cells lining that creature's intestinal tract. All plants contain lectins, but seeds—grains, beans, and some nuts—are notoriously high in gut-irritating lectins. Nightshade vegetables— potatoes, tomatoes, peppers, and eggplant—are also high in lectins.

If motility is normal and the mucus barrier is intact, the concentration of lectins in a healthy diet isn't a problem. They only become an issue if motility is slow and lectin-loaded foods are consumed in high concentrations. Unfortunately, the typical American diet is the very definition of lectin-loaded food. Damage to the intestinal lining caused by bacterial overgrowth and lectin damage slows motility even further, making a bad situation even worse.

Further down the line, slow motility and bacterial overgrowth cause chronic constipation associated with excessive gas and discomfort, a condition commonly called irritable bowel syndrome (IBS). IBS can also be associated with chronic loose stools or alternate between loose stools and constipation.

The overgrowth of certain "bad" bacteria can lead to more severe inflammation of the intestinal lining, deemed inflammatory bowel disease. When inflammation and ulceration primarily affect the colon, the condition is called ulcerative colitis. When the inflammation extends to the small intestine, the condition is termed Crohn's disease. Inflammation associated with gluten sensitivity is called celiac disease.

The Day It Started

I once met a patient who had to have his colon taken out because of severe ulcerative colitis. When I asked him how long he had suffered with it, he responded by telling me that he remembered exactly the day it started. He was a hunter and had eaten some tainted deer meat. The symptoms started that day, and he was miserable from then on. None of the medical therapies he had tried provided any benefit. Eventually his colon was removed. No doubt, he picked up a "bad" bacteria that ruined his colon and his life.

Diverticulitis is another common inflammatory condition of the colon. Chronic colon dysfunction leads to weakening in the wall of the colon, causing out-pouches to form. These pouches are called diverticula. If multiple diverticula are present, the condition is referred to as diverticulosis. Diverticulosis, by itself, causes no symptoms, but if food material and bacteria are trapped and stagnate within a diverticula, inflammation and infection occur.

While digestive issues can occur in isolation, it's more typical for people to experience a range of intestinal maladies all at once. Considering that all digestive dysfunction is rooted in similar causes, this shouldn't be surprising. The type and intensity of dysfunction is dependent on a person's genes, the spectrum of microbes present in the gut microbiome, and environmental factors, with food and stress being at the top of the list. Digestive dysfunction is closely linked to many chronic illnesses and shares symptoms with many chronic illnesses. Often digestive dysfunction is a factor in initiating other chronic illnesses.

What happens to all of that fiber from vegetables and fruit we're supposed to consume? When it gets to the end of the line—the colon—it feeds your gut flora (resident bacteria). They are able to convert some of that fiber into smaller molecules called short-chain fatty acids, which energize the gut wall. There is also indication that your gut bacteria can communicate (chemically) with your immune system and even with your brain. Dietary fiber plays important roles in maintaining good health, and it may help to prevent (and resolve) some types of digestive dysfunction.

Pathway for Restoring Digestive Health

The obvious pathway to enjoying healthy digestion is minimizing the factors that promote digestive dysfunction—namely, chronic stress and food loaded with starches and sugar. If those two factors are present, probiotics aren't going to prevent digestive dysfunction from happening. In cases of bacterial overgrowth, probiotics can even make intestinal dysfunction worse. Diets with high meat consumption can also be problematic. High meat intake promotes growth of bacteria in the colon that have been associated with colon cancer.

If you truly want to enjoy healthy digestion, the solution is to reduce stress in general, cultivate relaxed mealtimes, and incorporate plenty of vegetables into your meals. Vegetables provide everything the intestinal tract needs to function properly. Vegetable fiber promotes normal motility and growth of favorable bacteria. Vegetables are low in damaging lectins. They are also rich in nutrients and antioxidants to nourish your cells properly.

If you are struggling with any type of digestive issues, here's a simple plan that you can use to get back on track. It is fairly restrictive, but often all it takes is a week or two for digestive functions to start improving. Then, you can start adding other foods to round out a healthy diet that prevents digestive issues in the future. The list of supplements following the food guidelines can also be beneficial for healing the gut.

Foods you can have:

- Apples, berries
- White rice or puffed rice cereal for breakfast
- Chicken and/or mild, white fish (such as flounder or cod)
- Cabbage
- Sweet potatoes
- Squash (your choice: crookneck, zucchini, acorn squash, butternut squash, pumpkin)
- Green beans

- Mushrooms
- Peas
- Onions or leeks
- Avocados
- Yogurt or kefir
- Oat or rice milk
- Egg-free mayonnaise or mustard
- Vinegar
- Any culinary herbs and spices (except peppers)
- Sweeteners: stevia, honey, agave
- Herbal teas, green tea, roasted dandelion tea (coffee substitute)
- Grapeseed or olive oil for sauteing

Eat these foods in any combination for a week. All foods should be cooked, except for the apples and berries. They are all fairly easy to digest and, most importantly, promote favorable gut bacteria balance inside your intestines, while also providing key nutrients and some fiber to help keep things moving along. White rice is the best tolerated of all grains. It typically doesn't stimulate bacterial overgrowth and doesn't contain damaging lectins.

For breakfast, you can have yogurt and berries. For lunches and dinners, you can have different combinations of sautéed or steamed vegetables and chicken over rice. It is a bit monotonous, but it's only for a week or so.

Stay with the diet the best you can. After a week or so (depending on your digestive tract), you can start adding foods back in, one at a time as tolerated. The goal is ending up on a gut-friendly diet that is rich in vegetables and low in food products made from grain and meat.

Here's another key part: **fast overnight.** After your last meal of the day (usually dinner/supper), don't eat anything else for at least 12 hours. Allowing a gap of at least 12 hours that you don't eat anything gives your digestive tract an opportunity to digest the food you've already eaten and then heal and rest. Stick with this, and you will see a real improvement in your digestive function. (Note: If you are diabetic, you will need to seek advice from your health care provider to avoid hypoglycemia.)

Foods to avoid until your gut is healed:

- All food products made from flour (any type of flour)
- Acidic foods (citrus, tomatoes)
- Coffee and tea (until healing is complete)
- Spicy foods
- Dairy (with the exception of cultured yogurt/kefir)
- Pork and beef
- Broccoli, kale, cauliflower, Brussels sprouts, collards
- Nightshade family (tomatoes, potatoes, peppers, eggplant)
- Tropical fruits (oranges, pineapple, mangoes)
- Most beans (except mung beans and lentils, which are easier to digest)
- Nuts
- Soft drinks
- Alcohol

Natural Gut Support

The right restorative therapies go straight to the source of your digestive issues, so your body recovers its ability to heal itself, and symptoms subside. The goal is to restore homeostasis, optimize immune function, and control any threatening microbes.

- **Slippery elm.** Nearly everyone with gut issues could benefit from this gentle herbal supplement. Slippery elm contains mucilage, a slick, gel-like substance that naturally soothes sensitive or inflamed tissue in the gut lining. Mucilage also helps recreate the barrier in the gut lining that normally prevents leaky gut. Slippery elm can be found in capsules or chewable lozenges.

- **Digestive enzymes.** A dysfunctional gut can't produce enough digestive enzymes to break down food at a healthy rate; replacing those enzymes until you can restore your body's capability to produce them on its own can help reduce stagnant food in your gut and speed your recovery. Digestive enzymes also keep moving any toxins along that aren't absorbed by your tissues.

- **Cardamom and fennel supplements.** These have volatile oils that help ease inflammation and relieve painful spasms that contribute to abdominal cramps.

- **Digestive bitters.** Your tongue, stomach, pancreas, and colon have specific receptors that encourage digestion the minute they detect a bitter taste. They stimulate production of digestive enzymes, stomach acid, and bile. To help normalize your digestion, try taking bitters such as dandelion, goldenseal, berberine, coptis and Oregon grape. Bitters are taken undiluted as a tincture.

- **Berberine.** Berberine is an antimicrobial phytochemical found in many herbs, including goldenseal, coptis, barberry, and Oregon grape. Berberine disrupts the ability of bacteria to adhere to tissues and form colonies (biofilm). Though it is not absorbed well systemically, it provides exceptional antimicrobial coverage against many gut pathogens, including candida. The doses depend on the herb product used. Herbs that contain berberine are generally well tolerated. Berberine also provides blood-glucose lowering properties.

- **Chlorella.** Poor gut health usually translates to poor ability to absorb the essential nutrients your body needs to heal and function normally. Chlorella is a freshwater green algae that's brimming with beneficial nutrients to help replace those you're missing. Plus, chlorella is loaded with chlorophyll, a potent antioxidant that binds to toxins in the GI tract and holds them there so they don't get absorbed. That includes organic-type toxins (herbicides, pesticides, mycotoxins), as well as heavy metals and plastics. (See Chapter 12 for a complete profile on chlorella.)

- **Probiotics.** Probiotics provide concentrated live favorable bacteria. Special capsules ensure that the bacteria are not destroyed by stomach acid. The most common strains of favorable bacteria found in probiotics include lactobacilli and bifidobacteria species. If yeast overgrowth is a problem or overgrowth of *Clostridium difficile* (C. diff) has occurred after taking antibiotics, *Saccharomyces boulardii*, a favorable yeast, is also a good choice.

Note that use of probiotics can be tricky. Because every person's gut microbiome is unique, what works for one person may not work for another. Probiotics are most ideally suited for transient use after the gut microbiome has been acutely disrupted by antibiotics or by the introduction of a foreign bacteria from contaminated food. People with normal intestinal function do not need to take a probiotic every day. Herbs often do a better job of balancing the gut microbiome than probiotics. Use of probiotics when slow intestinal motility is present can actually worsen symptoms of gas, bloating, and abdominal discomfort.

Natural Liver Support

- **Dandelion (*Taraxacum officinale*).** Dandelion is excellent for protecting the liver and promoting bile flow. The fresh leaves are also rich in vitamin C. Though the leaves can be added to a salad or lightly sauteed with olive oil, most commonly, dandelion is taken as a supplement.

  Dandelion roots and leaves have long been revered in herbal medicine across Asia, Europe, and North America. Traditionally, dandelion has been used primarily to promote digestion and support the liver. The purest, most potent formulations are extracts of dandelion root or leaf or a combination of the two.

  Benefits of dandelion:

  ○ Supports digestion

  ○ Soothes the GI tract

  ○ Promotes a healthy gut microbiome (the root is a prebiotic)

  ○ Supports balanced blood sugar levels (root)

  ○ Supports liver function and a healthy urinary tract

  ○ High in antioxidants

  As a prebiotic, dandelion root promotes the growth of beneficial flora in the gut and helps to balance the gut microbiome. Dandelion is a bitter herb—the taste of bitter stimulates digestive functions. The compounds responsible for the bitter taste are also linked to promoting healthy liver function.

Several compounds in dandelion have been associated with balancing the inflammatory process, which helps promote the body's natural detoxification and elimination processes.

Suggested dosing: 100-300 mg, one to two times daily of a powdered extract or 3-5 mL, one to two times daily of a tincture.

Potential side effects and precautions: Dandelion is high in vitamin K, which affects blood clotting. If you are on a blood-thinning medication, consult your health care practitioner before taking dandelion.

Additional Tips for Gut Health

- **Chew thoroughly.** Digestion starts in your mouth. Chewing is the only part of the digestive process over which we have voluntary control.

- **Eat smaller, more frequent meals.** This allows an over-stretched stomach to return to normal size.

- **Eat mindfully.** Set aside time to relax and enjoy your food. This aids digestion.

- **Sip, don't chug.** Large amounts of cold liquids consumed with food may slow enzymatic function and impede digestion. Small sips of liquid during a meal are better. Europeans are one up on us with a habit of drinking water, wine, or beer at room temperature (though alcohol should be avoided until healing is complete). Large iced drinks should be reserved for quenching thirst after exercise.

- **Apple cider vinegar at meals.** Taking 1-2 tablespoons of apple cider vinegar (diluted in a 6-oz glass of water) with meals is a simple way to improve digestive function in the stomach. (Note: If stomach ulcers are a concern, digestive enzymes and vinegar should not be used unless instructed by a health care professional.)

- **Drink ginger tea.** Ginger's healing properties soothe an inflamed stomach and intestinal tract. Brew your own and drink it several times per day (see recipe in Chapter 15).

- **Keep stress in check.** Do whatever you can to reduce your stress. Regularly practicing relaxation techniques or getting out for a long walk may help. Some natural substances can help too. CBD oil may help to promote normal sleep, if stress is keeping you up at night.

- **Use medications sparingly.** Short-term use of medications to reduce acid is sometimes indicated, but long-term use should be avoided. Chronic use of acid-inhibiting drugs is associated with accelerated bone loss and increased allergies and food sensitivities. Such medications can allow healing of the lower esophagus, but acid-reducing drugs should never be your only strategy. Treatment with acid-reducing medications neutralizes acid and reduces symptoms of esophageal burning, but does not eliminate the actual reflux. These drugs actually compromise digestion.

  Tips for weaning off of an acid-inhibiting medication:

  ○ Follow a gut-friendly diet.

  ○ Adopt better eating habits.

  ○ Use the recommended supplements.

  ○ Very gradually wean off the drug.

  ○ Use over-the-counter (OTC) antacids for heartburn, as needed.

Recommended Reading:

The 2020 New York Times bestseller *Fiber Fueled* by gastroenterologist Will Bulsiewicz, MD offers a deep dive into the microbiome-balancing benefits of eating a wide diversity of plants, with insights into short-chain fatty acids and the roles they play in promoting gut health. Also included are recipes and guidance to incorporate more fiber-rich foods and plant diversity into your diet. This book is a terrific resource for anyone who is looking to correct gut issues.

Chapter Highlights

- Most digestive dysfunction can be linked to three primary factors: slow motility, bacterial overgrowth, and consumption of gut-offending foods.

- The type and intensity of digestive dysfunction are dependent on a person's genes, the spectrum of microbes present in the gut microbiome, and environmental factors (primarily diet and stress).

- Fiber–especially vegetable fiber–is essential for normal digestive function.

- Intermittent fasting allows your gut time to rest and heal between dinner and your first meal of the day.

- Herbs and other supplements can help protect the gut lining, promote optimal digestion, and balance the gut microbiome.

22

Joint Health

Throughout a lifetime, your joints get a lot of wear and tear. If it were not for the fact that joints are being constantly maintained, they wouldn't last very long. A team of cells maintain each joint's cartilage, fluids, membranes, ligaments, and tendons. As long as there are plenty of functional cells on the repair team, joint health is maintained. Unfortunately, some of these cell types have limited capacity to regenerate. With aging and injury, as the number of functional collagen-generating cells decline, joint health also declines.

Any type of arthritis can produce joint pain and swelling, joint stiffness, and immobility. But the onset of arthritis can be subtle; symptoms can come and go. Deformity of joints and relaxation of ligaments can occur as cartilage is worn away and synovial fluid dries up. Any joint can be affected, but hips, knees, and hands are particularly vulnerable. Shoulders, back (spine), and neck are also commonly affected. Fortunately, there are many things you can easily do to get more mileage out of your joints.

Factors Affecting Joint Health

What are the primary factors that compromise joint function and accelerate joint degeneration? You might have guessed them already: excessive physical stress, poor diet, chronic exposure to toxic substances, chronic stress with sleep deprivation, and, of course, microbes.

Let's start with the diet. Did you know that certain foods tend to promote inflammation in the body, which contributes to any type of arthritis? These foods include sugar (in any form), processed foods sourced from wheat and corn, grain-fed or soybean-fed meat and dairy, and red meat.

Do you eat a lot of sugar and starch? A process called glycation, associated with high carbohydrate consumption, is a contributor to arthritis of any type. Excess blood sugar sticks to proteins throughout the body. When it sticks to collagen (an abundant protein in joints), glycation is a notorious collagen cruncher that accelerates collagen breakdown. Many toxic substances are also collagen crunchers.

Another diet-related cause of arthritis is accumulation of uric acid crystals in joint tissues, a condition known as gout. It is often precipitated by consumption of a rich, meaty meal. Typically, a single joint is affected with sudden onset of severe pain, redness, and swelling. The big toe is the most common joint affected, but any joint can be involved.

Chronic mental stress can also factor into arthritis because it tends to adversely affect sleep, which all cells need to recover.

Microbes are a wild card. Growing evidence suggests that accelerated joint degeneration is associated with microbes in many cases. For example, Lyme disease has, among its many symptoms, the onset of arthritis (this was first noted in children). Lyme disease is associated with a bacteria called Borrelia.

Some other infectious diseases have microbial links and manifest as arthritis.

Links between rheumatoid arthritis and different species of bacteria called mycoplasma date back to the 1970s. One 2007 study found *Mycoplasma pneumoniae* in 90% of knee joint aspirations from patients with rheumatoid arthritis. Interestingly, in a different study, this same group of researchers found *Mycoplasma fermentans* in 89% of knee joint aspirations from patients with osteoarthritis. (Osteoarthritis is the garden-variety arthritis associated with aging.) This was surprising because knee joints are not where you'd expect to find microbes.

Though Mycoplasma and Borrelia are two prime examples, there are many microbes known to break down collagen. Autoimmune illnesses that involve joints (including lupus, scleroderma, ankylosing spondylitis, and Sjogren's syndrome) are increasingly being linked to various intracellular microbes.

Pathway to Healthy Joints

The herbal supplements, dietary guidelines, and lifestyle suggestions provided in Part Two and Part Three go a long way toward keeping your joints healthy for a lifetime, but if your joints aren't in top shape, you can do more.

Keep moving. Staying physically active is one of the most important ways to keep your joints healthy. Regular physical activity increases joint mobility and reduces joint stiffness. Increased muscle tone from athletic activity provides support and stability to joints. Staying physically active can also help you shed some pounds, which takes stress off your joints.

The 70% rule. Though being physically active is important for staying healthy, any exercise taken to an extreme can be damaging. Excessive movements cause friction and stress on cartilage and ligaments that hold joints together. Extreme sports, many competitive sports, triathlons, and long-distance running are really hard on joints. If one of those is your passion, it is important to train properly, respect your limits, eat well, and take adequate downtime to recover. One practical way to reduce excessive strain on your body and your joints is sticking with the 70% rule: Never exceed 70% of your maximum capacity, even if you feel you can tolerate more activity. In other words, don't push too hard.

Rest when your body needs it. Cells need downtime to regenerate, recover, and renew joint collagen. Get adequate sleep to speed recovery. If joint pain is keeping you up at night, try CBD oil. When taken orally, CBD oil helps reduce joint pain and also promotes better sleep.

Go low-impact. Low-impact exercises such as walking, yoga, Pilates, tai chi, qigong, swimming, casual biking, dancing, kayaking, and paddleboarding keep you in shape without overstressing your joints.

Stay smooth. Abrupt, jerky movements put a lot more strain on your joints.

Keep your core strong. Exercises that strengthen your core, such as Pilates and yoga, also protect your back while helping you maintain balance and good posture.

Pay attention to pain. Pain is a signal not to be ignored. It means that cells are stressed or injured and tissues are damaged. You know that healing is complete only when the pain is gone.

Add support when indicated. Joints that have been weakened by strain or injury need extra support. Neoprene supports that slide over the joint (knees, elbows) provide extra stability to the joint and braces prevent overextension. Extra stability and support allow cells to rework the joint to restore natural stability. This takes time, sometimes up to 6 months or a year.

Hot and cold. Apply warmth to joints that are stiff or chronically inflamed and cold (cool packs) to joints that have been acutely strained or injured to reduce swelling.

Natural Joint Support

Though loss of some joint cartilage is inevitable as cells age, it's amazing how much you can get back when the factors that drive joint inflammation and destruction of cartilage are addressed and minimized. Natural supplements can be really beneficial for reducing inflammation associated with arthritis.

- **Turmeric.** A common yellow spice found in Indian curries, turmeric is one of nature's most potent anti-inflammatory substances. Turmeric reduces inflammation by two different pathways. Rich in potent antioxidants, it neutralizes destructive free radicals and acids that account for the damage caused by inflammation. It also inhibits formation of COX-2, a key enzyme that drives inflammation, which allows joints to heal properly. The benefits of turmeric for reducing joint inflammation are well documented by clinical studies.

- **Boswellia.** Known in its native land as Indian frankincense, Boswellia has been used for thousands of years in India and Arabia for treatment of arthritic conditions. Boswellia offers potent anti-inflammatory properties and is often combined with turmeric for treatment of arthritis and other inflammatory conditions. Numerous clinical studies have demonstrated that Boswellia is not only effective but is also a very safe alternative to drug therapy for the long-term management of inflammatory conditions such as arthritis.

- **Eggshell membrane.** Combinations of glucosamine (from shellfish) and chondroitin (from animal sources such as shark or beef) have long been a go-to in joint supplements. However, eggshell membrane has been shown to be faster and more effective at promoting joint comfort. It also helps support healthy cartilage tissue. Eggshell membrane contains a natural matrix of beneficial nutrients and proteins such as collagen, peptides, and calcium that promote joint health.

- **Collagen.** Studies have documented benefits of taking hydrolyzed collagen for promoting joint health and reducing pain. About 20 mg of hydrolyzed collagen powder a day is all you need to promote joint health. (See the complete discussion on collagen and collagen supplements in Chapter 14.)

- **Glucosamine.** This is a precursor for protcoglycans, thc chcmicals necessary for smooth and slick joint linings. Glucosamine also stimulates the synthesis of collagen, the base substance for cartilage. With age, normal glucosamine synthesis decreases. This may be a contributing factor to arthritis.

- **Hyaluronic acid.** A naturally occurring substance in our connective tissues, skin, eyes, and synovial fluid (the thick liquid in joints). Hyaluronic acid helps keep joints lubricated and prevents bones from rubbing together and causing discomfort and pain. It's a tried-and-true ingredient for joint comfort.

- **Essential fatty acids (omega-3 fatty acids).** These reduce inflammation by shifting the chemical messengers of the immune system away from an inflammatory state. Essential fatty acids are found in many foods such as salmon, walnuts, and flaxseed. Numerous studies on fish oil support its acclaimed role and safety in reducing arthritis. Krill oil, another potent source of omega-3s, offers further advantage because it contains astaxanthin, a potent anti-inflammatory. (See the complete discussion of omega-3 fatty acids at the end of Chapter 11.)

- **Flaxseed** is a popular vegetable source of the essential fatty acid ALA (alpha-linolenic acid). You can add a tablespoon to a smoothie or to your morning cereal. Another beneficial essential fatty acid is GLA, most commonly found in borage oil, evening primrose oil, and black currant seed oil.

- **Vitamin D.** Individuals with optimal blood levels of vitamin D have lower rates of arthritis. Have your vitamin D levels checked by your health care provider.

- **Cat's claw.** This herb is derived from a vine native to the Amazon basin. Cat's claw may be particularly effective for arthritis because it offers both anti-inflammatory and antimicrobial properties. It is one of several antimicrobial herbs that can be beneficial for different forms of arthritis. (See complete profiles of antimicrobial herbs in Chapter 10.)

- **CBD oil from hemp.** Many people find that CBD oil helps to reduce pain and to improve sleep. This is worth trying if joint pain at night has been keeping you from getting the rest you need. CBD oil is best absorbed in the mouth. Place several drops under your tongue and hold for a few seconds, then swallow. (See a complete profile for CBD oil in Chapter 14.)

- **CBD/Essential oil rub.** This is a topical treatment that can provide benefits such as reducing overall joint discomfort, especially when used several times per day. Some formulations may include capsaicin, derived from chili pepper. Capsaicin is well known for reducing joint pain associated with arthritis. Clinical studies have shown benefit with applications to the affected joint four times daily with 0.025% cream.

Alternative Therapies

- **Massage therapy.** Very effective for reducing muscle tension that can compound the pain of arthritis.

- **Physical therapy.** Rehabilitative therapy can be very helpful in some situations.

- **Acupuncture.** Effective for decreasing pain associated with arthritis.

- **Application of heat.** Deep penetrating heat relieves joint discomfort like nothing else. Heat dilates blood vessels and flushes away inflammation. Heat can be applied locally to strained or injured joints or to the whole body by use of a sauna.

Surgical Therapies

- **Intra-articular injection of cortisone.** Offers short-term relief of pain associated with a severely inflamed joint. Side effects include increased appetite, insomnia, and increased blood glucose in diabetics. Evidence shows that repeated cortisone injections into the joint space may permanently break down cartilage.

- **Intra-articular injection of hyaluronic acid.** Hyaluronic acid is a component of cartilage consisting of acetyl-glucosamine and glucuronate. Primary therapeutic effects include lubrication and joint cushioning. Despite being approved by the FDA for intra-articular injection, hyaluronic acid is only variably effective.

- **Autologous stem cell therapy.** Stem cells are undifferentiated cells that have the potential to become any type of cell. Stem cells are distributed throughout the tissues in the body. Stem cells can be extracted from fatty tissue in the body (the spare tire around your middle) and injected into damaged parts of the body, such as worn-out knees or the spine after a spinal injury. The injected stem cells convert into cells that generate cartilage to repair the damaged joint. Although stem cell therapy has promise, the responses seem to be highly variable from person to person. That being said, it is less invasive and cheaper than a joint replacement. It may be worth considering as a first option.

- **Joint replacement.** A final option when damage to cartilage is severe and beyond healing. Hips are the most commonly replaced joint. Knee replacements are more complex and require more extensive rehabilitation, but are also commonly performed.

Chapter Highlights

- The primary factors that compromise joint health are inflammatory foods (especially sugars and starches) and poor sleep, which disrupts daily joint recovery.

- Emerging research suggests certain microbes likely also play a role by causing inflammation and breaking down collagen.

- Keys to protecting your joints include staying physically active, choosing low-impact activities when possible, listening to pain when you feel it, and taking recovery time seriously.

- Anti-inflammatory herbs, omega-3 fatty acids, CBD oil, and certain antimicrobial herbs can help promote joint health and comfort.

- Massage, physical therapy, acupuncture, and heat therapies can also be very beneficial.

23

Menopause

Menopause is a natural process that affects every woman in the world when she reaches middle age. Even so, the "change of life" catches many women by surprise. After decades of living in a predictable body, things start to change—physically and sometimes emotionally as well.

It helps to understand a bit about what's going on in the body during menopause. Menopause results from the fairly abrupt decline in estrogen levels associated with the natural cessation of ovarian function. Put more simply: when the ovaries run out of eggs, estrogen stops. A woman's ovaries typically contain a supply of eggs that last until midlife. Estrogen production is tied to ovulation (the monthly release of an egg from the ovaries). When the ovaries run out of eggs, estrogen levels decline sharply, along with reproductive function. When ovulation ceases, menstrual periods also stop.

Menopause, signaled by loss of menstrual periods, typically occurs between ages 45 and 55 (average age of menopause is 51 in the U.S.). Sometimes periods can come and go with increasing irregularity for years before they stop completely. The interval of irregular periods leading up to menopause is known as perimenopause. Hormonal fluctuations during perimenopause can also cause breast tenderness, bloating, and pelvic discomfort. Classic symptoms of menopause include hot flashes, night sweats, vaginal dryness, sleep disturbance, and mood imbalances. These symptoms can also occur during perimenopause and for years after the last menstrual period occurs.

Although menopause isn't a disease, sometimes it feels like a disease. That's because menopause can be the proverbial last straw. Stress that's been adding up for years—poor eating habits, the mental stress of navigating the complexities of modern life, not getting enough sleep, and not staying physically active—often go unnoticed until menopause comes along and tips the balance. Then, everything seems like it's falling apart.

However, there are a few significant health concerns that come along with menopause. One is cardiovascular disease. The cyclic production of estrogen associated with normal menstrual cycles has been linked to lower risk of cardiovascular events, as compared to men. After menopause, however, that protection is erased; postmenopausal women have about the same cardiovascular disease risk as men of the same age.

Postmenopausal women also need to be aware of their newly elevated risk of osteoporosis. Accelerated bone loss (up to 20% of total bone mass) occurs in the first seven years after menopause and then levels off as the body adapts to having minimal estrogen.

Tips for a Comfortable Transition

Health habits matter. Over many years of following women making the transition, it's been impossible to overlook the fact that women with poor health habits have more pronounced symptoms, and the symptoms go on longer. Smoking, poor dietary habits, chronic stress, poor sleep, and inactivity translate into greater menopausal symptoms. Better health habits reduce symptoms.

Get your diet squeaky clean! Walk right past those tempting processed foods, and pack your shopping cart with fruits and vegetables. Fill half of your plate with vegetables at every meal. Packed with fiber and phytonutrients, vegetables can help you maintain a healthy weight, especially during menopause and postmenopause, when weight gain is common. A diet high in veggies also helps to maintain a healthy cardiovascular system and good bones and brain health (for women and men of all ages!).

Prioritize self-care and relaxation. Menopause is a period of change, which can often feel stressful. That's why it's so important to manage your stress and make time for relaxing activities. Yoga, qigong, and other mind-body modalities are good for balancing stress, but choose any activity that brings you joy.

Stay active. Exercise can help you balance stress, maintain a healthy body weight, and keep your heart and lungs strong as you age. In response to such activity, your body generates endorphins, the "feel good" molecules that naturally help to elevate mood and sense of well-being while reducing pain. Aim for at least 30 minutes of moderate-intensity activity at least 5 days a week. The decline of estrogen after menopause tends to lead to an increase in visceral fat and a loss of muscle mass and bone density. But resistance training—including yoga and other weight-bearing activities—can help you maintain and build muscle and bone.

Establish a relationship with a health care provider. A health care provider, such as a gynecologist, can administer medical therapy when indicated and order or perform health screens such as PAP smears and mammograms.

Herbal Support for Menopause

In regard to menopause, you will often see the phrase "HPA axis" because reproductive function is closely tied to the hypothalamic-pituitary-adrenal axis (known as the HPA axis). As discussed in Chapter 13, the hypothalamus is a walnut-size gland at the base of the brain that controls sleep and wake cycles, body temperature, stress tolerance, energy and metabolism, body weight, and reproductive functions. It does so by regulating the pituitary gland, which in turn regulates the thyroid gland (metabolism), the adrenal glands (stress glands), and the ovaries (reproduction). Fluctuating estrogen levels disrupt the delicate balance of the HPA axis, resulting in many of the menopause symptoms.

Fortunately, Mother Nature has provided some very functional answers for balancing the HPA axis and reducing menopausal symptoms. Herbal options include both herbs that have estrogenic activity and others that act by non-estrogenic mechanisms. One of the best options is ashwagandha, already previously mentioned because, as an adaptogen, it has many applications.

- **Ashwagandha.** Ashwagandha balances the HPA axis, thus reducing menopausal symptoms, but without having any estrogenic effects. Ashwagandha has been used in India for thousands of years to treat symptoms that are indicative of hypothalamic imbalance, including menopausal symptoms.

  Over years of practicing gynecology and helping many women through menopause, I've found that ashwagandha pairs especially well with L-theanine (a natural substance that improves focus and concentration), along with some calming herbs such as extracts of the magnolia and phellodendron species from traditional Chinese medicine (known for supporting adrenal function and stress tolerance). This combination reduces all HPA axis–related symptoms, including hot flashes and anxiety, without being sedating. Because none of these herbs have estrogenic activity, they can be safely used along with estrogen replacement therapy when it is indicated. With use of the herbs, symptoms can typically be controlled with lower doses of estrogen.

(See Chapter 13 for complete profiles and dosing for ashwagandha and L-theanine.)

For irregular periods associated with perimenopausal women, the herb, vitex, also known as chaste tree berry is excellent for regulating periods and reducing PMS symptoms.

- **Vitex (*Vitex agnus-castus*).** Vitex acts as a tonic (hormonal modulator) specific for the female reproductive system. It is thought to work by normalizing ovarian function by affecting the pituitary gland. Vitex is effective for symptom management and regulation of periods during perimenopause and management of PMS symptoms. Note that it takes several months of taking vitex to see full benefit.

  Suggested dosing: 500 mg of standardized vitex extract twice daily. It can be combined with cyclic administration of natural progesterone cream (for 2 weeks before expected time of the period) for optimal benefit.

  Potential side effects and precautions: Vitex is generally well tolerated. Side effects are rare and include mild stomach upset, itching, rash, fatigue, and hair loss. Caution is advised if used with drugs that affect dopamine, but no other drug interactions are known.

Black cohosh is another herb commonly used to curb hot flashes without having estrogenic activity. My clinical experience is that ashwagandha is superior and covers a wider range of symptoms, but there's nothing wrong with taking black cohosh along with the herbs previously mentioned.

- **Black cohosh (*Actaea racemosa*).** This herb is derived from the roots of a shrub-like plant native to the Appalachian forests of North America. Though well known for treating hot flashes, black cohosh was traditionally used to treat rheumatism. Having well-documented anti-inflammatory properties, black cohosh is an effective remedy for joint aches exacerbated by menopause. The clinical response for treating hot flashes is variable among individuals. Response appears to be dose dependent and also dependent on the quality of the product.

  Suggested dosing: 20-80 mg per day of black cohosh standardized extract.

  Potential side effects and precautions: Black cohosh appears to be quite safe and is well tolerated at normal doses. Black cohosh has not been found to have significant estrogenic activity. There is a slight risk of adverse effects on liver function with use of black cohosh at very high doses.

Some herbal supplements used for menopause do have estrogenic activity. This shouldn't be a surprise because plants use many chemical messengers that are similar to ours. Phytochemicals with estrogenic activity (often called "phytoestrogens") come from a class of chemicals called isoflavones, which are very abundant in certain plants. Soy and red clover are common sources of isoflavones found in herbal supplements.

It's important to note that the estrogenic activity of phytoestrogens (isoflavones) is very weak. It's only about 1% of the activity of estrogens produced by the ovaries. Although it's common knowledge that estrogenic activity is equated with increased breast cancer risk, it doesn't work that way with phytoestrogens. Phytoestrogens compete with stronger estrogens in the body for the same receptors, so phytoestrogens actually reduce estrogenic stimulation of breast tissue.

Here's a fact worth considering: women in Japan consume large amounts of soy, which is very rich in isoflavones. Yet, women in Japan have a lower-than-average risk of breast cancer, which suggests that isoflavone consumption doesn't promote breast cancer. That being said, women with a high genetic risk of breast cancer or women who have had an estrogen-sensitive cancer (breast or uterine) would be wise to avoid supplements containing isoflavones or having any estrogenic activity.

Phytoestrogens are best obtained from dietary sources, and 40-80 mg of isoflavones are recommended daily. One cup of soymilk contains about 6 mg; ½ cup edamame, 16 mg; 3 oz of tofu, 20 mg; 3 oz of tempeh, 30 mg; 1 oz of dry-roasted soybeans, 40 mg.

Other Considerations

Women with symptomatic menopause will be confronted with whether or not to consider hormone replacement therapy (HRT). Symptoms of vaginal dryness and decreased libido are not benefited by herbal therapy. Properly administered HRT can help with those issues and protect against accelerated loss of bone mass and increased risk of cardiovascular disease.

Remember that the key to reducing symptoms of menopause is restoring balance in the HPA axis. One way to do that is by taking estrogen. When the ovaries stop working and estrogen secretion becomes erratic and eventually stops, abnormal feedback signals to the hypothalamus disrupt the entire HPA axis, including metabolic functions and management of the stress response. Administering estrogen restores balance to the HPA axis. For women who have a uterus, progesterone must be administered along with estrogen to prevent uterine bleeding.

Though HRT can dramatically reduce all symptoms of menopause and lower risk of osteoporosis, the type of HRT is important to consider. Pharmaceutical preparations of conjugated equine estrogen and medroxyprogesterone have been linked to increased risk of breast cancer, uterine cancer, and cardiovascular incidents (heart attack and stroke). This may be less true with low doses of transdermal (patches or cream) preparations of bioidentical estrogen and progesterone (identical to the natural hormones produced by the body). The greatest benefit of HRT appears to be within the first 7 years after menopause. The decision of whether or not to do HRT must be carefully weighed between the patient and a qualified health care provider.

You may choose to combine HRT with carefully selected herbal supplements. In almost all women, the hormonal imbalances of menopause gradually equilibrate over time. However, in the interim, nutritional and herbal therapies and/or properly dosed bioidentical hormone therapy can be safe, effective, and sometimes almost lifesaving.

As with any medical therapies, it's important to open the lines of communication with your health care provider, discuss the risks and benefits of all possible therapies, and then be ready to adjust those therapies as needed to confidently transition through this phase of life.

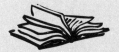

Recommended Reading:

Aviva Romm MD, *Botanical Medicine for Women's Health*, 2nd Edition, 2018

An authoritative resource by herbalist, midwife, and physician Aviva Romm on longevity, gynecologic health, menopausal health, fertility and childbearing. Supporting women with botanicals at every stage of life, this resource includes the latest scientific research as well as deep-rooted traditional wisdom on the use of herbs for women's health.

Chapter Highlights

- While menopause is a completely natural process, it can include sleep disruption, hot flashes, and other unsettling symptoms. Post-menopausally, women have an increased risk of cardiovascular disease and osteoporosis.

- Keys to a more comfortable transition through menopause include eating a clean diet, prioritizing self-care and relaxation, and staying active with moderate-intensity and weight-bearing activities.

- Certain herbs help normalize hormone function and minimize menopause symptoms.

- Bioidentical hormone replacement therapy may be beneficial for some women.

24

Prostate Health

P rostate disease is the most common uniquely male disorder in the world. Changes in the prostate gland produce symptoms that are almost universal after the age of fifty. Most symptoms of benign prostate disease are manageable with dietary modifications, lifestyle changes, and nutritional supplements.

The male prostate is a walnut-size gland that wraps around the urethra, the tube that allows urine to pass from the bladder through the penis. The prostate is located inside the body just above where the penis starts. It can be easily felt by a health care provider on a rectal examination. The purpose of the prostate is to produce the nourishing liquid that carries sperm during ejaculation.

Common Prostate Conditions

Most men are completely unaware of the presence of their prostate until midlife, when changes start to occur. Three different types of conditions can occur in the prostate: benign prostatic hypertrophy, prostatitis, and prostate cancer. All have similar symptoms. The most concerning and pronounced symptom is decreased urine flow and incomplete bladder emptying caused by constriction of the urethra from progressive enlargement of the prostate gland. This symptom is so common that virtually every male over the age of fifty will experience decreased urine flow.

Benign Prostatic Hyperplasia (BPH)

BPH is caused by progressive and symmetric growth of the prostate tissue. It is by far the most common of the three prostate disorders. More than half of men between ages 50 and 70 are affected and by age 90, 90% are affected. The cause is still being debated, but it appears that an abnormal ratio of estrogen to testosterone is a contributing factor to the disease process.

Other symptoms of BPH include leaking or dribbling from urethral constriction and an overdistended bladder, urgency to void, and frequent voiding at night. Occasionally, a crisis with complete obstruction can be precipitated by the use of over-the-counter cold medicines, alcohol consumption, sitting for a long period of time, or prolonged exposure to cold temperatures.

Chronic Prostatitis

Prostatitis is associated with inflammation of the prostate gland that causes enlargement and constriction of the urethra. Pain is the defining factor of prostatitis. It occurs most frequently in men younger than 45 years old. Though only 10% of cases are recognized as being caused by a bacterial infection, the rate of infection in prostatitis is probably higher than that. Studies are now showing that a wide range of intracellular bacteria maintain a permanent presence in the prostate, though the full range of bacteria that can cause symptoms of prostatitis has not yet been defined. Prostatitis can be acute or chronic. Acute cases are more likely to respond to conventional antibiotic therapy; chronic prostatitis can usually be managed with herbal therapy (see list below).

Prostate Cancer

Prostate cancer is, of course, the most concerning of the three. Fortunately, prostate cancer is almost 100% survivable if detected early. The main ways of screening for prostate cancer include the PSA (prostate-specific antigen) blood test and palpation of the prostate gland by rectal exam.

Other than skin cancer, prostate cancer is the most common cancer in males over fifty. Risk factors include race, family history, high intake of animal fat and refined oils, low intake of vegetables, obesity, sedentary lifestyle, and exposure to toxic substances. Men of African descent have higher risk than average. The lowest rate of prostate cancer in the world occurs in Asian men living in Japan, possibly related to high intake of soy and fish and low intake of meat. Symptoms of prostate cancer mimic those of benign prostate disease, but in early stages, there may be no symptoms at all.

The Microbe Connection

Increasingly, chronic infections are being linked to all conditions of the prostate. It shouldn't be surprising because the nutrient-rich cells of the prostate are likely magnets for microbes, and the barriers that protect the prostate are vulnerable, especially as a person ages. A wide spectrum of bacteria and other microbes from the gut, gums, skin, and other sources (including mycoplasma, ureaplasma, and chlamydia species) are being linked to all prostate diseases, especially prostate cancer. *P. acnes*, a skin bacterial species mentioned previously, has been closely associated with prostate cancer.

Emerging Prostate Research

A study[119] published in 2020 detailed the spectrum of microbes found in the prostate, which included dozens of species of bacteria from the gut, skin, urinary tract, and new infections. The researchers speculated that the microbes may play a role in prostate diseases, including prostate cancer. They also recognized that certain friendly flora were associated with reduced incidence of prostate disease. This study went on to suggest a possible role of protective plant phytochemicals in reducing the incidence of prostate disease.

Natural Prostate Support

As with any illness, the incidence of symptomatic prostate disease is decreased with good health habits and enhanced cellular protection with daily herbs. When prostate disease occurs, natural supplements should not be seen as a replacement for conventional medical therapies, but can be an important complement that promotes healing and reduces the need for drug therapy or invasive surgical therapies.

---

119 Crocetto F, Boccellino M, Barone B, et al. The crosstalk between prostate cancer and microbiota inflammation: nutraceutical products are useful to balance this interplay? *Nutrients*. 2020;12(9):2648.

Benign prostatic hyperplasia

Supplements commonly used for benign prostate disease have similar actions to drugs but work more comprehensively on the entire urogenital system and are associated with a much lower incidence of side effects. While it's important to have any persistent symptoms evaluated and monitored by a urologist (physician specializing in disorders of the genitourinary tract), herbal supplements, combined with appropriate lifestyle and dietary modifications, can often ameliorate symptoms without side effects. In Europe, the majority of men affected by benign prostate disease manage their symptoms without drug therapy using herbs. These supplements may also reduce the risk of prostate cancer.

- **Saw palmetto (*Serenoa repens*).** Extract derived from a dwarf palm native to the southeastern United States. Inhibits conversion of testosterone to dihydrotestosterone (DHT) and prevents adherence of DHT to prostate tissues. Also has potent anti-inflammatory properties. Effectively increases urine flow rate, decreases residual urine volume, and shrinks the prostate gland. This supplement takes 1-2 months of regular use to see benefit, therefore it should be started as soon as symptoms become evident. It is important to choose a supplement of saw palmetto berries with the extract standardized to 85%-95% of the active fatty acids and sterols.

  Suggested dosing: Average dosage is two 160-mg capsules twice daily.

  Potential side effects and precautions: Side effects are unusual and include gastrointestinal upset, headache, dizziness, and decreased libido.

- **Nettle (*Urtica dioica*).** An herb with anti-inflammatory properties commonly used for arthritis and respiratory problems. Nettle has also been commonly used for treatment of prostate disorders and has been shown in numerous studies to reduce all symptoms of benign prostate disease and reduce the size of the prostate gland. Felt to be most effective when synergistically combined with pygeum and saw palmetto.

Suggested dosing: Average dosage is 300-600 mg twice daily.

Potential side effects and precautions: Side effects are unusual and include gastrointestinal upset.

- **Rye grass pollen.** Flower pollen from rye grass has been used successfully to treat benign prostate disorders in Europe for many years. It relaxes smooth muscle and increases bladder contractility, reducing symptoms associated with benign prostate disease (effective for both BPH and prostatitis). Rye grass pollen has anti-inflammatory properties and is also useful for treating arthritis. Rye grass pollen contains beta-sitosterols, which not only reduce prostate symptoms but also naturally lower cholesterol.

Suggested dosing: Average dosage of standardized preparations is 50-120 mg two to three times daily.

Potential side effects and precautions: Side effects are uncommon. Note that flower pollen extracts typically do not cause allergic reactions, even in sensitive individuals, because the allergens are removed in the extraction process.

- **Beta-sitosterols.** These are plant compounds similar to cholesterol known to reduce symptoms of benign prostate disease. This supplement is also commonly used as an adjunct to dietary modifications for lowering blood cholesterol levels. Beta-sitosterols are naturally found in many foods, with significant amounts in avocados, raw pistachios, raw almonds, raw walnuts, and canola oil.

Prostatitis

Pain associated with urinary tract symptoms is a hallmark sign of prostatitis. The onset is usually before age 50. Treatment is multifaceted and includes dietary modifications, supplements, relaxation techniques involving the pelvic floor muscles, and acupuncture. Antibiotics may be indicated for acute prostatitis. Supplements that reduce inflammation and/or have antimicrobial actions can be beneficial for chronic prostatitis. Therapy should be guided by a urologist.

- **Cranberry.** Cranberry juice (unsweetened) is commonly used to support a healthy urinary tract. It prevents adherence of bacteria to tissues. One study suggests that a more concentrated form, cranberry powder (*Vaccinium macrocarpon*), may be of greater benefit for prostatitis than juice.[120]

- **Nettle, saw palmetto, and rye grass pollen.** These herbs commonly used for prostate issues may improve urinary flow, reduce pain, and aid in resolution of infection. (See descriptions of these in the previous section on BPH.)

- **Antimicrobial herbs.** The possible association between intracellular microbes and any type of prostate condition shouldn't be ignored. Though antimicrobial herbs have not been as widely studied as drugs for treatment of prostate conditions, they are very safe to use and do not interfere with other therapies. Any of the antimicrobial herbs mentioned in Chapter 10 have value, but my top picks among the antimicrobial herbs in regard to prostatitis are anamu and berberine.

- **Anamu (*Petiveria alliacea*).** An herb native to tropical regions of Central and South America that features potent medicinal

---

120 Vidlar A, Vostalova J, Ulrichova J, et al. The effectiveness of dried cranberries (*Vaccinium macrocarpon*) in men with lower urinary tract symptoms. *Br J Nutr.* 2010;104(8):1181-1189.

properties. Also known as guinea hen weed, anamu has been traditionally used for colds, flu, pain relief, pneumonia, and arthritis. Potent sulfur compounds give anamu a garlic-like odor. These and other chemical compounds offer potent broad-spectrum antimicrobial properties against bacteria, viruses, yeast, and fungi. Anamu is also immune enhancing and offers potent anti-inflammatory properties (inhibits COX-1) and anticancer properties. It increases cellular immunity and increases NK cells. Anamu is a good choice for prostatitis because it is concentrated in the urine and because it provides good coverage against mycoplasma and ureaplasma.

Suggested dosing: 1-2 grams (1000-2000 mg) of the whole herb, twice daily. Note that use of anamu will give urine and feces a distinct odor.

Potential side effects and precautions: Safe and well tolerated. It should be avoided in pregnancy.

- **Berberine.** Berberine is an antimicrobial phytochemical found in many herbs, including goldenseal, Coptis, barberry, and Oregon grape. Berberine disrupts the ability of bacteria to adhere to tissues and form colonies (biofilm). The doses depend on the herb product used. Berberine-containing herbs are generally well tolerated.

Dietary and Lifestyle Considerations

- Diets high in vegetables, fruit, beans, and soy but low in animal fat are associated with lower incidence of prostate disease. Ground flaxseed is also an important dietary inclusion.

- Cruciferous vegetables (cabbage, cauliflower, kale, Brussels sprouts, broccoli) increase estrogen metabolism and are very favorable for prostate health. Try to consume a vegetable from this family daily!

- An anti-inflammatory diet is the first step toward relieving pain and suffering associated with chronic prostate discomfort. The primary inflammatory foods are sugar, wheat (whether white flour or whole grain), red meat, processed corn products, and dairy. These foods should be minimized or avoided with prostate disease because they aggravate inflammation of the prostate gland.

- Lycopene is the compound responsible for the red color in tomatoes. It is concentrated and made more bioavailable upon cooking, so it is abundant in cooked tomatoes such as in cooked salsa, tomato sauce, and ketchup. It is also found in watermelons. Lycopene has antioxidant activity and has been associated with decreased risk of prostate disease. Countries with high intake of cooked tomatoes (Italy, Spain, and Mexico), have very low rates of prostate cancer as compared to the U.S. and UK.[121]

- Exposure to estrogen increases risk of prostate disease. Estrogens have been found in public water supplies as a result of the female population using pharmaceutical products containing estrogens. Many pesticides used in agriculture are estrogenic. Many by-products of the plastic industry, called xenoestrogens, display strong estrogenic activity.

- Soy contains phytochemicals, called isoflavones, that have very weak estrogenic activity. Though the estrogenic activity in soy isoflavones may be a concern for individuals who have an estrogen-sensitive cancer of the reproductive organs (prostate, breast), for healthy individuals, isoflavones in soy

121 Story EN, Kopec RE, Schwartz SJ, Harris GK. An update on the health effects of tomato lycopene. *Annu Rev Food Sci Technol.* 2010;1:189-210.

and soy products actually partially block estrogen receptors and decrease stimulation by more potent estrogens in the body. This may explain why, despite high soy consumption, Japanese men have low rates of prostate cancer.

- Regular exercise lowers risk of benign prostatic hypertrophy.

- Adequate hydration is a must in the presence of prostate dysfunction.

- Progressive relaxation: because prostatitis is often associated with tension and contraction of the pelvic floor muscles, the regular practice of total body relaxation techniques can offer effective pain relief.

- Acupuncture: may offer significant improvement of pain symptoms associated with prostatitis. Benefit may be predominantly related to relaxation of pelvic floor muscles.

Additional Supplement Support

- **Omega-3 fatty acids.** Omega-3 fatty acids reduce general body inflammation. Fish oil and krill oil are both terrific sources of omega-3s, with lots of supporting science behind them. Notably, krill oil also contains the antioxidant astaxanthin. Krill oil is especially beneficial because it is in a phospholipid form that is easily incorporated into cell membranes.

- **Pumpkin seed oil.** Pumpkin seed oil is rich in linoleic acid (an essential fatty acid) and minerals, especially zinc. It is also a good source of beta-sitosterols. Lower rates of prostate disease are found in parts of the world where pumpkin and other winter squash seeds are consumed regularly.

- **Flax seeds and oil.** Flaxseed oil has anti-inflammatory properties, and flax seeds contain chemicals called lignans, known to block the effects of estrogen on prostate tissues; this may reduce symptoms associated with prostate disease.

- **Ginger.** Ginger is a potent anti-inflammatory associated with a decreased cancer risk in general.

- **Turmeric.** As touted earlier in this book, turmeric has potent anti-inflammatory and anticancer properties and is a terrific all-around herb.

Chapter Highlights

- Prostate disease is the most common uniquely male disorder in the world.

- Changes to the prostate start to occur around midlife.

- Three different types of conditions can occur in the prostate: benign prostatic hypertrophy, prostatitis, and prostate cancer.

- Chronic infections are being linked to all conditions of the prostate.

- When paired with an anti-inflammatory diet, herbal therapy using saw palmetto, nettle, and rye grass pollen can be an important complement that promotes prostate healing and reduces the need for drug therapy or surgery.

25

Skin Health

While you may not have thought of it this way, your skin is considered the largest organ in your body. Skin provides many important functions. It plays an essential role in regulating body temperature. It protects you from the sun's radiation and toxic substances. It's also a barrier to invading microbes. Skin keeps you dry on the outside, but holds moisture inside.

Skin is composed of layers. Under a microscope, a section of skin looks something like a thin sponge. That outer layer, called the epidermis, is composed of thin, flat cells stacked one on top of another like a deck of cards. New cells form at the bottom, and old cells (dead and dehydrated) flake off at the outer top surface. A waxy coat on the outer surface of the skin provides waterproofing and also acts as a barrier to microbes.

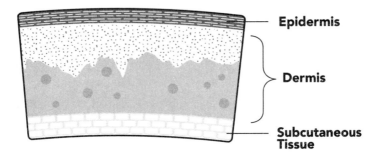

The deeper spongy layer, called the dermis, contains a network of blood vessels that nourish the skin. It's supported by interlaced strands of collagen, a specialized protein that holds skin cells and blood vessels in place. Another protein, elastin, provides flexibility and elasticity to skin. The health of your skin is dependent on the health of your dermis. The drying, wrinkling, and thinning that occurs in skin with aging is a direct result of the gradual destruction and collapse of the collagen and the tiny blood vessels in the dermis.

Most topical skin care products only affect the epidermis and do not penetrate into the dermis. Even topical products containing collagen do not penetrate deeply into the dermis and therefore have minimal effect. Cleansers and moisturizers mainly affect the outer surface of skin. Although anti-wrinkle creams artificially tighten and temporarily improve the appearance of skin, they do not actually improve the integrity of the skin itself or slow skin aging.

Your skin's appearance can be a window into your overall health. The best way to take care of your skin is actually from the inside out, starting with **collagen-friendly foods.** Fresh, whole foods in general are a good choice, but certain ones are especially good for your collagen. Kale and other deep-green leafy vegetables, fermented soy (tempeh and miso), cucumbers, salmon, eggs, celery, and olives stand out as being beneficial for protecting collagen in the body. They contain antioxidants that protect existing collagen and nutrients that are important for building new collagen. And because you have an abundance of collagen not only in skin but also in blood vessels, joints, eyes, and more, dietary antioxidants protect those other parts of the body, too!

Sun Damage to Skin

When most people think of skin damage, they think of sun damage. No doubt, prolonged exposure to sunlight, especially to intense sunlight, can result not only in painful sunburn but also in the destruction of some skin collagen (by free-radical formation). This is a major contributor to skin wrinkling. Invest in a good sunscreen with an SPF (sun protection factor) of 30 or higher. Clothing and a hat provide even more protection. The Environmental Working Group (ewg.org) regularly posts lists of sunscreens that are free of harmful chemicals.

But don't stop there. Build internal skin protection by consuming specific vegetables and fruits which contain potent antioxidants that build up in our skin layers. In particular, the antioxidants lutein and zeaxanthin (found in carrots, squash, pumpkin, collards, kale) and anthocyanins (from blueberries, blackberries, red cabbage, and pomegranate) directly protect against the damaging effects of sunlight. In addition to getting plenty of these tasty foods in your diet, you might also consider supplemental lutein, zeaxanthin, and berry extracts.

It's important to note that your eyes, which have abundant collagen and other proteins, are as susceptible to sun damage as your skin. Invest in good anti-glare sunglasses that screen out UV light and provide sufficient coverage around the sides of the eyes. Did you know that cumulative sun damage is one of the causes of cataracts in the eyes?

The Glucose Connection

A major collagen cruncher may be right in your cereal bowl! Recall that glucose tends to stick to proteins. This includes collagen, which is a protein. So, the glucose from a high- starch and high-sugar diet sticks to collagen strands in your skin and causes them to collapse over time. If you make a habit of eating a high-carb diet, plan on wrinkling at double the normal rate. If you smoke cigarettes, double that rate again.

Other factors that accelerate skin aging include:

- Excessive alcohol consumption (alcohol is both a toxin and an oxidant)

- Low vitamin C levels (vitamin C is a cofactor in collagen formation)

- High stress level, which uses up antioxidants such as vitamin C faster

- Lack of sleep, which inhibits cellular repair

Toxic Substances That Accelerate Skin Damage

Many toxins are also collagen crunchers. Your skin is the first line of defense between you and threats from the outside environment. As your body's largest organ, your skin takes on a significant amount of the toxin load you encounter each day.

Become toxin aware. We accidentally take in substances that are toxic to skin cells by ingesting them along with food and water, breathing them in, or absorbing them through our skin. Many harmful chemicals are hidden in fabrics and personal care products that you might use every day, including perfumes, cosmetics, hair dye, soap, lotion, shaving cream, deodorant, and shampoo. They can cause health concerns ranging from skin irritation to endocrine system disruption to liver problems or even to an increased risk of cancer.

Did I mention wrinkles? As collagen breaks down, the result can be sagging, thinning skin and easy bruising. Therefore, avoiding toxins and taking additional steps to protect your collagen are an important part of maintaining healthy skin. Moreover, toxins can have far-reaching damage not only to skin collagen but also to the liver and nearly all other organs.

The list of potential toxins is dizzying (formaldehyde, phthalates, triclosan, and thousands more). One great resource to help you find safe brands for personal care products, cleaners, and more is the Environmental Working Group (ewg.org). Be sure to also filter your water, maintain a clean indoor air-filtering system, eat fresh vegetables and fruits, and don't smoke. Houseplants help to absorb some air impurities as well.

Natural Supplements for Skin Health

Many vitamins have antioxidant properties and other values regarding skin health, including these frontrunners:

- Vitamin A plays several roles in skin, stimulating cell growth and differentiation.

- Beta-carotene, which is the precursor to vitamin A, protects against oxidative damage to DNA.

- Vitamin C is especially important for collagen synthesis, but also aids in wound healing.

- Vitamin D allows the body to protect itself against some sun damage and prompts the formation of melanin, which provides longer term protection.

- Vitamin E protects all cell membranes and also prevents oxidation of vitamin A.

A healthy diet rich in vegetables and fruit is the absolute best way to get your vitamins and minerals, but you can also supplement with a multivitamin. See the discussion at the end of Chapter 11 for guidelines on choosing a multivitamin product.

Here are some other natural supplements that support optimal skin health:

- Joint supplements with glucosamine and natural anti-inflammatory substances such as turmeric and boswellia also support healthy skin collagen. See Chapter 22 for further discussion about these important nutrients.

- Omega-3 fatty acids help maintain hydration of skin layers. Fish oil and krill oil are concentrated sources of omega-3s. Krill oil is an especially good source for skin because it also contains astaxanthin, a potent antioxidant. See Chapter 11 for a complete profile of omega-3 supplements.

- Other important nutrients for skin health (complete discussions in Chapter 11):

    ○ Lutein and zeaxanthin (antioxidants that protect both skin and eyes)

- ◦ Blueberry or bilberry extracts

- ◦ Resveratrol (from grapes or Japanese knotweed) supports blood vessel health

- ◦ Pine bark extract also supports blood vessel health

- Taking collagen supplements is another important way to support skin collagen. In a 2021 double-blind, placebo-controlled study published in the *Journal of Dermatological Treatment* found that participants who took collagen supplements over a 4-week period significantly improved different parameters of skin health.[122] For a complete discussion on collagen supplements, see Chapter 14.

---

122 Sangsuwan W, Asawanonda P. Four-weeks daily intake of oral collagen hydrolysate results in improved skin elasticity, especially in sun-exposed areas: a randomized, double-blind, placebo-controlled trial. *J Dermatolog Treat.* 2021;32(8):991-996.

Chapter Highlights

- Healthy skin is supported by collagen, a specialized protein that holds skin cells and blood vessels in place.

- With aging, you may notice drying, wrinkling, and thinning of the skin due to the gradual collapse of collagen.

- Most topical skin care products don't penetrate deep enough to improve the skin's integrity or slow skin aging.

- The best way to take care of your skin is from the inside out, starting with collagen-friendly foods such as kale and other deep-green leafy vegetables, fermented soy (tempeh and miso), chicken, salmon, eggs, celery, and olives.

- Natural supplements of collagen, as well as vitamins A, C, D, E and beta-carotene, may support skin health.

26

Sleep

A good night's sleep is an essential component of health. Sleep is when cells of the body have downtime to recover from the stress of working all day; it's an essential part of the healing process. During that downtime, the operating systems of the body are being fine-tuned, general maintenance functions are being performed, and the immune system is functioning at peak level. It's also when the brain clears built-up metabolic waste, sorts files, and stores memories.

Without at least 7½-8 hours of good sleep every night (including at least 4 hours of deep sleep), all systems of the body suffer, and the incidence of chronic illness increases.

Sleep Drivers

In humans, sleep is governed by two primary forces: **circadian rhythm** and **sleep pressure**. These two forces are independent but intimately tied together.

Circadian Rhythm

Circadian rhythm is the continuous series of physiological changes between sleeping and waking hours. It's led by **cortisol**, one of the primary hormones produced by the adrenal gland. Your cortisol levels are normally at low ebb in the middle of the night, when you are most relaxed. Cortisol kicks in first thing in the morning, around sunrise, with a surge of stimulating hormones to wake you and get you going. In effect, cortisol revs your engine.

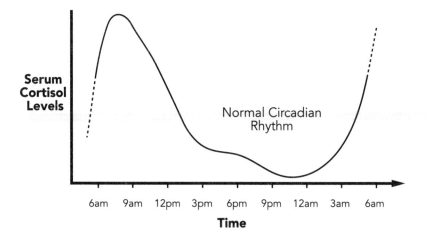

Dropping cortisol levels in the evening hours reverse the changes of the day. Waking activities are quieted, and the body is allowed to rest and repair. Under natural circumstances, declining cortisol levels correspond to dwindling daylight. Onset of darkness stimulates secretion of **melatonin**, which initiates a tide of hormones that flow into the brain and trigger sleep. Once sleep is initiated, secretion of melatonin gradually declines until early morning light brings flow of melatonin to a halt.

The tide of chemical messengers associated with sleep is both dynamic and complex. The brain and neurological system are kept in harmony by a balance of exciting and calming neurotransmitters. The main calming neurotransmitter of the brain is called **gamma-aminobutyric acid (GABA)**. GABA balances neurotransmitters of wakefulness including dopamine, norepinephrine, serotonin, histamine, orexin, and glutamate. The flux of brain chemistry flows back and forth through the waking and sleeping hours.

Adenosine and Sleep Pressure

Circadian rhythm isn't the only force that affects sleep. Because sleep is so important, the body also relies on a chemical called **adenosine** for promoting sleep. Adenosine accumulates naturally in the brain throughout the day. The longer you stay awake, the more adenosine levels build. The effect of adenosine buildup is called **sleep pressure**. The only way to fully clear adenosine from the brain is by sleeping. The better you sleep, the more adenosine is cleared, and the more awake you will feel the next morning. (If you're still dragging at 11:00 in the morning, you didn't clear enough adenosine the night before.)

Interestingly, exercise builds increased sleep pressure by increasing adenosine buildup. We've all experienced it: being physically active during the day usually ensures restful sleep at night.

Sleep Stages

In humans, sleep takes on two distinctly different forms that alternate throughout the night. The two different types of sleep are defined experimentally by measuring eye movements, muscle tone, and brain wave activity. One of the most well-known sleep characteristics is related to eye movements. **Rapid eye movement sleep, called REM sleep**, is associated with eyes darting rapidly back and forth. This is the sleep where most dreaming occurs. Eye movements are not present in **non-REM (NREM) sleep**, of which there are three stages from light to deep. Adequate amounts of both forms of sleep are essential for normal health and well-being.

The brain cycles between NREM sleep and REM sleep all night, with each full cycle lasting at approximately 90 minutes. The first half of the night is dominated by NREM sleep, and the second half of the night is dominated by REM sleep. When we awaken in the morning, we may think we've been dreaming all night, but most dreaming has actually been clustered closer to morning.

NREM Sleep

As sleep begins, the brain and body gradually slip into a state of light NREM sleep. Light dreams float through your evaporating consciousness. External awareness is lost as sensory input from the outside world is selectively blocked. As you progressively enter into the deeper stages of NREM sleep, brain activity decreases further; brain waves become slow and synchronized. Breathing becomes slow and regular. Heart rate slows too, and blood pressure drops. Body temperature falls. You enter a dreamless state of sleep, but there are important things going on. Deep sleep is when healing jumps into high gear! Cellular "housekeeping" is done, and damage that has accumulated from an active day is repaired.

During NREM sleep, your brain also consolidates memories. Thoughts you collect during the day are placed in a short-term memory bank in a part of the brain called the hippocampus. NREM sleep frees up space in the short-term memory bank by sorting files and storing them in long-term memory banks located in the cortex of the brain.

REM Sleep

Eventually, the sleeper will cycle into REM sleep. Interesting things happen in the brain during REM sleep. Brain waves begin to resemble that of the awakened state. It is when dreams happen most intensely. Just before you enter REM sleep, all motor commands to the brainstem are blocked, and you become completely but reversibly paralyzed (except for your eyes, of course, which dart back and forth under closed lids). This prevents exertion during very active dreams.

Memory formation and cellular healing continue during REM sleep, but REM is also important for learning. Furthermore, dreams may help us work through challenging problems. It turns out that the old adage "sleep on it" actually works quite well. Almost everyone has wrestled with some problem all day without resolution, only to wake up the next morning with the obvious solution. That's REM dream sleep working for you!

Considering that the majority of REM sleep comes during the second half of the night, if you habitually go to bed late and then get up with an alarm clock before you awaken naturally, you may be dramatically compromising your learning and problem-solving abilities.

Sleep Dysfunction

At the very core of most sleep problems is an overactive sympathetic nervous system. This is the fight or flight part of the nervous system that's driven by adrenaline. Adrenaline increases alertness, primes muscles for a quick getaway or confrontation, and, most importantly, overrides sleep by blocking adenosine. It's an essential survival mechanism—you wouldn't want to be nodding off during a middle of the night emergency, such as your house burning down.

About 25% of people are born with a hypersensitive sympathetic nervous system. If you are one of these people, like me, know it is built into the fabric of your being. In ancient times, hyperalert individuals were the members of the tribe who were the first to awaken when danger threatened, and they could alert others. Today, however, being hypervigilant in a world teeming with stimuli is a sure recipe for sleep trouble.

Sleep Disruptors

- **Adrenaline-driven days** lead to sleep disturbances at night. If you're still amped up at bedtime from an overly stressful day, the chances of getting a restful night's sleep are marginal. This is partly due to the fact that a cortisol surge tends to follow adrenaline release, and cortisol can override the normal sleep-inducing signals to your brain.

- **Not allowing enough time to sleep?** If you have a regular habit of staying up late and then getting up with an alarm clock before you awaken naturally the next morning, you are missing out on some important REM sleep. Without 7½-8 hours of restful sleep every night, you can't expect to feel sharp the next day.

- **Chronic worry and emotional stress** push the sympathetic nervous system into overdrive. The thinking brain often gets in the way of the sleeping brain. This means that you lie awake—and often, your agitated mind blows things out of proportion, making it tough to get to sleep.

- **Excessive consumption of refined carbohydrates** may cause insulin resistance, which has been linked to increased sympathetic nervous system activity and disturbed sleep.

- **Gastrointestinal issues such as heartburn (reflux)** can disturb sleep. Eating a big meal late in the evening can set the stage for heartburn. If you are prone to it, try to eat your last meal early in the evening, and keep the meal small.

- **Caffeine** and other stimulants found in food and drink disrupt normal sleep. Caffeine promotes alertness by blocking adenosine receptors in the brain. The "half-life" of caffeine is about 6 hours. This means that if you drink two cups of coffee in the morning, half of that caffeine is still with you at lunch and a quarter of it is still in your system at dinnertime. So, you probably don't need that after-dinner coffee.

- **Many drugs disrupt sleep.** The list includes heart medications, antidepressants, corticosteroids, some antibiotics, and (ironically) sleep medications, which are highly habituating and actually cause insomnia after tolerance to the drug develops.

- **Alcohol.** Many people ritually consume an alcoholic evening drink (or two) and swear that it helps them get to sleep, but then they are wide awake in the middle of the night. Alcohol is a depressant of the nervous system. It may lull you to sleep but the alcohol is metabolized by your liver, and the metabolites then work in the opposite way: they keep you from sleeping. Habitual alcohol use also tends to suppress REM sleep.

- **Environmental factors** such as noise, artificial lighting (including LED lighting and blue light from computer screens), or a snoring bed partner can keep you from getting a good night's sleep.

- **Nicotine**, associated with cigarette smoking or vaping, is a stimulant that may inhibit sleep.

- **Late work hours and/or working night shifts** disrupts our circadian rhythm. This includes caregivers who may need to get up several times during the night, which deprives them of restorative deep sleep.

- **Being sedentary through the day** is a ticket to a sleepless night. The body needs regular physical activity during daylight hours to help build up enough sleep pressure before bedtime.

- **Chronic illness** stresses the body, which activates the sympathetic nervous system and contributes to chronic sleep dysfunction. Inflammation associated with chronic illness causes pain and irritates the nervous system, both of which disrupt sleep. It's hard to sleep when stressed cells throughout the body are continually bombarding the brain with distress signals.

- **Aging** is also associated with sleep dysfunction. Specifically, NREM sleep deteriorates with advanced age.

Tips for Better Sleep

Sleep is often an afterthought that comes well behind all the other, more important things in our lives. But if your sleep is getting squeezed, you'll need to figure out how to change that to protect your long-term health. You have to be proactive about your sleep habits. Good sleep habits take practice to become established. No matter where you are—at home or traveling—following the same routine every night will help ensure a consistent good night's sleep.

Address sleep disruptors such as digestive dysfunction, menopausal issues, sleep apnea, chronic illness, or other concerns. If you've been told that you are a heavy snorer, see a neurologist or visit a sleep center for sleep apnea testing. Though they aren't aware of it, people suffering from sleep apnea are awakened many times during the night and are subsequently tired during the day.

A calm day is the best recipe for a restful night. The key to restful sleep is low adrenaline levels during the day. Being stressed during the day ultimately impacts your sleep at night. Getting out for some exercise during the day can help. Life restructuring or a job change may be in order, but the reality is that many people have some stressors in their lives that they can't change. A suggestion, then, is to seek and master some simple breathing and relaxation exercises and meditation techniques. The regular practice of these helps to purge built-up adrenaline. There are books and other instructional materials that can get you started. Some are as close as your phone; some apps for guided meditation are quite good.

Minimize caffeine. If you're struggling with sleep issues, caffeine is best avoided. Look for decaffeinated (most caffeine removed) or caffeine-free alternatives. If you are a big caffeine consumer and decide to abandon caffeine, wean slowly to prevent withdrawal symptoms (headache, fatigue). If you are a tea drinker, green tea (which has some caffeine) is a good choice because it also contains L-theanine, which helps block the detrimental effects of caffeine.

Take a short midday nap. If you can, make a midday power nap or meditation a regular habit. Even nodding off for a few minutes normalizes stress hormones. Most people who are able to nap regularly during the day sleep better at night.

Stay physically active during daylight hours. The best way to increase sleep pressure and promote normal sleep at night is by being active during the day. In general, the more physically tired you are by the end of the day, the better you will sleep at night. Physical activity that is too intense, however, can generate inflammation, which irritates your brain and keeps you awake. It's helpful to incorporate moderate exercise throughout the day—say, a workout in the morning, a walk at lunch, and another moderate activity in the afternoon.

Eat an early dinner. In the evenings, it is preferred to eat early and light. This allows plenty of time for digestion before you lie down to sleep. Especially avoid a heavy meal late in the evening. If you are hungry before bedtime, a banana is a digestible evening snack.

Ease built-up tension. Vigorous exercise should be avoided after 8 pm. If you need to work out pent-up muscle tension, use stretching routines such as yoga or qigong. The gentle relaxing movements of qigong are perfect for promoting a relaxed state before bedtime.

Wind down in the evening. Remember that cortisol follows adrenaline, and if you've had a stressful day, those cortisol levels will still be elevated in the evening. Start purging the stress of the day in the late afternoon or early evening. Reading Is a tried-and-true way to wind down in the evening. Avoid watching stimulating shows on television or working on your computer. I know it sounds boring, but the sleep improvement will be worth it.

Don't use alcohol to wind down. Alcohol initially is a sedative, but the metabolites are stimulants. Expect to be awake about 3-4 hours later if alcohol is consumed in the evening. This may surprise many people, but alcohol, in any amount, always disrupts normal sleep.

Take a shower or bath before bedtime. This relaxes muscle tension and is a great way to unwind. Warm water dilates blood vessels in the skin. When you get out of the bath, water evaporating from your skin accelerates cooling. Your body must cool down before sleep can happen naturally.

Respect normal day and night cycles. If you work an odd shift and must sleep during the day, use darkening shades to completely darken the room where you sleep. Allow yourself a full 8 hours of isolated sleep time to get enough sleep.

Avoid screen time after 9 pm. Light from computers, tablets, cell phones, and television screens suppresses melatonin, blocking the initiation of sleep. Blue-light filters can help, but the flickering light of the screen itself still keeps the brain buzzing. Take a break in the evening and enjoy some other relaxing activity. Some people find that drawing or other art helps them relax. This may work because it is a right-brain activity. Most of the things we do involve more of the left side of the brain. By switching brain hemispheres, it may help us alleviate some of the day's other concerns.

Allow plenty of time for sleep. Ideally, your sleep window should include time to wind down and fall asleep, and then adequate time for sleep, such that you don't have to rely on an alarm clock to wake up in the morning. In other words, you may have to allow 9 hours each night to get 8 hours of quality sleep. It will be worth it; your days will be amazing!

Turn down the lights. LED lights may be saving the planet, but they wreak havoc on sleep. Have a bedside lamp with a single, soft white, low-light bulb. After the sun goes down, use just enough light to get by. Have a few lights that can be dimmed. Always sleep in a dark room, but not a room that is totally sealed from light because, ideally, you want to wake in the morning with natural light coming in.

Sleep comfortably. A comfortable mattress is essential for a good night's sleep. If it's time for a new mattress, shop around, and try before you buy. Memory foam is comfortable, but can sleep hot. Comfortable pillows are equally important. If you're a side sleeper, get an extra-long (king-sized) pillow to place between your knees while sleeping. Note that sleeping on your back encourages sleep apnea.

Sleep cool (but not too cold). Turn the thermostat down several degrees before bedtime. Your body temperature must normally drop several degrees before deep sleep can be initiated. Turn the thermostat down—65 to 72 is ideal for most people—but find what works for you. Ceiling fans can help the room stay cool, and some people even find benefit from cooling mats. Cover lightly as needed, but avoid being hot. Let your body purge the heat of the day. Have extra covers in case you need them during the night because your body will continue to cool toward morning.

Limit noise pollution. Irregular noise such as traffic or howling wind can disrupt sleep. Consider obtaining an electronic device that produces "white noise" to drown out surrounding sounds. One of the best white noise generators on the market is a product called LectroFan. You can also use your smartphone as a white noise generator. There are numerous apps for white noise or relaxing sounds.

If you wake up in the middle of the night, keep the lights low. Many sleep experts recommend that upon waking in the middle of the night, you should get up, turn on the light, and read or do some other type of activity until you become sleepy. While this may work for some people, bright lights stimulate your brain. As an alternative, keep the lights off and start practicing relaxation techniques before the stream of thoughts starts pouring in.

When necessary, isolate yourself. Be aware that your bed partner may be keeping you awake. If you are sensitive to the movement and snoring of your partner or a pet in the room, consider sleeping in a separate location until sleep is improved.

If possible, avoid alarm clocks. The best alarm clock is natural sunlight, which drives our normal circadian rhythm. If work obligations force you to rise before the sun, use a waking device that gently but persistently awakens you. Avoid startling alarms.

Natural Support

In many cases, the stress factors causing insomnia will work themselves out over time, and you just need something to ride out the storm. In situations where the stress is not severe, natural therapy is the best and safest option for restoring normal sleep. Any of the following supplements can be taken individually or together. They are all very mild and non-habit-forming. If you're looking for a "hammer" to put you to sleep, however, these supplements will not meet your expectations. But you can't get in trouble with them either. All the following substances can be combined, but if combined, the lower dose range should be used for each ingredient.

- **Passionflower.** For someone suffering from nervous tension and poor sleep, passionflower can be a real lifesaver. Passionflower has been long revered for its characteristic sedative properties. It has a reputation for restoring restful sleep without causing a next-day hangover. It also offers muscle-relaxing and pain-relieving qualities.

  Suggested dosing: 150 mg of a 10:1 passionflower extract at bedtime to promote restful sleep. Passionflower can also be used as a tincture or enjoyed as a bedtime tea.

  Potential side effects and precautions: Passionflower is generally well tolerated and associated with few reported side effects. (General precautions for natural substances with the potential for causing sedation can be found at the end of Chapter 9.)

- **Lemon balm.** This multipurpose herb is a gentle, yet effective ally for a variety of mental, emotional, and digestive ailments. Its relaxing and grounding qualities make it well suited for clearing the mind and relaxing the body for quality sleep. Unwinding periodically throughout the day is a crucial step in preparing for sound sleep. Lemon balm is thought to naturally increase a neurotransmitter called GABA, which helps turn down the dial on incoming stimuli.

  Suggested dosing: 200 mg of lemon balm extract before bedtime. Lemon balm can also be used as a tincture or enjoyed as a before-bedtime tea.

  Potential side effects and precautions: At the recommended doses, lemon balm has a very good safety profile and long history of safe use. (General precautions for natural substances with the potential for causing sedation can be found at the end of Chapter 9.)

- **Melatonin.** Melatonin is a sleep initiator, not a sleep sustainer. The fading light of day (or turning the lights off at bedtime) stimulates release of melatonin, which initiates a cascade of hormones in the brain, which promotes and maintains sleep. Once sleep is established, melatonin levels go down. Avoid time-released melatonin because it doesn't mimic the normal secretion of melatonin in the body.

  Suggested dosing: At bedtime, take ½ -1 mg of melatonin to initiate sleep. This low dose of melatonin can be repeated one to two times during the night to reinitiate sleep after middle of the night awakening (up to 3 mg total).

  Potential side effects and precautions: Use of higher doses of melatonin can be associated with disturbed sleep or depression.

Melatonin should be avoided in elderly individuals with dementia. (General precautions for natural substances with the potential for causing sedation can be found at the end of Chapter 9.)

- **L-theanine.** L-theanine has a wonderful calming effect with little potential for side effects. At the same time, it improves focus and concentration. Consumption of L-theanine is also associated with a positive mood. It counters the negative effects of caffeine and stress-induced adrenaline secretion. It does not cause sedation during the day, making it ideal for daytime use, but it does promote natural sleep at night.

Suggested dosing: 100-200 mg before bedtime.

Potential side effects and precautions: L-theanine is very safe and has a low potential for side effects. (General precautions for natural substances with the potential for causing sedation can be found at the end of Chapter 9.)

- **GABA.** GABA (gamma-aminobutyric acid) is the primary neurotransmitter in the central nervous system associated with inhibiting neuron signaling, effectively calming the body by turning down the dial on incoming messages and stimuli. Taken as a dietary supplement, GABA is useful for promoting sleep, relaxation, and stress reduction by interacting with the calming GABA neuroreceptors in the human body. (GABA supplements should not be confused with gabapentin, a prescription drug.)

In an animal study, a mixture of GABA and L-theanine had a positive synergistic effect in decreasing the time it took to fall asleep as well as the sleep duration.

Suggested dosing: 100-300 mg before bedtime.

Potential side effects and precautions: GABA is generally well tolerated and is associated with a low incidence of side effects. Some clinical studies have shown that consuming GABA can cause a modest drop in blood pressure, so it theoretically could interact with blood pressure medications. (General precautions for natural substances with the potential for causing sedation can be found at the end of Chapter 9.)

- **Cannabidiol (CBD) oil from hemp.** CBD is the primary chemically active component of hemp. Unlike its alter ego, marijuana, it only contains trace amounts of THC, and therefore it doesn't cause euphoria and is not habituating. Many people find that CBD oil is excellent for promoting restful sleep. (See a complete profile for CBD oil in Chapter 14.)

- **Magnesium glycinate.** When taken as a supplement, the mineral magnesium provides an overall calming effect and relaxes muscles. It may help to lessen leg cramps at night and a condition called restless legs. Magnesium glycinate is a form of magnesium that contains the amino acid, glycine, which also has a calming effect on the brain. Response to magnesium increases with dosage, but dosage is limited by gastrointestinal symptoms, predominantly loose stools.

  Suggested dosing: The average therapeutic dose is 400 mg of magnesium citrate or magnesium glycinate taken a couple of hours before bedtime.

  Potential side effects and precautions: Magnesium glycinate is well-absorbed magnesium and is typically associated with a lower incidence of causing loose stools than other forms of magnesium. (General precautions for natural substances with the potential for causing sedation can be found at the end of Chapter 9.)

- **Lavender essential oil.** Put a few drops on your pillow to enhance normal sleep.

- **Chamomile tea.** The classic bedtime tea for promoting calm and restful sleep. Note that chamomile works great for some people, but causes stimulation for others.

When to Call Your Doctor

Sometimes stress gets out of hand and in these cases, medications can be beneficial for breaking a vicious cycle. Medical therapy can also have a role when chronic insomnia is severe and unrelenting. Even so, drug therapy is always best used cautiously and intermittently. All drugs have side effects, and most drugs with sedative properties carry the potential for habituation.

Out of desperation, many patients with insomnia understandably turn to pharmaceuticals (benzodiazepines or modern sleep medications) for relief. While this would seem like a legitimate course of action, sleep-inducing medications can actually worsen the problem in the long run, as they adversely affect the normal calming neurotransmitters and their receptors in the brain.

Be aware that medications you may be taking for anxiety or depression can cause insomnia. Serotonin-reuptake inhibitors (Prozac, Zoloft, Effexor, Wellbutrin, many others) are notorious for inhibiting sleep in certain individuals.

In addition, certain other situations are best addressed by a health care professional:

- Chronic pain

- Restless legs

- Sleep apnea, commonly associated with excessive weight

- Medical conditions in general

- Medications that may cause sleep disturbances

- Habituation to sleep medications

Recommended Reading:

For a deeper dive into the intricacies of sleep, *Why We Sleep*, by Matthew Walker, PhD., is a fascinating read. It provides a new understanding of the science of sleep and dreaming.

Chapter Highlights

- During sleep, the cells of the body have downtime to recover from the stress of working all day and to engage in cellular "housekeeping" and healing. The brain clears built-up metabolic waste, sorts files, and stores memories.

- To decrease the incidence of chronic disease, you need 7½-8 hours of good sleep every night, including 4 hours of deep sleep.

- Sleep is governed by two primary forces: circadian rhythm and sleep pressure.

- To improve your sleep, address sleep disruptors such as digestive dysfunction, menopausal issues, sleep apnea, chronic illness, or other concerns.

- Natural therapy is the best and safest option for restoring normal sleep.

- Passionflower and lemon balm are non-habit-forming herbs that calm and relax the body to promote restful sleep.

27

Final Thoughts

While life is filled with ups and downs, and good times don't always roll, life does have the potential to improve with age. At least that's been my experience. I've enjoyed better health in my sixties than I did in midlife. It's a true testament to the resiliency of the human body.

Though I've had to make some compromises to ensure good health, somehow they don't feel like compromises. I surround myself with fresh whole foods and take great pleasure in the act of preparing fresh meals from scratch. I make time for long walks or a yoga class every day and generally stay as physically active as daily work on a computer permits. I search for balance that allows me to maintain a productive life without being compromised by stress.

Achieving that kind of balance requires keeping life simpler than it was 20 years ago. That's taken time and effort to arrange, but it's been worth it.

While there isn't much doubt that I still harbor the same microbes in my tissues that I've had for most of my life, I've made peace with them. They're there, but contained, and therefore don't cause symptoms. For that I can give partial credit to good health habits for keeping my immune system strong, but herbs have given me an edge that I wouldn't have had otherwise.

Herbs have made an enormous difference in my life. I don't think that I would enjoy the robust health that I do today without them. They've also given me a new purpose. In my wildest dreams, I never expected to spend a third of my career as a physician researching and promoting the benefits of natural herbal therapy. Sometimes, however, it's the unexpected twists that make life so special.

It's been my pleasure to share the knowledge I've gained in this book. Through it, I hope you'll feel inspired to adopt new habits that will make a difference for your health and your life. **Being alive is a gift. Living well is an even greater gift, but wellness isn't a given.** How well you take care of your body will greatly influence the quality of your total life experience. The changes you make now can make all the difference in your health as time evolves.

In that respect, I hope you'll give herbs a chance. In my opinion, herbs are an unrecognized resource that could dramatically alter the landscape of health worldwide. For that, the future is bright: the world is reawakening to the remarkable benefits of herbal phytochemicals.

I see many signs that we are shifting in the right direction as a society. My hope is that the information contained in this book will move us there faster. While I don't expect to see major changes in health care delivery resulting from this book, my hope is to reach individuals. For every person who makes a shift after reading this book or shares it with a friend, that will create a ripple effect of change. I believe the concepts presented in this book have the power to change lives, and I hope that change will start with you.

Appendix A

Getting the Most out of the Healthcare System

Everyone needs access to the healthcare system. Even with insurance, however, using the healthcare system is costly. So ideally, you want to save it for when you really need it.

Getting the most out of the healthcare system is a matter of having the right expectations. The healthcare system's greatest strength is acute intervention for a sudden or unexpected event. If you were in an automobile accident or had a heart attack, the services offered by the healthcare system can stabilize the injury and possibly can even save your life. Note, however, that healing comes from inside your body. The healthier your body is, the faster you will recover from the injury or bodily insult.

Having access to the healthcare system is also important for screening. Labs and other types of diagnostic tests can sometimes pick up hidden signs of chronic illnesses before you would notice symptoms. While there are hundreds of different types of tests that can be performed, only certain tests are done routinely and covered by insurance.

Following are some of the routine diagnostic tests commonly ordered by health care providers:

- **Complete blood count (CBC):** screens for anemia and abnormal white blood cell count, which can indicate infection or blood cancers, such as leukemia

- **Blood chemistries:** generally normal unless you're really sick

- **Liver function tests:** screens for the rate of loss of liver cells, but not liver functional capacity. It does not test for the presence of fatty liver disease or define the ability of your liver to process toxic substances.

- **Blood glucose:** screens for prediabetes and diabetes

- **Kidney function tests:** screens for certain kidney diseases

- **Screening colonoscopy at age 50:** screens for precancerous polyps and early cancer. Less invasive DNA stool testing is also available, but is less accurate.

- **Mammogram in women:** for detection of early breast cancer

- **PAP smear:** screens for cancerous and precancerous lesions on the cervix

- **Prostate-specific antigen (PSA) in men:** screens for prostate cancer

These types of tests, however, are designed to pick up early disease, not disease before it happens. There are few other tests worth knowing about that can indicate other health parameters. Although these tests can be ordered through a doctor's office, they typically aren't covered by insurance. Fortunately, they are available as at-home tests that can be ordered through the internet or purchased at a pharmacy.

At-home testing:

- **Hemoglobin A1c (HbA1c):** tests for the rate of glycation in the body. Glycation is a significant risk factor for chronic illness. The lower your rate, the better off you are. See Chapter 17 for more information about HbA1c.

- **Vitamin D level:** measures the body's level of vitamin D. Vitamin D is important for many functions in the body. Though you get some vitamin D from a healthy diet containing fish, your body makes most of it from exposure to sunlight. If you live in northern latitudes and have reduced exposure to sunlight in the winter, having your vitamin D level checked once or twice a year is a good practice.

- **Omega-3 fatty acid level:** indicates balance of omega-3 vs. omega-6 fatty acids in the body. An ideal ratio for a normal inflammatory response is a ratio of 1:6 omega-3 to omega-6. See Chapter 11 for more information about omega-3 fatty acids.

Although testing can be an important part of preventing chronic illness, staying healthy is your responsibility. The healthcare system has little capacity to prevent chronic illness from happening or restore you back to wellness if you become chronically ill.

Symptoms are your best indication of changing health status. Pay attention to what your body is telling you. At the first sign of any symptoms, you should become proactive. Go down the list of the stress factors, and look for deficiencies.

- Could your diet use an upgrade, or have you been taking too many dietary liberties?

- Are you being exposed to hidden toxic substances, such as mold growing in a basement?

- Are you pushing the stress button too much or not sleeping enough?

- Have you picked up an infection of some type?

- Have you been taking herbs every day?

Acting early might save you a trip to the doctor's office. Even with the best intentions, however, sometimes life's events can't be controlled. Stress adds up while you're not paying attention, and suddenly symptoms come out of nowhere. And then you start to worry about what type of chronic illness might be brewing inside. Worst of all, is it cancer?

This is another place where the healthcare system is valuable. Diagnostic tests can rule out possibilities such as cancer. If cancer is present, conventional cancer therapies are important for eradicating the cancer cells. For other chronic illnesses, drug therapy and surgical procedures can reduce symptoms and stabilize the processes of illness, which can help set the stage for recovery.

What these conventional therapies can't do, however, is promote healing. That part is up to you. It's all about creating an environment inside your body to allow your cells to recover. If you are chronically ill or you become chronically ill, the guidelines in this book are your pathway back to wellness. Always remember, 90% of recovery from any chronic illness is a result of self-care.

Access to the Healthcare System

In the United States, physicians undergo 4 years of training in medical school and then 3 or more years of training in a specialty. The primary care specialties include family medicine, pediatrics, internal medicine, obstetrics/gynecology, or emergency medicine. Some physicians choose to specialize in more advanced surgical or medical specialties, such as cardiovascular surgery or neurology, which are typically accessed only by referral from a primary care provider (PCP).

Your connection to the system is a PCP. That can be a physician from one of the primary care specialties, but it also can be a nurse practitioner or physician's assistant who works under a PCP.

There are three different types of encounters with a PCP. The first is a routine screening exam, often called a well visit. In other words, you're not sick. It's an opportunity to connect with your PCP, have a basic screening physical that may include a breast exam, prostate exam, or PAP smear (depending on your sex), and they may order screening labs or other diagnostic screening tests. This type of exam occurs every 1-2 years.

The second is a sick visit. It's scheduled if you develop concerning symptoms or become ill in some way. Your PCP will take a history, do a physical exam, and order appropriate tests to evaluate your symptoms and determine a diagnosis. If your situation is straightforward, your PCP may be able to administer treatment or prescribe drug therapy, depending on the nature of the problem. Otherwise, you may be referred to a specialist for further evaluation.

As you've learned, chronic illnesses are typically associated with stressed cells throughout the body, and therefore all chronic illnesses can be associated with a diverse range of possible symptoms. Medical specialties, however, are compartmentalized. In other words, you may end up being referred to multiple specialists—one for each type of symptom—who each may have different opinions about your condition and what therapies to offer.

The third type of visit is a follow-up exam. Once you've been diagnosed and receive treatment, you return to define whether the treatment is working properly and receive prescriptions for ongoing therapy. Initially, this may include follow-up visits with multiple specialists and your PCP. Because medical therapies for chronic illness typically only suppress symptoms and inhibit the processes of illness, follow-up visits are typically scheduled on an ongoing basis. In fact, medication refills make up the majority of office visits for many PCPs.

It's important to keep in mind that all medical providers are trained exclusively in treatment of illness with pharmaceutical and surgical therapies. They receive little training in nutrition or prevention of illness. Information about herbal therapy, nutritional therapy, or other alternative therapies is not part of the medical curriculum. If a provider happens to know about those things, it's because they have sought out education beyond what the medical system offers.

It's also important to note that conventional medicine is highly procedure driven. Even an office visit is defined as a procedure. The bigger and more complex the procedure, the greater the reimbursement to the provider and health care facility. Of all procedures, office visits garner the lowest reimbursement. This provides a huge incentive for health care providers to turn over office visits rapidly and order diagnostic and therapeutic procedures whenever possible.

The key to making the best use of the healthcare system is to respect its limitations and learn how to work with practitioners within those limitations. The following guidelines will help you cultivate a more positive relationship with any health care provider you might encounter.

Establishing a Good Relationship with a Health Care Provider

Here are a few guidelines to help you establish a positive, productive relationship with your general health care provider:

1. **Be specific about the goals of the visit.** If it's a routine screening exam, there isn't time allotted to discuss symptoms or issues that may be bothering you. Touch on the highlights of your concerns, and schedule another visit to go into the details.

2. **Be respectful of your provider's time.** The system is designed around strict time limitations. Your provider only has about 15-30 minutes (depending on the type of visit) to spend with you. If you press for more, then you will throw the provider's schedule off, and nobody is going to be happy.

3. **Be organized.** Have information readily available, such as previous lab results and/or personal observations, which may be helpful in achieving the goal of the visit.

4. **Accept that your provider will likely offer only drugs and possibly surgical procedures.** Your provider's knowledge and training generally does not extend beyond conventional medical therapies. If you expect more, you will be disappointed.

5. **Don't be afraid to ask questions.** If something isn't clear, make sure it is clear before moving forward. Many doctors know less about the long-term side effects of the drugs they prescribe than they should. Also, many doctors take a "shotgun" approach to ordering labs or other diagnostic tests with little regard to cost or whether the results will actually influence your outcome. All surgical procedures are associated with potential risks and adverse outcomes. It's up to you to make decisions about risk vs. benefit.

6. **Remember, you always have the last word.** Do your own research. The internet provides a wealth of information (but sometimes misinformation) about medical therapies, but also alternatives to medical therapies. Before making decisions about your health, you should be as informed as possible.

Types of Medical Providers

Doctor of Osteopathy (DO): DOs are the equivalent of MDs. They go through similar medical training as MDs, but some DOs have more training in natural approaches to healing. DOs can go through the same specialty training as MDs. Specialty-trained DOs function the same as specialty-trained MDs. Both are considered physicians.

Nurse Practitioner/Physician's Assistant (NP/PA): NPs and PAs work under the license of a medical doctor. Generally, they work in the same office as the doctor who sponsors them, but they can also work in free-standing offices. They can, within certain restrictions, write prescriptions and order labs or diagnostic procedures. In general, NPs and PAs are able to take more time with you than a doctor and can tap into the knowledge of the doctor when necessary.

Integrative Medical Doctor: Integrative physicians are defined by the use of alternative therapies or alternative applications of drug therapies. They typically do more extensive laboratory evaluations than conventional doctors, with the hope of picking up subtle abnormalities that can be corrected. They commonly offer alternative medicine procedures, such as IV nutrient therapy, IV chelation, IV ozone therapy, and hyperbaric oxygen. While these procedures can improve patient well-being, they come with a hefty price tag and typically aren't covered by insurance. If you decide to work with an integrative physician, know upfront the purpose of each lab and procedure, the overall cost to you, and how the information will guide your treatment plan.

Functional Medical Doctor: Providers trained in functional medicine take a holistic approach to therapy. They look for underlying causes that can be reversed with diet, lifestyle changes, and supplements. They typically spend a generous amount of time with patients and use less in the way of invasive procedures. Seeing a functional medical doctor can be a best-of-all-worlds situation, short of one big drawback: the out-of-pocket cost. Because the healthcare system does not pay them to practice this way, most functional medicine providers are only found in larger cities, typically do not take insurance, and can be quite expensive.

Naturopathic Doctor: Naturopathic doctors operate much like functional or integrative medical doctors, except they generally have more extensive training in herbal therapy. Naturopaths can also write prescriptions for drugs in states where they are licensed, but this is limited to select states.

Chiropractor: Most chiropractors rely on realignment of the musculoskeletal system to reduce symptoms of pain and discomfort. A chiropractor can be valuable for relieving musculoskeletal symptoms without the use of drug therapy. Some chiropractors also offer care much like functional medical doctors, but they cannot write prescriptions. Many chiropractors are far more knowledgeable about natural therapy options than conventional physicians.

Acupuncturist: An acupuncturist uses specialized needles or pressure at specific points on the body (called meridians) to restore balance in the body's energy fields. Studies have documented benefits for many types of conditions. Achieving benefit generally requires multiple sessions and may fade when sessions are discontinued. Many acupuncturists are also trained in traditional Chinese medicine (TCM) with Chinese herbs.

Herbalist: To become certified as a practicing herbalist, the American Herbalist's Guild recommends 1,600 hours of didactic training and 400 hours of clinical training at a certified school of herbal medicine. That being said, there are some highly skilled practicing herbalists who have little formal training, but have accumulated years of practical experience. If you are fortunate to have a knowledgeable herbalist in your life, this person can add great value in tweaking and varying your herbal regimen. Many herbalists offer or partner with complementary wellness services such as energy healing, acupuncture, or massage therapy.

Health Coach: Rather than offering medical advice, a health coach is trained to help individuals be accountable, proactive, and remain motivated to improve their health habits. They are there to support the goals you've set with your health care practitioner. A health coach can keep you moving in a positive direction – wherever you are on your health journey. While health coaches are generally more accessible and affordable than other providers, know that most coaching services are not covered by insurance.

Appendix B

Extended Herbal Safety Spectrum Reference List

Most of the herbs mentioned in this book fall into the *green zone* of the Herbal Safety Spectrum outlined in Chapter 7. These herbs have the greatest potential to provide significant benefits while being the easiest and safest to use, assuming you follow the General Precautions for Taking Herbs found in Chapter 9.

That said, there are many other herbs available, and you may be wondering where they fall on the Herbal Safety Spectrum. Some are extremely low-risk to use on your own, and others are best avoided altogether or used only under professional guidance. Below, I've listed over 200 herbs and herbal phytochemicals categorized into the *green zone, yellow zone, or red zone*, depending on their safety profile. Refer to Chapter 7 for a refresher on the Herbal Safety Spectrum zones.

Green zone herbs have been separated into *everyday, antimicrobial,* and *targeted* subcategories. Most herbs have multiple actions and could be placed into many benefit categories. But to keep this reference simple, I've chosen the top 1 or 2 categories for each herb that is most representative of how they are typically used. For instance, since cat's claw is a great antimicrobial herb *and* has targeted benefits for joint and cognitive health, it is listed as both *antimicrobial* and *targeted.*

Of course, there are always exceptions. For example, just because an herb is classified as *targeted* doesn't always mean it's higher risk than an *everyday* herb. It may simply mean that it's typically taken for short periods for a specific reason rather than being taken daily for overall wellness.

Unless otherwise indicated, the herbs listed below should be assumed to be in the form that is most often used for their medicinal purposes. That would be a powdered extract or tincture for the vast majority, but for certain herbs, a tea, whole herb powder, topical ointment, or essential oil may be more commonly used.

Finally, please note that this appendix is for general reference only and will vary depending on the herbal sourcing quality, preparation method, and dosage used. It's always important to get herbal products from a reputable source and follow appropriate cautions and contraindications for your specific health concern. Refer to Chapters 8 and 9 for more information on finding quality herbal products and general cautions and contraindications for using herbs. When in doubt, ask a certified herbalist or herb-savvy health care provider for assistance.

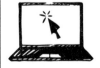

For a printable and updated version of this list as well as more information on making the most out of the *green zone* herbs mentioned in this book, visit **CellularWellness.com/Extras**

Herb	Green Zone			Yellow Zone	Red Zone
	Everyday	Antimicrobial	Targeted	Cautionary	Potentially Harmful
Achyranthes (*Achyranthes bidentata*) (root)			x		
Aconite / wolf's bane (*Aconitum spp.*) (processed root)					x
Agrimony (*Agrimonia eupatoria*) (leaf)			x		
Alfalfa (*Medicago sativa*) (leaf & seed)	x				
Aloe (*Aloe vera*) (inner leaf gel)			x		
American ginseng (*Panax quinquefolius*) (root & leaf)	x				
Amla (*Emblica officilanis*) (fruit)	x				
Amur cork tree (*Phellodenron amurense*) (bark)			x		
Angelica (*Angelica archangelica*) (root & seed)			x		
Anamu (*Petiveria alliacea*) (leaf & root)		x			
Andrographis (*Andrographis paniculata*) (leaf)		x	x		
Arnica (*Arnica montana*) (flower)				x	
Artemisia (*Artemisia annua*) (aerial parts)				x	
Artichoke (*Cynara scolymus*) (leaf)	x				
Ashwagandha (*Withania somnifera*) (leaf & root)	x				
Asian ginseng (*Panax ginseng*) (root)	x				
Astragulus (*Astragalus membranaceus*) (root)	x				
Bacopa (*Bacopa monnieri*) (leaf)	x		x		
Banaba (*Lagerstroemia speciosa*) (leaf)			x		

Herb	Green Zone			Yellow Zone	Red Zone
	Everyday	Antimicrobial	Targeted	Cautionary	Potentially Harmful
Barberry (*Berberis vulgaris*) (root bark, leaf, & berry)		x	x		
Berberine (phytochemical)		x	x		
Bitter melon (*Momordica charantia*) (unripe fruit, leaf, & seed)			x		
Bladderwrack (*Fucus vesiculosus*) (seaweed tips)			x		
Black cohosh (*Actaea racemosa*) (root)			x		
Blue cohosh (*Caulophyllum thalictroides*) (root)				x	
Blue flag (*Iris versicolor*) (rhizome)				x	
Black walnut (*Juglans nigra*) (hull)				x	
Blue vervain (*Verbena hastata*) (leaf & flower)			x		
Boneset (*Eupatorium perfoliatum*) (leaf & flower)				x	
Boswellia (*Boswellia serrata*) (gum-resin)			x		
Bupleurum (*Bupleurum falcatum*) (root)		x	x		
Burdock (*Arctium lappa*) (root)			x		
Calamus (*Acorus calamus*) (rhizome)				x	
California poppy (*Eschscholzia californica*) (root & herb)				x	
Calendula (*Calendula officinalis*) (flower)			x		
Cardamom (*Elettaria cardamomum*) (seed)			x		
Catnip (*Nepeta cataria*) (flowering herb)			x		
Cat's claw (*Uncaria tomentosa*) (inner bark)		x	x		

| Herb | Green Zone | | | Yellow Zone | Red Zone |
	Everyday	Antimicrobial	Targeted	Cautionary	Potentially Harmful
Cayenne (*Capsicum annum*) (fruit)			x		
CBD oil from hemp (*Cannabis sativa*) (flower)			x		
Celandine (*Chelidonium majus*) (whole plant)				x	
Celery (*Apium graveolens*) (seed)			x		
Chaga (*Inonotus obliquus*) (sclerotium)	x				
Chaste tree (*Vitex agnus-castus*) (berry)			x		
Chickweed (*Stellaria media*) (aerial parts)	x		x		
Chinese salvia (*Salvia miltiorrhiza*) (root)		x	x		
Chinese skullcap (*Scutelleria baicalensis*) (root)		x	x		
Chlorella (*Chlorella spp.*) (whole algae)	x		x		
Cinnamon (*Cinnamomum spp.*) (twig/bark)			x		
Cleavers (*Gallium aparine*) (aerial parts)			x		
Codonopsis (*Codonopsis pilosula*) (root)	x				
Coltsfoot (*Tussilaga farfara*) (leaf & flower bud)				x	
Comfrey (*Symphytum officinale*) (leaf & root, topically)			x		
Comfrey (*Symphytum officinale*) (leaf & root, internally)				x	
Chamomile (*Matricaria recutita*) (flower)			x		
Cordyceps (*Cordyceps spp.*) (fruiting body & mycelium)	x				
Corn silk (*Zea mays*) (stigma)			x		

Herb	Green Zone			Yellow Zone	Red Zone
	Everyday	Antimicrobial	Targeted	Cautionary	Potentially Harmful
Corydalis (*Corydalis yanhusuo*) (rhizome)			x		
Cranberry (*Vaccinium macrocarpon*) (berry)	x				
Cryptolepis (*Cryptolepis sanguinolenta*) (root)		x			
Cynomorium (*Cynomorium songariucum*) (stem)			x		
Dandelion (*Taraxacum officinale*) (leaf and root)	x		x		
Devil's claw (*Harpagophytum procumbens*) (root)			x		
Devil's club (*Oplopanax spp.*) (root & stem bark)			x		
Dong quai (*Angelica sinensis*) (root)			x		
Echinacea (*Echinacea spp.*) (root, seed, & flower head)			x		
Eclipta / bhringaraj (*Eclipta prostrata*) (aerial parts)	x				
Elder (*Sambuccus canadensis, S. nigra*) (flower & berry)		x			
Elecampane (*Inula helenium*) (root)		x	x		
Eleuthero (*Eleuthero senticosus*) (root & stem bark)	x				
Epimedium (*Epimedium grandiflorum*) (leaf)			x		
Ephedra (*Ephedra sinica*) (twig)				x	
Eucalyptus (*Eucalyptus globulus*) (leaf essential oil, topically)			x		
Eucalyptus (*Eucalyptus globulus*) (leaf essential oil, internally)				x	

Herb	Green Zone			Yellow Zone	Red Zone
	Everyday	Antimicrobial	Targeted	Cautionary	Potentially Harmful
Eucalyptus (*Eucalyptus globulus*) (leaf)		x			
Eucommia (*Eucommia ulmoides*) (bark)			x		
Evening primrose (*Oenothera biennis*) (seed oil)			x		
Fennel (*Foeniculum vulgar*) (seed)			x		
Fenugreek (*Trigonella foenum-graecum*) (seed)			x		
Feverfew (*Tanacetum parthenium*) (aerial parts)			x		
Fleeceflower / foti (*Fallopia multiflora*) (root)				x	
Foxglove (*Digitalis spp.*) (leaf)					x
Fragrant angelica / bai zhi (*Angelica dahurica*) (root)			x		
Frankincense (*Boswellia sacra*) (gum-resin)			x		
Garlic (*Allium sativum*) (bulb)	x	x			
Gentian (*Gentiana lutea*) (root)			x		
Ginger (*Zingiber officinale*) (rhizome)		x	x		
Ginkgo (*Ginkgo biloba*) (leaf)			x		
Goji (*Lycium chinensis*) (berry)	x				
Goldenrod (*Solidago spp.*) (flowering herb)			x		
Goldenseal (*Hydrastis canadensis*) (root & leaf)		x			
Gotu kola (*Centella asiatica*) (leaf)	x				
Grape (*Vitis vinifera*) (seed)	x				

Herb	Green Zone			Yellow Zone	Red Zone
	Everyday	Antimicrobial	Targeted	Cautionary	Potentially Harmful
Gravel root (*Eutrochium purpreum*) (leaf & root)				x	
Guduchi (*Tinospora cordifolia*) (stem & leaf)	x				
Guarana (*Paullinia cupana*) (seed)			x		
Gum guggul (*Commiphora mukul*) (gum resin)			x		
Gymnema (*Gymnema sylvestre*) (leaf)			x		
Hawthorn (*Crataegus spp.*) (leaf, flower, & berry)			x		
Hibiscus (*Hibiscus sabdariffa*) (flower)	x				
Honeysuckle (*Lonicera japonica*) (flower)		x			
Hops (*Humulus lupulus*) (strobilus)			x		
Horehound (*Marrubium vulgare*) (aerial parts)			x		
Horse chestnut (*Aesculus hippocastanum*) (seed)				x	
Horsetail (*Equisetum arvense*) (aerial parts)			x		
Houttuynia (*Houttuynia cordata*) (leaf & root)		x			
Indian pipe (*Monotropa uniflora*) (root and plant tops)				x	
Isatis (*Isatis tinctoria*) (leaf & root)		x	x		
Jamaica dogwood (*Piscidia piscipula*) (bark)				x	
Japanese knotweed (*Polygonum cuspidatum*, syn: *Fallopia japonica*) (root)		x			
Jiaogulan (*Gynostemma pentaphyllum*) (aerial parts)	x				

Herb	Green Zone			Yellow Zone	Red Zone
	Everyday	Antimicrobial	Targeted	Cautionary	Potentially Harmful
Jujube (*Zizyphus jujuba*) (fruit & seed)			x		
Kava (*Piper methysticum*) (root)				x	
Kratom (*Mitragyna speciosa*) (leaf)					x
Kudzu (*Pueraria montana*) (root)			x		
L-theanine (phtyochemical)			x		
Lavender (*Lavendula spp.*) (flower)			x		
Lemon balm (*Melissa officinalis*) (aerial parts)			x		
Lemon verbena (*Aloysia citriodora*) (leaf)	x				
Licorice (*Glycyrrhiza glabra, G. uralensis*) (rhizome)				x	
Linden (*Tilia platyphyllos*) (flower)			x		
Lion's mane (*Hericium erinaceus*) (mycelium & fruiting body)	x				
Lobelia (*Lobelia inflata*) (herb & seed)				x	
Lomatium (*Lomatium dissectum*) (root)		x			
Magnolia (*Magnolia officinalis*) (bark & root bark)			x		
Maitake / hen of the woods (*Grifola frondosa*) (mycelium & fruiting body)	x				
Marijuana (*Cannabis sativa*) (flower)				x	
Marshmallow (*Althaea officinalis*) (root & leaf)	x		x		
Maqui berry (*Aristotelia chilensis*) (berry)	x				
Meadowsweet (*Filipendula ulmaria*) (flowering tops)			x		

Herb	Green Zone			Yellow Zone	Red Zone
	Everyday	Antimicrobial	Targeted	Cautionary	Potentially Harmful
Myrrh (*Commiphora myrrha*) (gum-resin)			X		
Milk thistle (*Silybum marianum*) (seed)	X				
Mimosa (*Albizia julibrissin*) (bark & flower)			X		
Motherwort (*Leonurus cardiaca*) (aerial parts)			X		
Morinda (*Morinda officinalis*) (root)	X				
Mullein (*Verbascum thapsus*) (leaf, flower (topically), & root)			X		
Neem (*Azadirachta indica*) (leaf & bark)		X			
Nettle (*Urtica dioica*) (leaf, root, & seed)			X		
Oats (*Avena sativa*) (fresh milky seed)			X		
Olive leaf (*Olea europaea*) (leaf)	X				
Orange (*Citrus spp.*) (peel)			X		
Oregon grape (*Mahonia aquifolium*) (root)		X			
Parsley (*Petroselinum sativum*) (leaf, root, & seed)			X		
Passionflower (*Passiflora incarnata*) (aerial parts)			X		
Pau d'arco (*Tabebuia impetiginosa*) (bark)				X	
Peppermint (*Mentha piperita*) (leaf)			X		
Pine (*Pinus spp.*) (bark)	X				
Pine (*Pinus spp.*) (pollen)				X	
Pinellia (*Pinellia ternata*) (prepared rhizome)				X	
Plantain (*Plantago major*) (leaf)			X		

Herb	Green Zone			Yellow Zone	Red Zone
	Everyday	Antimicrobial	Targeted	Cautionary	Potentially Harmful
Pokeweed (*Phytolacca americana*) (root & berry)					x
Poria (*Wolfiporia cocos*) (sclerotium)			x		
Prickly ash (*Zanthoxylum spp.*) (bark & berry)		x			
Prince seng (*Pseudostellaria heterphylla*) (root)	x				
Propolis (*Propolium*) (resin)			x		
Pasque flower (*Anemone patens*) (flowering herb)				x	
Red clover (*Trifolium pratense*) (flower)	x				
Red root (*Ceanothus americanus*) (root & leaf)				x	
Red yeast rice (*Monascus purpureus*) (cultured rice)				x	
Rehmannia (*Rehmannia glutinosa*) (root)	x				
Reishi (*Ganoderma lucidum*) (mycelium & fruiting body)	x				
Rhaponticum (*Rhaponticum carthamoides*) (root)	x				
Rhodiola (*Rhodiola rosea*) (root)	x				
Rosemary (*Salvia rosmarinus*) (aerial parts)	x				
Rye grass (*Secale cereale*) (pollen)			x		
Sage (*Salvia officinalis*) (leaf)		x			
Sarsaparilla (*Smilax spp.*) (root)		x			
Saw palmetto (*Serenoa repens*) (fruit)			x		
Schisandra (*Schisandra chinensis*) (root)	x				

Herb	Green Zone			Yellow Zone	Red Zone
	Everyday	Antimicrobial	Targeted	Cautionary	Potentially Harmful
Skullcap (*Scutellaria lateriflora*) (flowering aerial parts)			x		
Self heal (*Prunella vulgaris*) (flowers & leaves)			x		
Senna (*Senna alexandrina*) (leaf & pods)				x	
Shatavari (*Asparagus racemosus*) (root)	x				
Shiitake (*Lentinus edodes*) (mycelia & fruiting body)	x				
Shilajit (*Bituminous asphaltum*) (purified exudate)	x				
Slippery elm (*Ulmus rubra*) (bark)			x		
Solomon's seal (*Polygonatum biflorum*) (rhizome)			x		
Spilanthes (*Acmella oleracea*) (whole plant)		x			
St. John's wort (*Hypericum perforatum*) (flowering aerial parts)				x	
Stephania (*Stephania spp.*) (root)			x		
Stillingia (*Stillingia sylvatica*) (root)				x	
Tart cherry (*Prunus cerasus*) (fruit)	x				
Teasel (*Dipsacus spp.*) (root)			x		
Thuja (*Thuja occidentalis*) (leaf & cone)				x	
Tongkat ali (*Eurycoma longifola*) (root)			x		
Triphala (combination of *Terminella chebula*, *T. belerica*, *Phylanthus emblica*) (fruit)			x		
Tulsi / holy basil (*Ocimum tenuiflorum*) (leaf)	x				
Turkey tail (*Trametes versicolor*) (mycelium & fruiting body)	x				

Herb	Green Zone			Yellow Zone	Red Zone
	Everyday	Antimicrobial	Targeted	Cautionary	Potentially Harmful
Turmeric (*Curcuma longa*) (rhizome)	x				
Thyme (*Thymus vulgarus*) (leaf)		x			
Usnea (*Usnea barbata*) (lichen)		x			
Uva-ursi (*Arctostaphylos uva-ursi*) (leaf)		x			
Valerian (*Valeriana officinalis*) (root)				x	
Violet (*Viola soraria*) (leaf & flower)			x		
White peony (*Paeonia lactiflora*) (root cortex)			x		
White sage (*Salvia apiana*) (leaf)		x			
Wild cherry (*Prunus serotina*) (bark)			x		
Wild indigo (*Baptisia tinctoria*) (leaf & root)				x	
Wild lettuce (*Lactuca spp.*) (latex, leaf, & seed)			x		
Wild yam (*Dioscorea villosa*) (rhizome)			x		
Wormwood (*Artemisia absinthium*) (leaf & flowering top)				x	
Willow (*Salix spp.*) (bark)			x		
Yarrow (*Achillea millefolium*) (leaf & flower)		x	x		
Yellow dock (*Rumex crispus*) (root)			x		
Yellow root (*Xanthorhiza simplicissima*) (root)		x			
Yohimbe (*Pausinystalia johimbe*) (bark)				x	

Acknowledgments

First and foremost, I want to thank my daughter, Braden. You saw how important this book was to me and how important the information is to the world. By creating a flexible work schedule for me at our company, Vital Plan, you enabled me to spend the many hours necessary to research, write, and continually revise the contents of this book. Otherwise, it would not have happened.

I want to extend a special thanks to the team at Vital Plan. Working with you has challenged me in wonderful ways. I never imagined my sixties as a time to learn new skills in technology and social media, but it has been a pleasure. You are all bright and incredibly talented. Thank you for the passion you bring each day to make the lives of other people better.

In particular, I want to thank Tim Yarborough and Paulette Bennett for meticulously reviewing the herbal content in the book. It is inspiring to see your passion for the study of herbs and herbal medicine. I especially want to thank Tim for the extra hours spent helping to refine the *Herbal Spectrum* concept and create the extended list of herbs in Appendix B. This will be an extraordinary resource for people new to herbs. In addition, I want to thank Ryan Burke for checking doses and the standardization of supplement recommendations. Your attention to detail is critical to this work.

Many thanks to Jenny Buttaccio for a thorough review of the final version of the book and suggestions on improving its readability. Your ongoing willingness to drop everything to help out and endless enthusiasm to keep people informed are commendable. Beyond the book, your work at making RawlsMD.com a remarkable resource that serves so many people is much appreciated.

To Mark Casey: Your eye for design truly brings this text to life. Thank you for working diligently together on the many diagrams and illustrations contained throughout, which illuminate important concepts and remove barriers to understanding technical information. In particular, the *Wellness Spectrum* at the beginning of the book and the *Herbal Spectrum* later in the book would have been incomplete without your touch. Kudos also on the brilliant cover design, which will help get this essential information into a wider number of hands.

To Jon Hudson, digital marketing expert: I am grateful for your efforts in setting up the online presence to make sure this book reaches the people who need it most. Thank goodness to be surrounded by a team of tech-savvy folks. I appreciate your deep passion for wanting to help people and the marketing skills you bring to the table to make it happen. You are a true leader and a pleasure to work with. I am especially grateful for the guidance you offered in structuring the book. Because of your efforts, everything ended up in the right place.

No book is possible without a team of professionals in the field. A special thanks to the editing team who helped to make this book a reality: Brooke-Sidney Harbour for helping me see things that I couldn't see and putting things in an order that worked, Susan Strecker for helping to add structure to the content at an early stage, and Ashley Cullen for a meticulous final copy edit. Each of you helped make the technical content more accessible and more enjoyable. This book will have a wider reach because of your efforts.

A special word of appreciation to early readers, who provided invaluable comments and feedback at a critical stage in the writing process—the final book is better because of you.

To our extended Vital Plan community: Serving you has been a highlight of my life. Whenever I wasn't sure about this new path I was taking as a physician, you would remind me of the importance. The groundswell has been truly amazing.

In particular, to those struggling with Lyme disease and chronic illness: I want to give you a shout-out. You are stronger than you may know at this moment. It is such a challenging condition. You are not alone, despite how you may feel at this moment.

To the herbalists who have done such incredible work for bringing herbal medicine into the 21st century: Stephen Buhner, David Winston, Donald Yance, and many others—your hard-won research laid the foundation for me to build on.

To my brother, Jimmy Rawls: Even though we've had very different paths as physicians, I am grateful to have your respect and interest. Thank you for reading early book drafts and giving honest feedback. Because of you, this book is less technical and, I hope, more accessible.

Last, but certainly not least, my deepest thanks to my wife, Meg Rawls: For being my partner for over four decades. For hanging in there with me through the Lyme years. For being a constant sounding board for the concepts echoed in this book. Your professional insights and inputs as a trained biologist have been invaluable. Having someone close at hand with training in science helped me stay true to the science. I am also indebted to your patience for the many long hours in evenings and weekends that I spent heads down on the computer.

Lastly, I want to recognize the people behind the PUBMED search engine sponsored by NIH. This incredible resource places peer-reviewed scientific research from sources around the world at every person's fingertips. Without it, this book would have been less credible. With it, I was able to validate everything in the book with scientific evidence.

Author Profile

For over 30 years, Dr. Bill Rawls has dedicated his life to medicine. When a health crisis in his early forties abruptly changed his quality of life, he came face to face with the limitations of modern medicine and began to explore the vast possibilities of alternative treatments. Restoring his health through holistic and herbal therapies inspired him to share his revelations on the importance of cellular wellness. Today, he works to bring health and vitality to others as he helps them establish their own paths to wellness through modern herbology.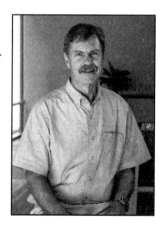

Dr. Rawls has two grown children and lives on the North Carolina coast with his wife and golden retriever. He enjoys cooking, biking, hiking, and any activity that gets him out on the water.

References

Introduction

Centers for Disease Control and Prevention. cdc.gov

Mikulic M. Global pharmaceutical industry–statistics & facts. https://www.statista.com/topics/1764/global-pharmaceutical-industry/#dossierKeyfigures

Light DW. New prescription drugs: a major health risk with few offsetting advantages. https://ethics.harvard.edu/blog/new-prescription-drugs-major-health-risk-few-offsetting-advantages

Light DW, Lexchin J, Darrow JJ. Institutional corruption of pharmaceuticals and the myth of safe and effective drugs (June 1, 2013). *J Law Med*. 2013;14(3):590-610.

Chapter 1: Wellness / Chapter 2: Cells

Bianconi E, Piovesan A, Facchin F, et al. An estimation of the number of cells in the human body. *Ann Hum Biol*. 2013;40(6):463-71.

Cooper GM. *The Cell: A Molecular Approach*, 2nd ed. Sinauer Associates; 2000.

Fridlyanskaya I, Alekseenko L, Nikolsky N. Senescence as a general cellular response to stress: a mini-review. *Exp Gerontol*. 2015;72:124-128.

Plopper G, Ivankovic DB. *Principles of Cell Biology,* 3rd ed. Jones & Bartlett Learning: 2021.

Dietary

Al-Shaar L, Satija A, Wang DD, et al. Red meat intake and risk of coronary heart disease among US men: prospective cohort study. *BMJ.* 2020;371:m4141.

American Diabetes Association. Economic costs of diabetes in the U.S. in 2012. *Diabetes Care.* 2013;36(4):1033-1046.

Bernstein AM, Sun Q, Hu FB, Stampfer MJ, Manson JE, Willett WC. Major dietary protein sources and risk of coronary heart disease in women. *Circulation.* 2010;122(9):876-883.

Byun K, Yoo Y, Son M, et al. Advanced glycation end-products produced systemically and by macrophages: a common contributor to inflammation and degenerative diseases. *Pharmacol Ther.* 2017;177:44-55.

Dehghan M, Mente A, Zhang X, et al. Associations of fats and carbohydrate intake with cardiovascular disease and mortality in 18 countries from five continents (PURE): a prospective cohort study. *Lancet.* 2017;390(10107):2050-2062.

Flegal KM, Kruszon-Moran D,Carroll MD. Trends in obesity among adults in the United States, 2005 to 2014. *JAMA.* 2016;315(21):2284-2291.

González N, Marquès M, Nadal M, Domingo JL. Meat consumption: which are the current global risks? A review of recent (2010-2020) evidences. *Food Res Int.* 2020;137:109341.

Higdon J, Delage B, Williams DE, Dashwood RH. Cruciferous vegetables and human cancer risk: epidemiologic evidence and mechanistic basis. *Pharmacol Res.* 2007;55(3):224-236.

Keating ST, El-Osta A. Epigenetics and metabolism. *Circ Res.* 2015;116(4):715-736.

Lang UE, Beglinger C, Schweinfurth N, Walter M, Borgwardt S. Nutritional aspects of depression. *Cell Physiol Biochem.* 2015;37(3):1029-1043.

Lankinen M, Uusitupa M, Schwab U. Genes and dietary fatty acids in regulation of fatty acid composition of plasma and erythrocyte membranes. *Nutrients.* 2018;10(11):1785.

Lim U, Song MA. Dietary and lifestyle factors of DNA methylation. *Methods Mol Biol.* 2012;863:359-376.

Myles IA. Fast food fever: reviewing the impacts of the Western diet on immunity. *Nutr J.* 2014;13:61.

Ott C, Jacobs K, Haucke E, Navarrete Santos A, Grune T, Simm A. Role of advanced glycation end products in cellular signaling. *Redox Biol.* 2014;2:411-429.

Pan A, Sun Q, Bernstein AM, et al. Red meat consumption and mortality: results from 2 prospective cohort studies. *Arch Intern Med.* 2012;172(7):555-563.

Pham-Huy LA, He H, Pham-Huy C. Free radicals, antioxidants in disease and health. *Int J Biomed Sci*. 2008;4(2):89-96.

Robblee MM, Kim CC, Porter Abate J, et al. Saturated fatty acids engage an IRE1α-dependent pathway to activate the NLRP3 inflammasome in myeloid cells. *Cell Rep*. 2016;14(11):2611-2623.

Rosen ED. Epigenomic and transcriptional control of insulin resistance. *J Intern Med*. 2016;280(5):443-456.

Song M, Fung TT, Hu FB, et al. Association of animal and plant protein intake with all-cause and cause-specific mortality. *JAMA Intern Med*. 2016;176(10):1453-1463.

Turesky RJ. Mechanistic evidence for red meat and processed meat intake and cancer risk: a follow-up on the International Agency for Research on Cancer Evaluation of 2015. *Chimia (Aarau)*. 2018;72(10):718-724.

Wang J, Wu Z, Li D, et al. Nutrition, epigenetics, and metabolic syndrome. *Antioxid Redox Signal*. 2012;17(2):282-301.

Wolk A. Potential health hazards of eating red meat. *J Intern Med*. 2017;281(2):106-122.

Toxic Environment

A Baccarelli, V. Bollati. Epigenetics and environmental chemicals. *Curr Opin Pediatr*. 2009; 21(2):243-251.

Ahsan H, Ali A, Al R. Oxygen free radicals and systemic autoimmunity. *Clin Exp Immunol*. 2003;131(3):398-404.

Aiko V, Mehta A. Occurrence, detection and detoxification of mycotoxins. *J Biosci*. 2015;40(5):943-954.

Baja ES, Schwartz JD, Coull AA, et al. Structural equation modeling of parasympathetic and sympathetic response to traffic air pollution in a repeated measures study. *Environ Health*. 2013;12(1):81.

Bollati V, Baccarelli A. Environmental epigenetics. *Heredity (Edinb)*. 2010;105(1):105-112.

Collotta M, Bertazzi PA, Bollati V. Epigenetics and pesticides.*Toxicology*. 2013;307:35-41.

Eckelman MJ, Sherman J. Environmental impacts of the U.S. health care system and effects on public health. *PLoS One*. 2016;11(6):e0157014.

Fleisch AF, Wright RO, Baccarelli AA. Environmental epigenetics: a role in endocrine disease? *J Mol Endocrinol*. 2012;49(2):R61-67.

Francque SM, Marchesini G, Kautz A, et al. Non-alcoholic fatty liver disease: a patient guideline. *JHEP Rep*. 2021;3(5):100322.

Gilbert J. Environmental contaminants and pesticides in animal feed and meat. In: Sofos JN, ed. *Improving the Safety of Fresh Meat.* 2005:132-155.

Gray J, Rasanayagam S, Engel C, Rizzo Jl. State of the evidence 2017: an update on the connection between breast cancer and the environment. *Environ Health.* 2017;16(1):94.

Hou L, Zhang X, Wang D, Baccarelli A. Environmental chemical exposures and human epigenetics. *Int J Epidemiol.* 2012;41(1):79-105.

Kim M, Bae M, Hyunkyung N, Yang M. Environmental toxicants--induced epigenetic alterations and their reversers. *J Environ Sci Health C Environ Carcinog Ecotoxicol Rev.* 2012;30(4):323-367.

Logan S, Spencer N. Smoking and other health related behaviour in the social and environmental context. *Arch Dis Child.* 1996;74(2):176-179.

Marshall J. Environmental health: megacity, mega mess. *Nature.* 2005;437(7057):312-314.

Middlekauff HR, Park J, Moheimani RS. Adverse effects of cigarette and noncigarette smoke exposure on the autonomic nervous system: mechanisms and implications for cardiovascular risk. *J Am Coll Cardiol.* 2014;64(16):1740-1750.

Mitra S, De A, Chowdhury A. Epidemiology of non-alcoholic and alcoholic fatty liver diseases. *Transl Gastroenterol Hepatol.* 2020;5:16.

Malhotra P, Gill RK, Saksena S, Alrefai WA. Disturbances in cholesterol homeostasis and non-alcoholic fatty liver diseases. *Front Med.* 2020;7:467.

Myers JP, Zoeller RT, vom Saal FS. A clash of old and new scientific concepts in toxicity, with important implications for public health. *Environ Health Perspect.* 2009;117(11):1652-1655.

Perez CM, Hazari MS, Farraj AK. Role of autonomic reflex arcs in cardiovascular responses to air pollution exposure. *Cardiovasc Toxicol.* 2015;15(1):69-78.

Runnels MT. Impure water and its dangers. *Public Health Pap Rep.* 1881;7:283-290.

Sanborn M, Kerr KJ, Sanin LH, Cole DC, Bassil KL, Vakil C. Non-cancer health effects of pesticides: systematic review and implications for family doctors. *Can Fam Physician.* 2007;53(10):1712-1720.

Sears ME, Genuis SJ. Environmental determinants of chronic disease and medical approaches: recognition, avoidance, supportive therapy, and detoxification. *J Environ Public Health.* 2012;2012:356798.

Suk WA, Davis EA. Strategies for addressing global environmental health concerns. *Ann N Y Acad Sci.* 2008;1140:40-44.

Sullivan D, Schmitt HJ, Calloway EE, et al. Chronic environmental contamination: a narrative review of psychosocial health consequences, risk factors, and pathways to community resilience. *Soc Sci Med*. 2021;276:113877.

Vandegehuchte MB, Janssen CR. Epigenetics in an ecotoxicological context. *Mutat Res Genet Toxicol Environ Mutagen*. 2014;764-765:36-45.

Mental Stress

Champagne FA. Interplay between social experiences and the genome: epigenetic consequences for behavior. *Adv Genet*. 2012;77:33-57.

Cohen S, Janicki-Deverts D, Doyle WJ, et al. Chronic stress, glucocorticoid receptor resistance, inflammation, and disease risk. *Proc Natl Acad Sci U S A*. 2012;109(16):5995-5999.

Gudsnuk K, Champagne F. Epigenetic influence of stress and the social environment. *ILAR J*. 2012;53(3-4):279-288.

Househam AM, Peterson CT, Mills PJ, Chopra D. The effects of stress and meditation on the immune system, human microbiota, and epigenetics. *Adv Mind Body Med*. 2017;31(4):10-25.

Rittschof C, Hughes K. Advancing behavioural genomics by considering timescale. *Nat Commun*. 2018;9:489.

Physical Factors

Arocha Rodulfo JI. Sedentary lifestyle a disease from xxi century. *Clin Investig Arterioscler*. 2019;31(5):233-240.

Di Liegro CM, Schiera G, Proia P, Di Liegro I. Physical activity and brain health. *Genes (Basel)*. 2019;10(9):720.

Friedenreich CM, Ryder-Burbidge C, McNeil J. Physical activity, obesity and sedentary behavior in cancer etiology: epidemiologic evidence and biologic mechanisms. *Mol Oncol*. 2021;15(3):790-800.

Spólnicka M, Pospiech E, Adamczyk JG, et al. Modified aging of elite athletes revealed by analysis of epigenetic age markers. *Aging (Albany NY)*. 2018;10(2):241-252.

Whitham M, Parker BL, Friedrichsen M, et al. Extracellular vesicles provide a means for tissue crosstalk during exercise. *Cell Metab*. 2018;27(1):237-251.e4.

Zhang Y, Ren J. Epigenetics and obesity cardiomyopathy: from pathophysiology to prevention and management. *Pharmacol Ther*. 2016;161:52-66.

Chapter 3: Microbes

Gangwe Nana GY, Ripoll C, Cabin-Flaman A, et al. Division-based, growth rate diversity in bacteria. *Front Microbiol.* 2018;9:849.

Janeway CA, et al. *Immunobiology: The Immune System in Health and Disease*, 5th ed. Garland Science; 2001.

Levin PA, Angert ER. Small but mighty: cell size and bacteria. *Cold Spring Harb Perspect Biol.* 2015;7(7):a019216.

Martin WF, Sousa FL. Early microbial evolution: the age of anaerobes. *Cold Spring Harb Perspect Biol.* 2015;8(2):a018127.

Murray P, Rosenthal K, Pfaller M. *Medical Microbiology*, 8th ed. Elsevier; 2016.

Norris V. Why do bacteria divide? *Front Microbiol.* 2015;6:322

Protozoa: structure, classification, growth, and development. In: Yaeger RB, Baron S, eds. *Medical Microbiology*, 4th ed. University of Texas Medical Branch at Galveston; 1996. Chapter 77.

Woese CR. Bacterial evolution. *Microbiol Rev.* 1987;51(2):221-271.

Intracellular microbes

Broz P. Immune response: intracellular pathogens under attack. *Elife.* 2016;5:e14729.

Colonne PM, Winchell CG, Voth DE. Hijacking host cell highways: manipulation of the host actin cytoskeleton by obligate intracellular bacterial pathogens. *Front Cell Infect Microbiol.* 2016;6:107.

Das K, Garnica O, Dhandayuthapani S. Modulation of host miRNAs by intracellular bacterial pathogens. *Front Cell Infect Microbiol.* 2016;6:79.

Dehio C, Berry C, Bartenschlager R. Persistent intracellular pathogens. *FEMS Microbiol Rev.* 2012;36(3):513.

Eisenreich W, Rudel T, Heesemann J, Goebel W. To eat and to be eaten: mutual metabolic adaptations of immune cells and intracellular bacterial pathogens upon infection. *Front Cell Infect Microbiol.* 2017;7:316.

Fabrik I, Härtlova A, Rehulka P, Stulik J. Serving the new masters - dendritic cells as hosts for stealth intracellular bacteria. *Cell Microbiol.* 2013;15(9):1473-1483.

Garib FY, Rizopulu AP, Kuchmiy AA, Garib VF. Inactivation of inflammasomes by pathogens regulates inflammation. *Biochemistry (Mosc).* 2016;81(11):1326-1339.

Gray WT, Govers SK, Xiang Y, et al. Nucleoid size scaling and intracellular organization of translation across bacteria. *Cell.* 2019;177(6):1632-1648.e20.

Han B, Lin CJ, Hu G, Wang MC. 'Inside Out'- a dialogue between mitochondria and bacteria. *FEBS J*. 2019;286(4):630-641.

Hugon P, Dufour JC, Colson P, Fournier PE, Sallah K, Raoult D. A comprehensive repertoire of prokaryotic species identified in human beings. *Lancet Infect Dis*. 2015;15(10):1211-1219.

Kwon DH, Song HK. A structural view of xenophagy, a battle between host and microbes. *Mol Cells*. 2018;41(1):27-34.

Lamason RL, Welch MD. Actin-based motility and cell-to-cell spread of bacterial pathogens. *Curr Opin Microbiol*. 2017;35:48-57.

Liu Y, Jia Y, Yang K, Wang Z. Heterogeneous strategies to eliminate intracellular bacterial pathogens. *Front Microbiol*. 2020;11:563.

Lluch J, Servant F, Paisse S, et al. The characterization of novel tissue microbiota using an optimized 16S metagenomic sequencing pipeline. *PLoS One*. 2015;10(11):e0142334.

McClure EE, Chavez ASO, Shaw DK, et al. Engineering of obligate intracellular bacteria: progress, challenges and paradigms. *Nat Rev Microbiol*. 2017;15(9):544-558.

McCutcheon JP. From microbiology to cell biology: when an intracellular bacterium becomes part of its host cell. *Curr Opin Cell Biol*. 2016;41:132-136.

Mitchell G, Chen C, Portnoy DA. Strategies used by bacteria to grow in macrophages. *Microbiol Spectr*. 2016;4(3):10.1128/microbiolspec.MCHD-0012-2015.

Odendall C, Dixit E, Stavru F, et al. Diverse intracellular pathogens activate type III interferon expression from peroxisomes. *Nat Immunol*. 2014;15(8):717-726.

Rüter C, Lubos ML, Norkowski S, Schmidt MA. All in-multiple parallel strategies for intracellular delivery by bacterial pathogens. *Int J Med Microbiol*. 2018;308(7):872-881.

Saldova R. Cause of cancer and chronic inflammatory diseases and the implications for treatment. *Discov Med*. 2016;22(120):105-119.

Schulz F, Horn M. Intranuclear bacteria: inside the cellular control center of eukaryotes. *Trends Cell Biol*. 2015;25(6):339-346.

Snyder DT, Hedges JF, Jutila MA. Getting "inside" type I IFNs: type I IFNs in intracellular bacterial infections. *J Immunol Res*. 2017;2017:9361802.

Stenger S, Röllinghoff M. Role of cytokines in the innate immune response to intracellular pathogens. *Ann Rheum Dis*. 2001;60 Suppl 3(Suppl 3):iii43-46.

Stewart MK, Cookson BT. Evasion and interference: intracellular pathogens modulate caspase-dependent inflammatory responses. *Nat Rev Microbiol*. 2016;14(6):346-359.

Strle K, Drouin EE, Shen S, et al. Borrelia burgdorferi stimulates macrophages to secrete higher levels of cytokines and chemokines than Borrelia afzelii or Borrelia garinii. *J Infect Dis.* 2009;200(12):1936-1943.

Winchell CG, Steele S, Kawula T, Voth DE. Dining in: intracellular bacterial pathogen interplay with autophagy. *Curr Opin Microbiol.* 2016;29:9-14.

Wu YW, Li F. Bacterial interaction with host autophagy. *Virulence.* 2019;10(1):352-362.

Young D, Hussell T, Dougan G. Chronic bacterial infections: living with unwanted guests. *Nat Immunol.* 2002;3(11):1026-1032.

Specific Microbes

Ahmed W, Zheng K, Liu ZF. Establishment of chronic infection: brucella's stealth strategy. *Front Cell Infect Microbiol.* 2016;6:30.

Bayramova F, Jacquier N, Greub G. Insight in the biology of Chlamydia-related bacteria. *Microbes Infect.* 2018;20(7-8):432-440.

Ben-Tekaya H, Gorvel JP, Dehio C. Bartonella and brucella--weapons and strategies for stealth attack. *Cold Spring Harb Perspect Med.* 2013;3(8):a010231.

Brunke S, Hube B. Two unlike cousins: Candida albicans and C. glabrata infection strategies. *Cell Microbiol.* 2013;15(5):701-708.

Celli J. The intracellular life cycle of *Brucella* spp. *Microbiol Spectr.* 2019;7(2):10.1128/microbiolspec.BAI-0006-2019.

Chernova OA, Medvedeva ES, Mouzykantov AA, Baranova NB, Chernov VM. Mycoplasmas and their antibiotic resistance: the problems and prospects in controlling infections. *Acta Naturae.* 2016;8(2):24-34.

Elwell C, Mirrashidi K, Engel J. Chlamydia cell biology and pathogenesis. *Nat Rev Microbiol.* 2016;14(6):385-400.

Fichorova R, Fraga J, Rappelli P, Fiori PL. Trichomonas vaginalis infection in symbiosis with Trichomonasvirus and Mycoplasma. *Res Microbiol.* 2017;168(9-10):882-891.

Jha H, Pei Y, Robertson E. Epstein–Barr virus: diseases linked to infection and transformation. *Front Microbiol.* 2016;7:1602.

Kashyap S, Sarkar M. Mycoplasma pneumonia: clinical features and management. *Lung India.* 2010;27(2):75-85.

Pulliainen AT, Dehio C. Persistence of Bartonella spp. stealth pathogens: from subclinical infections to vasoproliferative tumor formation. *FEMS Microbiol Rev.* 2012;36(3):563-599.

Razin S, Yogev D, Naot Y. Molecular biology and pathogenicity of mycoplasmas. *Microbiol Mol Biol Rev*. 1998;62(4):1094-1156.

Microbes in Tissues

Achermann Y, Goldstein EJ, Coenye T, Shirtliff ME. Propionibacterium acnes: from commensal to opportunistic biofilm-associated implant pathogen. *Clin Microbiol Rev*. 2014;27(3):419-440.

Emery DC, Shoemark DK, Batstone TE, et al. 16S rRNA next generation sequencing analysis shows bacteria in Alzheimer's post-mortem brain. *Front Aging Neurosci*. 2017;9:195.

Koren O, Spor A, Felin J, et al. Human oral, gut, and plaque microbiota in patients with atherosclerosis. *Proc Natl Acad Sci U S A*. 2011;108 Suppl 1(Suppl 1):4592-4598.

Lanter BB, Davies DG. Propionibacterium acnes recovered from atherosclerotic human carotid arteries undergoes biofilm dispersion and releases lipolytic and proteolytic enzymes in response to norepinephrine challenge in vitro. *Infect Immun*. 2015;83(10):3960-3971.

Marques da Silva R, Caugant DA, Eribe ER, et al. Bacterial diversity in aortic aneurysms determined by 16S ribosomal RNA gene analysis. *J Vasc Surg*. 2006;44(5):1055-1060.

Ott SJ, El Mokhtari NE, Musfeldt M, et al. Detection of diverse bacterial signatures in atherosclerotic lesions of patients with coronary heart disease. *Circulation*. 2006;113(7):929-937.

Potgieter M, Bester J, Kell DB, Pretorius E. The dormant blood microbiome in chronic, inflammatory diseases. *FEMS Microbiol Rev*. 2015;39(4):567-591.

Roberts RC, Farmer CB, Walker CK. The human brain microbiome; there are bacteria in our brains! Psychiatry and Behavioral Neurobio., Univ. of Alabama Birmingham, Birmingham, AL. Program no. 594.08. 2018 Neuroscience Meeting Planner. San Diego, CA: Society for Neuroscience; 2018. Online.

Sun W, Dong L, Kaneyama K, Takegami T, Segami N. Bacterial diversity in synovial fluids of patients with TMD determined by cloning and sequencing analysis of the 16S ribosomal RNA gene. *Oral Surg Oral Med Oral Pathol Oral Radiol Endod*. 2008;105(5):566-571.

Microbe-Disease Connections

Abu-Shakra M, Shoenfeld Y. Chronic infections and autoimmunity. *Immunol Ser*. 1991;55:285-313.

Alam MZ, Alam Q, Kamal MA, et al. Infectious agents and neurodegenerative diseases: exploring the links. *Curr Top Med Chem*. 2017;17(12):1390-1399.

Bae Y, Ito T, Iida T, et al. Intracellular propionibacterium acnes infection in glandular epithelium and stromal macrophages of the prostate with or without cancer. *PLoS One*. 2014;9(2):e90324.

Balin BJ, Hammond CJ, Little CS, et al. Chlamydia pneumoniae: an etiologic agent for late-onset dementia. *Front Aging Neurosci*. 2018;10:302.

Bayani M, Riahi SM, Bazrafshan N, Ray Gamble H, Rostami A. Toxoplasma gondii infection and risk of Parkinson and Alzheimer diseases: a systematic review and meta-analysis on observational studies. *Acta Trop*. 2019;196:165-171.

Bayram A, Erdogan MB, Eksi F, Yamak B. Demonstration of Chlamydophila pneumoniae, Mycoplasma pneumoniae, Cytomegalovirus, and Epstein-Barr virus in atherosclerotic coronary arteries, nonrheumatic calcific aortic and rheumatic stenotic mitral valves by polymerase chain reaction. *Anadolu Kardiyol Derg*. 2011;11(3):237-243.

Berer K, Mues M, Koutrolos M, et al. Commensal microbiota and myelin autoantigen cooperate to trigger autoimmune demyelination. *Nature*. 2011;479(7374):538-541.

Branton WG, Lu JQ, Surette MG, et al. Brain microbiota disruption within inflammatory demyelinating lesions in multiple sclerosis. *Sci Rep*. 2016;6:37344.

Capoor MN, Ruzicka F, Schmitz JE, et al. Propionibacterium acnes biofilm is present in intervertebral discs of patients undergoing microdiscectomy. *PLoS One*. 2017;12(4):e0174518.

Carter JD, Inman RD, Whittum-Hudson J, Hudson AP. Chlamydia and chronic arthritis. *Ann Med*. 2012;44(8):784-792.

Casadevall A1, Pirofski LA. Host-pathogen interactions: basic concepts of microbial commensalism, colonization, infection, and disease. *Infect Immun*. 2000;68(12):6511-6518.

Chen J, Zhu M, Ma G, Zhao Z, Sun Z. Chlamydia pneumoniae infection and cerebrovascular disease: a systematic review and meta-analysis. *BMC Neurol*. 2013;13:183.

Choi YS, Kim Y, Yoon H-J, et al. The presence of bacteria within tissue provides insights into the pathogenesis of oral lichen planus. *Sci Rep*. 2016;6:29186.

Czaja AJ. Examining pathogenic concepts of autoimmune hepatitis for cues to future investigations and interventions. *World J Gastroenterol*. 2019;25(45):6579-6606.

Dance A. Inner workings: How bacteria cause pain and what that reveals about the role of the nervous system. *Proc Natl Acad Sci U S A*. 2019;116(26):12584-12586.

De Chiara G, Marcocci ME, Sgarbanti R, et al. Infectious agents and neurodegeneration. *Mol Neurobiol*. 2012;46(3):614-638.

Delogu LG, Deidda S, Delitala G, Manetti R. Infectious diseases and autoimmunity. *J Infect Dev Ctries*. 2011;5(10):679-687.

Dittfeld A, Gwizdek K, Michalski M, Wojnicz R. A possible link between the Epstein-Barr virus infection and autoimmune thyroid disorders. *Cent Eur J Immunol*. 2016;41(3): 297-301.

Draborg AH, Duus K, Houen G. Epstein-Barr virus in systemic autoimmune diseases. *Clin Dev Immunol*. 2013;2013:535738.

Dunmire SK, Hogquist KA, Balfour HH. Infectious mononucleosis. *Curr Top Microbiol Immunol*. 2015; 390:211-240.

Endresen GK. Mycoplasma blood infection in chronic fatigue and fibromyalgia syndromes. *Rheumatol Int*. 2003;23(5):211-215.

Fierz W. Multiple sclerosis: an example of pathogenic viral interaction? *Virol J*. 2017;14(1):42.

Gadila SK, Rosoklija G, Dwork AJ, et al. Detecting Borrelia spirochetes: a case study with validation among autopsy specimens. *Front Neurol*. 10 May 2021.

Godkin A, Smith KA. Chronic infections with viruses or parasites: breaking bad to make good. *Immunology*. 2017;150(4):389-396.

Harley JB, Chen X, Pujato M, et al. Transcription factors operate across disease loci, with EBNA2 implicated in autoimmunity. *Nat Genet*. 2018;50(5):699-707.

Ivanova MV, Kolkova NI, Morgunova EY, et al. Role of chlamydia in multiple sclerosis. *Bull Exp Biol Med*. 2015;159(5):646-648.

Johnson S, Sidebottom D, Bruckner F, Collins D. Identification of Mycoplasma fermentans in synovial fluid samples from arthritis patients with inflammatory disease. *J Clin Microbiol*. 2000;38(1):90-93.

Johnson SM, Bruckner F, Collins D. Distribution of Mycoplasma pneumoniae and Mycoplasma salivarium in the synovial fluid of arthritis patients. *J Clin Microbiol*. 2007;45(3):953-957.

Kelly CJ, Colgan SP, Frank DN. Of microbes and meals: the health consequences of dietary endotoxemia. *Nutr Clin Pract*. 2012;27(2):215-225.

Kriesel JD, Bhetariya P, Wang Z-M, et al. Spectrum of microbial sequences and a bacterial cell wall antigen in primary demyelination brain specimens obtained from living patients. *Sci Rep*. 2019;9(1):1387.

Leech MT, Bartold PM. The association between rheumatoid arthritis and periodontitis. *Best Pract Res Clin Rheumatol*. 2015;29(2):189-201.

Libbey JE, Cusick MF, Fujinami RS. Role of pathogens in multiple sclerosis. *Int Rev Immunol*. 2014;33(4):266-283.

Lossius A, Johansen JN, Torkildsen O, et al. Epstein-Barr virus in systemic lupus erythematosus, rheumatoid arthritis and multiple sclerosis—association and causation. *Viruses*. 2012;4(12):3701-3730.

Mickiewicz KM, Kawai Y, Drage L, et al. Possible role of L-form switching in recurrent urinary tract infection. *Nat Commun*. 2019;10(1):4379.

Nayeri Chegeni T, Sarvi S, Moosazadeh M, et al. Is Toxoplasma gondii a potential risk factor for Alzheimer's disease? A systematic review and meta-analysis. *Microb Pathog*. 2019;137:103751.

Pender M, Burrows S. Epstein-Barr virus and multiple sclerosis: potential opportunities for immunotherapy. *Clin Transl Immunology*. 2014;3(10):e27.

Pender M. The essential role of Epstein-Barr virus in the pathogenesis of multiple sclerosis. *Neuroscientist*. 2011;17(4):351-367.

Pianta A, Arvikar SL, Strle K, et al. Two rheumatoid arthritis-specific autoantigens correlate microbial immunity with autoimmune responses in joints. *J Clin Invest*. 2017;127(8):2946-2956.

Proal AD, Albert PJ, Marshall TG, Blaney GP, Lindseth IA. Immunostimulation in the treatment for chronic fatigue syndrome/myalgic encephalomyelitis. *Immunol Res*. 2013;56(2-3):398-412.

Rasa S, Nora-Krukle Z, Henning N, et al. Chronic viral infections in myalgic encephalomyelitis/chronic fatigue syndrome (ME/CFS). *J Transl Med*. 2018;16(1):268.

Rashid T, Ebringer A. Autoimmunity in rheumatic diseases is induced by microbial infections via cross reactivity or molecular mimicry. *Autoimmune Dis*. 2012;2012:539282.

Saikku P. Chlamydia pneumoniae in atherosclerosis. *J Intern Med*. 2000;247(3):391-396.

Saikku P, Leinonen M, Mattila K, et al. Serological evidence of an association of a novel Chlamydia, TWAR, with chronic coronary heart disease and acute myocardial infarction. *Lancet*. 1988;2(8618):983-986.

Samanta D, Mulye M, Clemente TM, Justis AV, Gilk SD. Manipulation of host cholesterol by obligate intracellular bacteria. *Front Cell Infect Microbiol*. 2017;7:165.

Schrijver IA, van Meurs M, Melief MJ, et al. Bacterial peptidoglycan and immune reactivity in the central nervous system in multiple sclerosis. *Brain*. 2001;124(Pt 8):1544-1554.

Sebastian S, Stein LK, Dhamoon MS. Infection as a stroke trigger. *Stroke*. 2019;50(8):2216-2218.

Siala M, Gdoura R, Fourati H, et al. Broad-range PCR, cloning and sequencing of the full 16S rRNA gene for detection of bacterial DNA in synovial fluid samples of Tunisian patients with reactive and undifferentiated arthritis. *Arthritis Res Ther*. 2009;11(4):R102.

Soldan SS, Berti R, Salem N, et al. Association of human herpes virus 6 (HHV-6) with multiple sclerosis: increased IgM response to HHV-6 early antigen and detection of serum HHV-6 DNA. *Nat Med*. 1997;3(12):1394-1397.

Sriram S, Stratton CW, Yao S, et al. Chlamydia pneumoniae infection of the central nervous system in multiple sclerosis. *Ann Neurol*. 1999;46(1):6-14.

Sriram S, Ljunggren-Rose A, Yao S-Y, et al. Detection of chlamydial bodies and antigens in the central nervous system of patients with multiple sclerosis. *J Infect Dis*. 2005;192(7):1219-1228.

Taylor-Robinson D, Thomas BJ. Chlamydia pneumoniae in atherosclerotic tissue. *J Infect Dis*. 2000;181 (Suppl 3):S437-S440.

Underhill RA. Myalgic encephalomyelitis, chronic fatigue syndrome: an infectious disease. *Med Hypotheses.* 2015;85(6):765-773.

van der Meulen TA, Harmsen H, Bootsma H, et al. The microbiome-systemic diseases connection. *Oral Dis.* 2016;22(8):719-734.

Wu H, Zhao M, Yoshimura A, et al. Critical link between epigenetics and transcription factors in the induction of autoimmunity: a comprehensive review. *Clin Rev Allergy Immunol.* 2016;50(3):333-344.

Zeidler H, Hudson AP. Coinfection of Chlamydiae and other bacteria in reactive arthritis and spondyloarthritis: need for future research. *Microorganisms.* 2016;4(3):30.

Zhou L, Miranda-Saksena M, Saksena NK. Viruses and neurodegeneration. *Virol J.* 2013;10:172.

Bacterial Persistence

Amato SM, Fazen CH, Henry TC, et al. The role of metabolism in bacterial persistence. *Front Microbiol.* 2014;5:70.

Astrauskiene D, Bernotiene E. New insights into bacterial persistence in reactive arthritis. *Clin Exp Rheumatol.* 2007;25(3):470-479.

Harms A, Maisonneuve E, Gerdes K. Mechanisms of bacterial persistence during stress and antibiotic exposure. *Science.* 2016;354(6318):aaf4268.

Kaldalu N, Hauryliuk V, Tenson T. Persisters-as elusive as ever. *Appl Microbiol Biotechnol.* 2016;100(15):6545-6553.

Michiels JE, van den Bergh B, Verstraeten N, Michiels J. Molecular mechanisms and clinical implications of bacterial persistence. *Drug Resist Updat.* 2016;29:76-89.

Miyaue S, Suzuki E, Komiyama Y, et al. Bacterial memory of persisters: bacterial persister cells can retain their phenotype for days or weeks after withdrawal from colony-biofilm culture. *Front Microbiol.* 2018;9:1396.

Radzikowski JL, Schramke H, Heinemann M. Bacterial persistence from a system-level perspective. *Curr Opin Biotechnol.* 2017;46:98-105.

Renbarger TL, Baker JM, Sattley WM. Slow and steady wins the race: an examination of bacterial persistence. *AIMS Microbiol.* 2017;3(2):171-185.

Verstraeten N, Knapen W, Fauvart M, Michiels J. A historical perspective on bacterial persistence. *Methods Mol Biol.* 2016;1333:3-13.

Wood TK, Knabel SJ, Kwan BW. Bacterial persister cell formation and dormancy. *Appl Environ Microbiol.* 2013;79(23):7116-7121.

Gut Microbiome and Disease

Brown GC. The endotoxin hypothesis of neurodegeneration. *J Neuroinflammation*. 2019;16(1):180.

Dinan TG, Cryan JF. The microbiome-gut-brain axis in health and disease. *Gastroenterol Clin North Am*. 2017;46(1):77-89.

Foster JA, McVey Neufeld KA. Gut-brain axis: how the microbiome influences anxiety and depression. *Trends Neurosci*. 2013;36(5):305-312.

Jie Z, Xia H, Zhong SL, et al. The gut microbiome in atherosclerotic cardiovascular disease. *Nat Commun*. 2017;8(1):845.

Köhler CA, Maes M, Slyepchenko A, et al. The gut-brain axis, Including the microbiome, leaky gut and bacterial translocation: mechanisms and pathophysiological role in Alzheimer's disease. *Curr Pharm Des*. 2016;22(40):6152-6166.

Lach G, Schellekens H, Dinan TG, Cryan JF. Anxiety, depression, and the microbiome: a role for gut peptides. *Neurotherapeutics*. 2018;15(1):36-59.

Li Y, Hao Y, Fan F, Zhang B. The role of microbiome in insomnia, circadian disturbance and depression. *Front Psychiatry*. 2018;9:669.

Lima-Ojeda JM, Rupprecht R, Baghai TC. "I am I and my bacterial circumstances": linking gut microbiome, neurodevelopment, and depression. *Front Psychiatry*. 2017;8:153.

Mulak A, Bonaz B. Brain-gut-microbiota axis in Parkinson's disease. *World J Gastroenterol*. 2015;21(37):10609-10620.

Peirce JM, Alviña K. The role of inflammation and the gut microbiome in depression and anxiety. *J Neurosci Res*. 2019;97(10):1223-1241.

Chapter 4: Aging

Barbi E, Lagona F, Marsili M, Vaupel JW, Wachter KW. The plateau of human mortality: demography of longevity pioneers. *Science*. 2018;360(6396):1459-1461.

Buettner D. *The Blue Zones*, 2nd ed. National Geographic Society; 2008, 2012.

Clayton P, Rowbotham J. How the mid-Victorians worked, ate and died. *Int J Environ Res Public Health*. 2009;6(3):1235-1253.

Davidovic M, Sevo G, Svorcan P, Milosevic DP, Despotovic N, Erceg P. Old age as a privilege of the "selfish ones". *Aging Dis*. 2010;1(2):139-146.

Diaconeasa AG, Rachita M, Stefan-van Staden RI. A new hypothesis of aging. *Med Hypotheses*. 2015;84(3):252-257.

Dolgin E. There's no limit to longevity, says study that revives human lifespan debate. *Nature*. 2018;559(7712):14-15.

Finch CE. Evolution in health and medicine Sackler colloquium: evolution of the human lifespan and diseases of aging: roles of infection, inflammation, and nutrition. *Proc Natl Acad Sci U S A*. 2010;107(Suppl 1):1718-1724.

Gavrilov LA, Gavrilova NS. Evolutionary theories of aging and longevity. *ScientificWorldJournal*. 2002;2:339-356.

Goldsmith TC. Modern evolutionary mechanics theories and resolving the programmed/non-programmed aging controversy. *Biochemistry (Mosc)*. 2014t;79(10):1049-1055.

Griffin JP. Changing life expectancy throughout history. *J R Soc Med*. 2008;101(12):577.

Jeune B. Living longer--but better? *Aging Clin Exp Res*. 2002;14(2):72-93.

Kunlin J. Modern biological theories of aging. *Aging Dis*. 2010;1(2):72-74.

Macieira-Coelho A. Cell division and aging of the organism. *Biogerontology*. 2011;12(6):503-515.

Paganini-Hill A, Kawas C, Corrada M. Lifestyle factors and dementia in the oldest-old: the 90+ study. *Alzheimer Dis Assoc Disord*. 2016; 30(1):21-26.

Passarino G, De Rango F, Montesanto A. Human longevity: genetics or lifestyle? It takes two to tango. *Immun Ageing*. 2016;13:12.

Peng C, Wang X, Chen J, et al. Biology of ageing and role of dietary antioxidants. *Biomed Res Int*. 2014;2014:831841.

Preston JD, Reynolds LJ, Pearson KJ. Developmental origins of health span and life span: a mini-review. *Gerontology*. 2018;64(3):237-245.

Robin-Champigneul F. Jeanne Calment's unique 122-rear life span: facts and factors; longevity history in her genealogical tree. *Rejuvenation Res*. 2020;23(1):19-47.

Rowbotham J, Clayton P. An unsuitable and degraded diet? Part three: Victorian consumption patterns and their health benefits. *J R Soc Med*. 2008;101(9):454-462.

Sebastiani P, Solovieff N, Dewan AT, et al. Genetic signatures of exceptional longevity in humans. *PLoS One*. 2012;7(1):e29848.

Tosato M, Zamboni V, Ferrini A, Cesari M. The aging process and potential interventions to extend life expectancy. *Clin Interv Aging*. 2007;2(3):401-412.

Young R. If Jeanne Calment were 122, that is all the more reason for biosampling. *Rejuvenation Res*. 2020;23(1):48-64.

Mitochondria

Apostolova N, Victor VM. Molecular strategies for targeting antioxidants to mitochondria: therapeutic implications. *Antioxid Redox Signal.* 2015;22(8):686-729.

Bukowiecki R, Adjaye J, Prigione A. Mitochondrial function in pluripotent stem cells and cellular reprogramming. *Gerontology.* 2014;60(2):174-182.

Deelen J, Evans DS, Arking DE, et al. A meta-analysis of genome-wide association studies identifies multiple longevity genes [published correction appears in *Nat Commun.* 2021;12(1):2463]. *Nat Commun.* 2019;10(1):3669.

Emelyanov VV. Evolutionary relationship of Rickettsiae and mitochondria. *FEBS Lett.* 2001;501(1):11-18.

Jiang Q, Yin J, Chen J, et al. Mitochondria-targeted antioxidants: a step towards disease treatment. *Oxid Med Cell Longev.* 2020;2020:8837893.

Liochev SI. Free radicals: how do we stand them? Anaerobic and aerobic free radical (chain) reactions involved in the use of fluorogenic probes and in biological systems. *Med Princ Pract.* 2014;23(3):195-203.

Manini TM. Energy expenditure and aging. *Ageing Res Rev.* 2010;9(1):1-11.

Menshikova EV, Ritov VB, Fairfull L, et al. Effects of exercise on mitochondrial content and function in aging human skeletal muscle. *J Gerontol A Biol Sci Med Sci.* 2006;61(6):534-540.

Prunuske AJ, Ullman KS. The nuclear envelope: form and reformation. *Curr Opin Cell Biol.* 2006;18(1):108-116.

Sun N, Youle RJ, Finkel T. The mitochondrial basis of aging. *Mol Cell.* 2016;61(5):654-666.

Senescence/Immunosenescence

Aspinall R, Goronzy JJ. Immune senescence. *Curr Opin Immunol.* 2010;22(4):497-499.

Burton DG. Cellular senescence, ageing and disease. *Age (Dordr).* 2009;31(1):1-9.

Burton DG, Krizhanovsky V. Physiological and pathological consequences of cellular senescence. *Cell Mol Life Sci.* 2014;71(22):4373-4386.

Camous X, Pera A, Solana R, Larbi A. NK cells in healthy aging and age-associated diseases. *J Biomed Biotechnol.* 2012;2012:195956.

Childs BG, Baker DJ, Kirkland JL, Campisi J, van Deursen JM. Senescence and apoptosis: dueling or complementary cell fates? *EMBO Rep.* 2014;15(11):1139-1153.

Freund A, Orjalo AV, Desprez PY, Campisi J. Inflammatory networks during cellular senescence: causes and consequences. *Trends Mol Med.* 2010;16(5):238-246.

Gonzalez LC, Ghadaouia S, Martinez A, Rodier F. Premature aging/senescence in cancer cells facing therapy: good or bad? *Biogerontology.* 2016;17(1):71-87.

Blazkova H, Krejcikova K, Moudry P, et al. Bacterial intoxication evokes cellular senescence with persistent DNA damage and cytokine signalling. *J Cell Mol Med.* 2010;14(1-2):357-367.

Hazeldine J, Lord JM. The impact of ageing on natural killer cell function and potential consequences for health in older adults. *Ageing Res Rev.* 2013;12(4):1069-1078.

Hohensinner PJ, Goronzy JJ, Weyand CM. Targets of immune regeneration in rheumatoid arthritis. *Mayo Clin Proc.* 2014;89(4):563-575.

Iannello A, Raulet DH. Immune surveillance of unhealthy cells by natural killer cells. *Cold Spring Harb Symp Quant Biol.* 2013;78:249-257.

Kaczanowski S. Apoptosis: its origin, history, maintenance and the medical implications for cancer and aging. *Phys Biol.* 2016;13(3):031001.

Lutz CT, Quinn LS. Sarcopenia, obesity, and natural killer cell immune senescence in aging: altered cytokine levels as a common mechanism. *Aging (Albany NY).* 2012;4(8):535-546.

Minamino T, Miyauchi H, Yoshida T, Tateno K, Kunieda T, Komuro I. Vascular cell senescence and vascular aging. *J Mol Cell Cardiol.* 2004;36(2):175-183.

Muñoz-Espín D, Serrano M. Cellular senescence: from physiology to pathology. *Nat Rev Mol Cell Biol.* 2014l;15(7):482-496.

Pooja Shivshankar, Boyd AR, Le Saux CJ, et al. Cellular senescence increases expression of bacterial ligands in the lungs and is positively correlated with increased susceptibility to pneumococcal pneumonia. *Aging Cell.* 2011;10(5):798-806.

Sagiv A, Krizhanovsky V. Immunosurveillance of senescent cells: the bright side of the senescence program. *Biogerontology.* 2013;14(6):617-628.

Sikora E. Rejuvenation of senescent cells-the road to postponing human aging and age-related disease? *Exp Gerontol.* 2013;48(7):661-666.

Solana R, Alonso MC, Peña J. Natural killer cells in healthy aging. *Exp Gerontol.* 1999;34(3):435-443.

Nyström T. A bacterial kind of aging. *PLoS Genet.* 2007;3(12):e224.

van Deursen JM. The role of senescent cells in ageing. *Nature.* 2014;509(7501):439-446.

Vicente R, Mausset-Bonnefont AL, Jorgensen C, Louis-Plence P, Brondello JM. Cellular senescence impact on immune cell fate and function. *Aging Cell.* 2016;15(3):400-406.

von Kobbe C. Targeting senescent cells: approaches, opportunities, challenges. *Aging (Albany NY).* 2019;11(24):12844-12861.

Weyand CM, Yang Z, Goronzy JJ. T-cell aging in rheumatoid arthritis. *Curr Opin Rheumatol.* 2014;26(1):93-100.

Stem Cells

Beerman I, Rossi DJ. Epigenetic control of stem cell potential during homeostasis, aging, and disease. *Cell Stem Cell.* 2015;16(6):613-625.

Behfar A, Terzic A. Stem cells versus senescence: the yin and yang of cardiac health. *J Am Coll Cardiol.* 2015;65(2):148-150.

Cable J, Fuchs E, Weissman I, et al. Adult stem cells and regenerative medicine-a symposium report. *Ann N Y Acad Sci.* 2020;1462(1):27-36.

Chang KA, Lee JH, Suh YH. Therapeutic potential of human adipose-derived stem cells in neurological disorders. *J Pharmacol Sci.* 2014;126(4):293-301.

Cipriani P, Carubbi F, Liakouli V, et al. Stem cells in autoimmune diseases: implications for pathogenesis and future trends in therapy. *Autoimmun Rev.* 2013;12(7):709-716.

Doles J, Storer M, Cozzuto L, Roma G, Keyes WM. Age-associated inflammation inhibits epidermal stem cell function. *Genes Dev.* 2012;26(19):2144-2153.

Finch CE, McMahon AP. Stem cells for all ages, yet hostage to aging. *Stem Cell Investig.* 2016;3:11.

Goodell MA, Rando TA. Stem cells and healthy aging. *Science.* 2015;350(6265):1199-1204.

Liang G, Zhang Y. Embryonic stem cell and induced pluripotent stem cell: an epigenetic perspective. *Cell Res.* 2013;23(1):49-69.

Oh J, Lee YD, Wagers AJ. Stem cell aging: mechanisms, regulators and therapeutic opportunities. *Nat Med.* 2014;20(8):870-880.

Shin J, Mohrin M, Chen D. Reversing stem cell aging. *Oncotarget.* 2015;6(17):14723-14724.

Trounson A, McDonald C. Stem cell therapies in clinical trials: progress and challenges. *Cell Stem Cell.* 2015;17(1):11-22.

Telomeres

Artandi SE, DePinho RA. Telomeres and telomerase in cancer. *Carcinogenesis.* 2010;31(1):9-18.

Bernardes de Jesus B, Blasco MA. Telomerase at the intersection of cancer and aging. *Trends Genet.* 2013;29(9):513-520.

Harley CB, Liu W, Blasco M, et al. A natural product telomerase activator as part of a health maintenance program. *Rejuvenation Res.* 2011;14(1):45-56.

Anti-Aging Therapy

Díez JJ, Sangiao-Alvarellos S, Cordido F. Treatment with growth hormone for adults with growth hormone deficiency syndrome: benefits and risks. *Int J Mol Sci.* 2018;19(3):893.

Fahy GM, Brooke RT, Watson JP, et al. Reversal of epigenetic aging and immunosenescent trends in humans. *Aging Cell.* 2019;18(6):e13028.

Giannoulis MG, Martin FC, Nair KS, Umpleby AM, Sonksen P. Hormone replacement therapy and physical function in healthy older men. Time to talk hormones?. *Endocr Rev.* 2012;33(3):314-377.

Samaras N, Papadopoulou MA, Samaras D, Ongaro F. Off-label use of hormones as an antiaging strategy: a review. *Clin Interv Aging.* 2014;9:1175-1186.

Williams BR, Cho JS. Hormone replacement: the fountain of youth? *Prim Care.* 2017;44(3):481-498.

Microbes and Cancer

Chan CC. Molecular pathology of primary intraocular lymphoma. *Trans Am Ophthalmol Soc.* 2003;101:275-292.

Chen J, Domingue JC, Sears CL. Microbiota dysbiosis in select human cancers: evidence of association and causality. *Semin Immunol.* 2017;32:25-34.

Chmiel R. University of New Haven Professor Makes Great Strides in Lyme Disease, Cancer Research. Sept 15, 2020, Office of Marketing and Communications, University of New Haven.

https://www.newhaven.edu/news/blog/2020/eva-sapi-research.php

Cimolai N. Do mycoplasmas cause human cancer? *Can J Microbiol.* 2001;47(8):691-697.

Dong Q, Xing X. Cancer cells arise from bacteria. *Cancer Cell Int.* 2018;18:205.

Dudgeon LS, Dunkley EV. The Micrococcus neoformans: its cultural characters and pathogenicity and the results of the estimation of the opsonic and agglutinative properties of the serum of patients suffering from malignant disease on this organism and on the Staphylococcus albus. *J Hyg (Lond).* 1907;7(1):13-21.

Erturhan SM, Bayrak O, Pehlivan S, et al. Can mycoplasma contribute to formation of prostate cancer? *Int Urol Nephrol.* 2013;45(1):33-38.

Faden AA. The potential role of microbes in oncogenesis with particular emphasis on oral cancer. *Saudi Med J.* 2016;37(6):607-612.

Gyémánt N, Molnár A, Spengler G, Mándi Y, Szabó M, Molnár J. Bacterial models for tumor development. mini-review. *Acta Microbiol Immunol Hung.* 2004;51(3):321-332.

Hieken TJ, Chen J, Hoskin TL, et al. The microbiome of aseptically collected human breast tissue in benign and malignant disease. *Sci Rep.* 2016;6:30751.

Hornsby PJ. Cellular aging and cancer. *Crit Rev Oncol Hematol.* 2011;79(2):189-195.

Huang S, Li JY, Wu J, Meng L, Shou CC. Mycoplasma infections and different human carcinomas. *World J Gastroenterol.* 2001;7(2):266-269.

Iizasa H, Nanbo A, Nishikawa J, et al. Epstein-Barr virus (EBV)-associated gastric carcinoma. *Viruses.* 2012;4(12):3420-3439.

Laumbacher B, Fellerhoff B, Herzberger B, Wank R. Do dogs harbour risk factors for human breast cancer? *Med Hypotheses.* 2006;67(1):21-26.

Meng S, Chen B, Yang J, et al. Study of microbiomes in aseptically collected samples of human breast tissue using needle biopsy and the potential role of *in situ* tissue microbiomes for promoting malignancy. *Front Oncol.* 2018;8:318.

Nejman D, Livyatan I, Fuks G, et al. The human tumor microbiome is composed of tumor type-specific intracellular bacteria. *Science.* 2020;368(6494):973-980.

Nené NR, Reisel D, Leimbach A, et al. Association between the cervicovaginal microbiome, BRCA1 mutation status, and risk of ovarian cancer: a case-control study. *Lancet Oncol.* 2019; S1470-2045(19):30340-30347.

Rous P. A sarcoma of the fowl transmissible by an agent separable from the tumor cells. *J Exp Med.* 1911;13(4):397-411.

Rowe M, Fitzsimmons L, Bell A. Epstein-Barr virus and Burkitt lymphoma. *Chin J Cancer.* 2014;33(12):609-619.

Shen DF, Herbort CP, Tuaillon N, Buggage RR, Egwuagu CE, Chan CC. Detection of Toxoplasma gondii DNA in primary intraocular B-cell lymphoma. *Mod Pathol.* 2001;14(10):995-999.

Singh N, Baby D, Rajguru JP, Patil PB, Thakkannavar SS, Pujari VB. Inflammation and cancer. *Ann Afr Med.* 2019;18(3):121-126.

Tsao S, Tsang CM, To K-F, Lo K-W. The role of Epstein-Barr virus in epithelial malignancies. *J Pathol.* 2015;235(2):323-333.

Vedham V, Verma M, Mahabir S. Early-life exposures to infectious agents and later cancer development. *Cancer Med.* 2015;4(12):1908-1922.

Vranic S, Cyprian FS, Akhtar S, Al Moustafa AE. The role of Epstein-Barr virus in cervical cancer: a brief update. *Front Oncol.* 2018;8:113.

Whisner CM, Athena Aktipis C. The role of the microbiome in cancer initiation and progression: how microbes and cancer cells utilize excess energy and promote one another's growth. *Curr Nutr Rep*. 2019;8(1):42-51.

Yang H, Qu L, Ma H, et al. Mycoplasma hyorhinis infection in gastric carcinoma and its effects on the malignant phenotypes of gastric cancer cells. *BMC Gastroenterol*. 2010;10:132.

Yow MA, Tabrizi SN, Severi G, et al. Detection of infectious organisms in archival prostate cancer tissues. *BMC Cancer*. 2014;14:579.

Zarei O, Rezania S, Mousavi A. Mycoplasma genitalium and cancer: a brief review. *Asian Pac J Cancer Prev*. 2013;14(6):3425-3428.

Autophagy

Batoko H, Dagdas Y, Baluska F, Sirko A. Understanding and exploiting autophagy signaling in plants. *Essays Biochem*. 2017;61(6):675-685.

Choi AM, Ryter SW, Levine B. Autophagy in human health and disease. *N Engl J Med*. 2013;368(7):651-662.

Glick D, Barth S, Macleod KF. Autophagy: cellular and molecular mechanisms. *J Pathol*. 2010;221(1):3-12.

Gomes LR, Menck CFM, Leandro GS. Autophagy roles in the modulation of DNA repair pathways. *Int J Mol Sci*. 2017;18(11):2351.

Guo F, Liu X, Cai H, Le W. Autophagy in neurodegenerative diseases: pathogenesis and therapy. *Brain Pathol*. 2018;28(1):3-13.

Ho J, Yu J, Wong SH, et al. Autophagy in sepsis: degradation into exhaustion? *Autophagy*. 2016;12(7):1073-1082.

Kim KH, Lee MS. Autophagy--a key player in cellular and body metabolism. *Nat Rev Endocrinol*. 2014;10(6):322-337.

Kohler LJ, Roy CR. Autophagic targeting and avoidance in intracellular bacterial infections. *Curr Opin Microbiol*. 2017;35:36-41.

Kroemer G. Autophagy: a druggable process that is deregulated in aging and human disease. *J Clin Invest*. 2015;125(1):1-4.

Lapaquette P, Guzzo J, Bretillon L, Bringer MA. Cellular and molecular connections between autophagy and inflammation. *Mediators Inflamm*. 2015;2015:398483.

Levine B, Kroemer G. Biological functions of autophagy genes: a disease perspective. *Cell*. 2019;176(1-2):11-42.

McEwan DG. Host-pathogen interactions and subversion of autophagy. *Essays Biochem.* 2017;61(6):687-697.

Mialet-Perez J, Vindis C. Autophagy in health and disease: focus on the cardiovascular system. *Essays Biochem.* 2017;61(6):721-732.

Mizushima N, Komatsu M. Autophagy: renovation of cells and tissues. *Cell.* 2011;147(4):728-741.

Mizushima N, Levine B, Cuervo AM, Klionsky DJ. Autophagy fights disease through cellular self-digestion. *Nature.* 2008;451(7182):1069-1075.

Ogawa M, Mimuro H, Yoshikawa Y, Ashida H, Sasakawa C. Manipulation of autophagy by bacteria for their own benefit. *Microbiol Immunol.* 2011;55(7):459-471.

Parzych KR, Klionsky DJ. An overview of autophagy: morphology, mechanism, and regulation. *Antioxid Redox Signal.* 2014;20(3):460-473.

Puleston DJ, Simon AK. Autophagy in the immune system. *Immunology.* 2014;141(1):1-8.

Rubinsztein DC, Bento CF, Deretic V. Therapeutic targeting of autophagy in neurodegenerative and infectious diseases. *J Exp Med.* 2015;212(7):979-990.

Chapter 5: Pathway to Wellness

Phytochemicals and Autophagy

Mosaddeghi P, Eslami M, Farahmandnejad M, et al. A systems pharmacology approach to identify the autophagy-inducing effects of Traditional Persian medicinal plants. *Sci Rep.* 2021;11(1):336.

Ohnishi K, Yano S, Fujimoto M, et al. Identification of dietary phytochemicals capable of enhancing the autophagy flux in HeLa and Caco-2 human cell lines. *Antioxidants (Basel).* 2020;9(12):1193.

Patra S, Pradhan B, Nayak R, et al. Apoptosis and autophagy modulating dietary phytochemicals in cancer therapeutics: current evidences and future perspectives. *Phytother Res.* 2021;35(8):4194-4214.

Rahman MA, Hannan MA, Dash R, et al. Phytochemicals as a complement to cancer chemotherapy: pharmacological modulation of the autophagy-apoptosis pathway. *Front Pharmacol.* 2021;12:639628.

Phytochemical Actions

Borges A, Saavedra MJ, Simões M. Insights on antimicrobial resistance, biofilms and the use of phytochemicals as new antimicrobial agents. *Curr Med Chem.* 2015;22(21):2590-2614.

Forni C, Facchiano F, Bartoli M, et al. Beneficial role of phytochemicals on oxidative stress and age-related diseases. *Biomed Res Int.* 2019;2019:8748253.

Ma ZF, Zhang H. Phytochemical constituents, health benefits, and industrial applications of grape seeds: a mini-review. *Antioxidants (Basel).* 2017;6(3):71.

Madrigal-Santillán E, Madrigal-Bujaidar E, Álvarez-González I, et al. Review of natural products with hepatoprotective effects. *World J Gastroenterol.* 2014;20(40):14787-14804.

Mahdavi A, Bagherniya M, Mirenayat MS, Atkin SL, Sahebkar A. Medicinal plants and phytochemicals regulating insulin resistance and glucose homeostasis in type 2 diabetic patients: a clinical review. *Adv Exp Med Biol.* 2021;1308:161-183.

Minich DM, Brown BI. A review of dietary (phyto)nutrients for glutathione support. *Nutrients.* 2019;11(9):2073.

Miryeganeh M. Plants' epigenetic mechanisms and abiotic stress. *Genes (Basel).* 2021;12(8):1106.

Panossian A. Understanding adaptogenic activity: specificity of the pharmacological action of adaptogens and other phytochemicals. *Ann N Y Acad Sci.* 2017;1401(1):49-64.

Parveen A, Sultana R, Lee SM, Kim TH, Kim SY. Phytochemicals against anti-diabetic complications: targeting the advanced glycation end product signaling pathway. *Arch Pharm Res.* 2021;44(4):378-401.

Patel S. Phytochemicals for taming agitated immune-endocrine-neural axis. *Biomed Pharmacother.* 2017;91:767-775.

Saleh HA, Yousef MH, Abdelnaser A. The anti-inflammatory properties of phytochemicals and their effects on epigenetic mechanisms involved in TLR4/NF-κB-mediated inflammation. *Front Immunol.* 2021;12:606069.

Shen CY, Lu CH, Wu CH, et al. The development of maillard reaction, and advanced glycation end product (AGE)-receptor for AGE (RAGE) signaling inhibitors as novel therapeutic strategies for patients with AGE-related diseases. *Molecules.* 2020;25(23):5591.

Smeriglio A, Denaro M, Trombetta D. Dietary phytochemicals and endocrine-related activities: an update. *Mini Rev Med Chem.* 2018;18(16):1382-1397.

Sun JQ, Jiang HL, Li CY. Systemin/Jasmonate-mediated systemic defense signaling in tomato. *Mol Plant.* 2011;4(4):607-615.

Vestergaard M, Ingmer H. Antibacterial and antifungal properties of resveratrol. *Int J Antimicrob Agents.* 2019;53(6):716-723.

Witzany G. Plant communication from biosemiotic perspective: differences in abiotic and biotic signal perception determine content arrangement of response behavior. Context determines meaning of meta-, inter- and intraorganismic plant signaling. *Plant Signal Behav.* 2006;1(4):169-178.

Yamagishi SI, Matsui T, Ishibashi Y, et al. Phytochemicals against advanced glycation end products (AGEs) and the receptor system. *Curr Pharm Des*. 2017;23(8):1135-1141.

Zhang YJ, Gan RY, Li S, et al. Antioxidant phytochemicals for the prevention and treatment of chronic diseases. *Molecules*. 2015;20(12):21138-21156.

History of Herbal Medicine and Herbal Usage

Petrovska BB. Historical review of medicinal plants' usage. *Pharmacogn Rev*. 2012;6(11):1-5.

Storl WD. *The Untold History of Healing: Plant Lore and Medicinal Magic from the Stone Age to Present*. North Atlantic Books; 2017.

Phytochemicals for Prevention of Chronic Illness

Arulselvan P, Fard MT, Tan WS, et al. Role of antioxidants and natural products in inflammation. *Oxid Med Cell Longev*. 2016;2016:5276130.

Esposito S, Bianco A, Russo R, Di Maro A, Isernia C, Pedone PV. Therapeutic perspectives of molecules from *Urtica dioica* extracts for cancer treatment. *Molecules*. 2019;24(15):2753.

Fernando WMADB, Somaratne G, Goozee KG, et al. Diabetes and Alzheimer's disease: can tea phytochemicals play a role in prevention? *J Alzheimers Dis*. 2017;59(2):481-501.

Firth J, Teasdale SB, Allott K, et al. The efficacy and safety of nutrient supplements in the treatment of mental disorders: a meta-review of meta-analyses of randomized controlled trials. *World Psychiatry*. 2019;18(3):308-324.

Ilhan M, Gürağaç Dereli FT, Akkol EK. Novel drug targets with traditional herbal medicines for overcoming endometriosis. *Curr Drug Deliv*. 2019;16(5):386-399.

Kim CS, Park S, Kim J. The role of glycation in the pathogenesis of aging and its prevention through herbal products and physical exercise. *J Exerc Nutrition Biochem*. 2017;21(3):55-61.

Ng CY, Yen H, Hsiao HY, Su SC. Phytochemicals in skin cancer prevention and treatment: an updated review. *Int J Mol Sci*. 2018;19(4):941.

Salehi B, Ata A, Kumar NVA, et al. Antidiabetic potential of medicinal plants and their active components. *Biomolecules*. 2019;9(10):551.

Sofowora A, Ogunbodede E, Onayade A. The role and place of medicinal plants in the strategies for disease prevention. *Afr J Tradit Complement Altern Med*. 2013;10(5):210-229.

Szczuka D, Nowak A, Zakłos-Szyda M, et al. American Ginseng (*Panax quinquefolium* L.) as a source of bioactive phytochemicals with pro-health properties. *Nutrients*. 2019;11(5):1041.

Zhang YJ, Gan RY, Li S, et al. Antioxidant phytochemicals for the prevention and treatment of chronic diseases. *Molecules*. 2015;20(12):21138-21156.

Anti-Aging Herbal Therapy

Almanaa TN, Geusz ME, Jamasbi RJ. Effects of curcumin on stem-like cells in human esophageal squamous carcinoma cell lines. *BMC Complement Altern Med.* 2012;12:195.

Efferth T. Stem cells, cancer stem-like cells, and natural products. *Planta Med.* 2012;78(10):935-942.

Haifeng Li, Ma F, Hu M, et al. Polysaccharides from medicinal herbs as potential therapeutics for aging and age-related neurodegeneration. *Rejuvenation Res.* 2014;17(2):201-204.

Hasan NM, Al Sorkhy M. Herbs that promote cell proliferation. *IJHM.* 2014;1(6):18-21.

Ho YS, So KF, Chang RC. Anti-aging herbal medicine--how and why can they be used in aging-associated neurodegenerative diseases? *Ageing Res Rev.* 2010;9(3):354-362.

Hu B, An H-M, Shen K-P, et al. Liver Yin deficiency tonifying herbal extract induces apoptosis and cell senescence in Bel-7402 human hepatocarcinoma cells. *Exp Ther Med.* 2012;3(1):80-86.

Hung CW, Liou YJ, Lu SW, et al. Stem cell-based neuroprotective and neurorestorative strategies. *Int J Mol Sci.* 2010;11(5):2039-2055.

Lin PC, Chang LF, Liu PY, et al. Botanical drugs and stem cells. *Cell Transplant.* 2011;20(1):71-83.

Mao J, Huang S, Liu S, et al. A herbal medicine for Alzheimer's disease and its active constituents promote neural progenitor proliferation. *Aging Cell.* 2015;14(5):784-796.

McCormack D, McFadden D. A review of pterostilbene antioxidant activity and disease modification. *Oxid Med Cell Longev.* 2013;2013:575482.

McCubrey JA, Lertpiriyapong K, Steelman LS, et al. Effects of resveratrol, curcumin, berberine and other nutraceuticals on aging, cancer development, cancer stem cells and microRNAs. *Aging (Albany NY).* 2017;9(6):1477-1536.

Rauf A, Imran M, Butt MS, et al. Resveratrol as an anti-cancer agent: a review. *Crit Rev Food Sci Nutr.* 2018;58(9):1428-1447.

Schwager J, Richard N, Widmer F, Raederstorff D. Resveratrol distinctively modulates the inflammatory profiles of immune and endothelial cells. *BMC Complement Altern Med.* 2017;17(1):309.

Udalamaththa VL, Jayasinghe CD, Udagama PV. Potential role of herbal remedies in stem cell therapy: proliferation and differentiation of human mesenchymal stromal cells. *Stem Cell Res Ther.* 2016;7(1):110.

Wang WW, Lu L, Bao TH, et al. Scutellarin alleviates behavioral deficits in a mouse model of multiple sclerosis, possibly through protecting neural stem cells. *J Mol Neurosci.* 2016;58(2):210-220.

Wu B, Chen Y, Huang J, et al. Icariin improves cognitive deficits and activates quiescent neural stem cells in aging rats. *J Ethnopharmacol.* 2012;142(3):746-753.

Anti-Cancer Properties of Herbs

Arora I, Sharma M, Tollefsbol TO. Combinatorial epigenetics impact of polyphenols and phytochemicals in cancer prevention and therapy. *Int J Mol Sci.* 2019;20(18):4567.

Hudson TS, Hartle DK, Hursting SD, et al. Inhibition of prostate cancer growth by muscadine grape skin extract and resveratrol through distinct mechanisms. *Cancer Res.* 2007;67(17):8396-8405.

Rahman MA, Hannan MA, Dash R, et al. Phytochemicals as a complement to cancer chemotherapy: pharmacological modulation of the autophagy-apoptosis pathway. *Front Pharmacol.* 2021;12:639628.

Ashwagandha

Choudhary B, Shetty A, Langade DG. Efficacy of Ashwagandha (Withania somnifera [L.] Dunal) in improving cardiorespiratory endurance in healthy athletic adults. *Ayu.* 2015;36(1):63-68.

Choudhary D, Bhattacharyya S, Bose S. Efficacy and safety of Ashwagandha (Withania somnifera (L.) Dunal) root extract in improving memory and cognitive functions. *J Diet Suppl.* 2017;14(6):599-612.

Dar NJ, Hamid A, Ahmad M. Pharmacologic overview of Withania somnifera, the Indian Ginseng. *Cell Mol Life Sci.* 2015;72(23):4445-4460.

Dar NJ, Ahmad M. Neurodegenerative diseases and Withania somnifera (L.): an update. *J Ethnopharmacol.* 2020;256:112769.

Deshpande A, Irani N, Balkrishnan R, Benny IR. A randomized, double blind, placebo controlled study to evaluate the effects of ashwagandha (Withania somnifera) extract on sleep quality in healthy adults. *Sleep Med.* 2020;72:28-36.

Gupta M, Kaur G. Withania somnifera (L.) Dunal ameliorates neurodegeneration and cognitive impairments associated with systemic inflammation. *BMC Complement Altern Med.* 2019;19(1):217.

Johnson A, Roberts L, Elkins G. Complementary and alternative medicine for menopause. *J Evid Based Integr Med.* 2019;24:2515690X19829380.

Lopresti AL, Smith SJ, Malvi H, Kodgule R. An investigation into the stress-relieving and pharmacological actions of an ashwagandha (Withania somnifera) extract: a randomized, double-blind, placebo-controlled study. *Medicine (Baltimore).* 2019;98(37):e17186.

Mishra LC, Singh BB, Dagenais S. Scientific basis for the therapeutic use of Withania somnifera (ashwagandha): a review. *Altern Med Rev.* 2000;5(4):334-346.

Pratte MA, Nanavati KB, Young V, Morley CP. An alternative treatment for anxiety: a systematic review of human trial results reported for the Ayurvedic herb ashwagandha (Withania somnifera). *J Altern Complement Med.* 2014;20(12):901-908.

Sharma AK, Basu I, Singh S. Efficacy and safety of Ashwagandha root extract in subclinical hypothyroid patients: a double-blind, randomized placebo-controlled trial. *J Altern Complement Med.* 2018;24(3):243-248.

Singh N, Bhalla M, de Jager P, Gilca M. An overview on ashwagandha: a Rasayana (rejuvenator) of Ayurveda. *Afr J Tradit Complement Altern Med.* 2011;8(5 Suppl):208-213.

Verma N, Gupta SK, Tiwari S, Mishra AK. Safety of Ashwagandha root extract: a randomized, placebo-controlled, study in healthy volunteers. *Complement Ther Med.* 2021;57:102642.

Hawthorn

Dahmer S, Scott E. Health effects of hawthorn. *Am Fam Physician.* 2010;81(4):465-468.

Holubarsch CJF, Colucci WS, Eha J. Benefit-risk assessment of Crataegus extract WS 1442: an evidence-based review. *Am J Cardiovasc Drugs.* 2018;18(1):25-36.

Orhan IE. Phytochemical and pharmacological activity profile of Crataegus oxyacantha L. (Hawthorn) - a cardiotonic herb. *Curr Med Chem.* 2018;25(37):4854-4865.

Tadić VM, Dobrić S, Marković GM, et al. Anti-inflammatory, gastroprotective, free-radical-scavenging, and antimicrobial activities of hawthorn berries ethanol extract. *J Agric Food Chem.* 2008;56(17):7700-7709.

Wang J, Xiong X, Feng B. Effect of crataegus usage in cardiovascular disease prevention: an evidence-based approach. *Evid Based Complement Alternat Med.* 2013;2013:149363.

Wu M, Liu L, Xing Y, Yang S, Li H, Cao Y. Roles and mechanisms of hawthorn and its extracts on atherosclerosis: a review. *Front Pharmacol.* 2020;11:118.

Chapter 6: Missing Phytochemicals

Adler CJ, Dobney K, Weyrich LS, et al. Sequencing ancient calcified dental plaque shows changes in oral microbiota with dietary shifts of the Neolithic and industrial revolutions. *Nat Genet.* 2013;45(4):450-455e1.

Forshaw R. Dental indicators of ancient dietary patterns: dental analysis in archaeology. *Br Dent J.* 2014;216(9):529-535.

Frąckowiak T, Groyecka-Bernard A, Oleszkiewicz A, Butovskaya M, Żelaźniewicz A, Sorokowski P. Difference in perception of onset of old age in traditional (Hadza) and modern (Polish) societies. *Int J Environ Res Public Health.* 2020;17(19):7079.

Jew S, AbuMweis SS, Jones PJ. Evolution of the human diet: linking our ancestral diet to modern functional foods as a means of chronic disease prevention. *J Med Food*. 2009;12(5):925-934.

Schnorr SL, Candela M, Rampelli S, et al. Gut microbiome of the Hadza hunter-gatherers. *Nat Commun*. 2014;5:3654.

Shelef O, Weisberg PJ, Provenza FD. The Value of Native Plants and Local Production in an Era of Global Agriculture. *Front Plant Sci*. 2017;8:2069.

Simmons AH, Köhler-Rollefson I, Rollefson GO, Mandel R, Kafafi Z. 'Ain ghazal: a major neolithic settlement in central jordan. *Science*. 1988;240(4848):35-39.

Smits SA, Leach J, Sonnenburg ED, et al. Seasonal cycling in the gut microbiome of the Hadza hunter-gatherers of Tanzania. *Science*. 2017;357(6353):802-806.

Warinner C, Speller C, Collins MJ, Lewis CM Jr. Ancient human microbiomes. *J Hum Evol*. 2015;79:125-136.

Chapter 7: Herbal Spectrum

Cappelletti S, Piacentino D, Sani G, Aromatario M. Caffeine: cognitive and physical performance enhancer or psychoactive drug? *Curr Neuropharmacol*. 2015;13(1):71-88. [published correction appears in *Curr Neuropharmacol*. 2015;13(4):554].

Carlin MG, Dean JR, Ames JM. Opium alkaloids in harvested and thermally processed poppy seeds. *Front Chem*. 2020;8:737.

Monteiro JP, Alves MG, Oliveira PF, Silva BM. Structure-bioactivity relationships of methylxanthines: trying to make sense of all the promises and the drawbacks. *Molecules*. 2016;21(8):974.

Pan L, Chai HB, Kinghorn AD. Discovery of new anticancer agents from higher plants. *Front Biosci (Schol Ed)*. 2012;4:142-156.

Pandey RC. Prospecting for potentially new pharmaceuticals from natural sources. *Med Res Rev*. 1998;18(5):333-346.

Rodríguez-Antona C. Pharmacogenomics of paclitaxel. *Pharmacogenomics*. 2010;11(5):621-623.

Adaptogens

Liao LY, He YF, Li L, et al. A preliminary review of studies on adaptogens: comparison of their bioactivity in TCM with that of ginseng-like herbs used worldwide. *Chin Med*. 2018;13:57.

Panossian A. Understanding adaptogenic activity: specificity of the pharmacological action of adaptogens and other phytochemicals. *Ann N Y Acad Sci*. 2017;1401(1):49-64.

Panossian AG, Efferth T, Shikov AN, et al. Evolution of the adaptogenic concept from traditional use to medical systems: pharmacology of stress- and aging-related diseases. *Med Res Rev*. 2021;41(1):630-703.

Ratan ZA, Youn SH, Kwak YS, et al. Adaptogenic effects of *Panax ginseng* on modulation of immune functions. *J Ginseng Res*. 2021;45(1):32-40.

Roumanille R, Vernus B, Brioche T, et al. Acute and chronic effects of Rhaponticum carthamoides and Rhodiola rosea extracts supplementation coupled to resistance exercise on muscle protein synthesis and mechanical power in rats. *J Int Soc Sports Nutr*. 2020;17(1):58.

Chapter 8: Making Herbs Part of Your Life

Bower A, Marquez S, Gonzalez de Mejia E. The health benefits of selected culinary herbs and spices found in the traditional Mediterranean diet. *Crit Rev Food Sci Nutr*. 2016;56(16):2728-2746.

Butt MS, Pasha I, Sultan MT, et al. Black pepper and health claims: a comprehensive treatise. *Crit Rev Food Sci Nutr*. 2013;53(9):875-886.

Hoffmann D. *Medical Herbalism, the Science and Practice of Herbal Medicine*. Healing Arts Press; 2003.

Guiné RP, Goncavles FJ. Bioactive compounds in some culinary aromatic herbs and their effects on human health. *Mini Rev Med Chem*. 2016;16(11):855-866.

Halvorsen BL, Carlsen MH, Phillips KM, et al. Content of redox-active compounds in foods consumed in the United States. *Am J Clin Nutr*. 2006;84:95-135.

Hamidpour R, Hamidpour S, Hamidpour M, Shahlari M, Sohraby M. Summer savory: from the selection of traditional applications to the novel effect in relief, prevention, and treatment of a number of serious illnesses such as diabetes, cardiovascular disease, Alzheimer's disease, and cancer. *J Tradit Complement Med*. 2014;4(3):140-144.

Kamath AB, Wang L, Das H, et al. Antigens in tea-beverage prime human Vγ2Vδ2 T cells in vitro and in vivo for memory and nonmemory antibacterial cytokine responses. *Proc Natl Acad Sci U S A*. 2003;100(10):6009-6014.

Li C, Tong H, Yan Q, et al. L-theanine improves immunity by altering TH2/TH1 cytokine balance, brain neurotransmitters, and expression of phospholipase C in rat hearts. *Med Sci Monit*. 2016;22:662-669.

Opara El, Chohan M. Culinary herbs and spices: their bioactive properties, the contribution of polyphenols and the challenges in deducing their true health benefits. *Int J Mol Sci*. 2014;15(10):19183-19202.

Rowe CA, Nantz MP, Bukowski JF, Percival SS. Specific formulation of Camellia sinensis prevents cold and flu symptoms and enhances gamma, delta T cell function: a randomized, double-blind, placebo-controlled study. *J Am Coll Nutr.* 2007;26(5):445-452.

Chapter 9: Foundational Herbs

Rhodiola

Ahmed M, Hensen DA, Sanderson MC, et al. Rhodiola rosea exerts antiviral activity in athletes following a competitive marathon race. *Front Nutr.* 2015;2:24.

Ait-Ghezala G, Hassan S, Tweed M, et al. Identification of telomerase-activating blends from naturally occurring compounds. *Altern Ther Health Med.* 2016;22(Suppl 2):6-14.

Al-Kuraishy HM. Central additive effect of Ginkgo biloba and Rhodiola rosea on psychomotor vigilance task and short-term working memory accuracy. *J Intercult Ethnopharmacol.* 2015;5(1):7-13.

Amsterdam JD, Panossian AG. Rhodiola rosea L. as a putative botanical antidepressant. *Phytomedicine.* 2016;23(7):770-783.

Brown R, Gerbarg P, Ramazanov Z. Rhodiola rosea: a phytomedicinal overview. *HerbalGram.* 2002; 56:40-52.

Chen M, Cai H, Yu C, et al. Salidroside exerts protective effects against chronic hypoxia-induced pulmonary arterial hypertension via AMPKα1-dependent pathways. *Am J Transl Res.* 2016;8(1):12-27.

Chiang HM, Chen HC, Wu CS, Wu PY, Wen KC. Rhodiola plants: chemistry and biological activity. *J Food Drug Anal.* 2015;23(3):359-369.

Cropley M, Banks AP, Boyle J. The effects of Rhodiola rosea L. extract on anxiety, stress, cognition and other mood symptoms. *Phytother Res.* 2015;29(12):1934-1939.

Darbinyan V, Kteyan A, Panossian A, Gabrielian E, Wikman G, Wagner H. Rhodiola rosea in stress induced fatigue--a double blind cross-over study of a standardized extract SHR-5 with a repeated low-dose regimen on the mental performance of healthy physicians during night duty. *Phytomedicine.* 2000;7(5):365-371.

De Bock K, Eijnde BO, Ramaekers M, Hespel P. Acute Rhodiola rosea intake can improve endurance exercise performance. *Int J Sport Nutr Exerc Metab.* 2004;14(3):298-307.

Duncan M, Clarke N. *An Overview on Rhodiola rosea in Cardiovascular Health, Mood Alleviation, and Energy Metabolism. Sustained Energy for Enhanced Human Functions and Activity.* Academic Press; 2017:173-186.

Gerbarg PL, Brown RP. Pause menopause with Rhodiola rosea, a natural selective estrogen receptor modulator. *Phytomedicine.* 2016;23(7):763-769.

Han J, Xiao Q, Lin Y-H, et al. Neuroprotective effects of salidroside on focal cerebral ischemia/reperfusion injury involve the nuclear erythroid 2-related factor 2 pathway. *Neural Regen Res.* 2015;10(12):1989-1996.

Hsu SW, Chang T-C, Wu Y-K, et al. Rhodiola crenulata extract counteracts the effect of hypobaric hypoxia in rat heart via redirection of the nitric oxide and arginase 1 pathway. *BMC Complement Altern Med.* 2017;17(1):29.

Hung SK, Perry R, Ernst E. The effectiveness and efficacy of Rhodiola rosea L.: a systematic review of randomized clinical trials. *Phytomedicine.* 2011;18(4):235-244.

Ishaque S, Shamseer L, Bukutu C, Vohra S. Rhodiola rosea for physical and mental fatigue: a systematic review. *BMC Complement Altern Med.* 2012;12:70.

Kang DZ, Hong HD, Kim KI, Choi SY. Anti-fatigue effects of fermented Rhodiola rosea extract in mice. *Prev Nutr Food Sci.* 2015;20(1):38-42.

Kasper S, Dienel A. Multicenter, open-label, exploratory clinical trial with Rhodiola rosea extract in patients suffering from burnout symptoms. *Neuropsychiatr Dis Treat.* 2017;13:889-898.

Khanna K, Mishra KP, Ganju L, Singh SB. Golden root: a wholesome treat of immunity. *Biomed Pharmacother.* 2017;87:496-502.

Kosakowska O, Bączek K, Przybył JL, et al. Antioxidant and antibacterial activity of Roseroot (Rhodiola rosea L.) dry extracts. *Molecules.* 2018;23(7):1767.

Lan KC, Chao S-C, Wu H-Y, et al. Salidroside ameliorates sepsis-induced acute lung injury and mortality via downregulating NF-κB and HMGB1 pathways through the upregulation of SIRT1. *Sci Rep.* 2017;7(1):12026.

Lekomtseva Y, Zhukova I, Wacker A. Rhodiola rosea in subjects with prolonged or chronic fatigue symptoms: results of an open-label clinical trial. *Complement Med Res.* 2017;24(1):46-52.

Li HX, Sze SC, Tong Y, Ng TB. Production of Th1- and Th2-dependent cytokines induced by the Chinese medicine herb, Rhodiola algida, on human peripheral blood monocytes. *J Ethnopharmacol.* 2009;123(2):257-266.

Li Y, Wu J, Shi R, et al. Antioxidative effects of Rhodiola genus: phytochemistry and pharmacological mechanisms against the diseases. *Curr Top Med Chem.* 2017;17(15):1692-1708.

Liu H, Lv P, Zhu Y, et al. Salidroside promotes peripheral nerve regeneration based on tissue engineering strategy using Schwann cells and PLGA: in vitro and in vivo. *Sci Rep.* 2017;7:39869.

Liu H, Lv P, Wu H, et al. The proliferation enhancing effects of salidroside on Schwann cells in vitro. *Evid Based Complement Alternat Med.* 2017;2017:4673289.

Liu SH, Hsaio Y-W, Chong E, et al. Rhodiola inhibits atrial arrhythmogenesis in a heart failure model. *J Cardiovasc Electrophysiol.* 2016;27(9):1093-1101.

Ma GP, Zheng Q, Xu MB, et al. *Rhodiola rosea* L. improves learning and memory function: preclinical evidence and possible mechanisms. *Front Pharmacol.* 2018;9:1415.

Mao JJ, Xie SX, Zee J, et al. Rhodiola rosea versus sertraline for major depressive disorder: a randomized placebo-controlled trial. *Phytomedicine.* 2015;22(3):394-399.

Megna M, Amico AP, Cristella G, Saggini R, Jirillo E, Ranieri M. Effects of herbal supplements on the immune system in relation to exercise. *Int J Immunopathol Pharmacol.* 2012;25(1 Suppl):43S-49S.

Miller SC, Delorme D, Shan JJ. CVT-E002 stimulates the immune system and extends the life span of mice bearing a tumor of viral origin. *J Soc Integr Oncol.* 2009;7(4):127-136.

Morgan LA, Grundmann O. Preclinical and potential applications of common Western herbal supplements as complementary treatment in Parkinson's disease. *J Diet Suppl.* 2017;14(4):453-466.

Nabavi SF, Braidy N, Orhan IE, et al. Rhodiola rosea L. and Alzheimer's disease: from farm to pharmacy. *Phytother Res.* 2016;30(4):532-539.

Olsson EM, von Schéele B, Panossian AG. A randomised, double-blind, placebo-controlled, parallel-group study of the standardised extract shr-5 of the roots of Rhodiola rosea in the treatment of subjects with stress-related fatigue. *Planta Med.* 2009;75(2):105-112.

Panossian A, Wikman G. Evidence-based efficacy of adaptogens in fatigue, and molecular mechanisms related to their stress-protective activity. *Curr Clin Pharmacol.* 2009;4(3):198-219.

Panossian A, Wikman G, Kaur P, Asea A. Adaptogens exert a stress-protective effect by modulation of expression of molecular chaperones. *Phytomedicine.* 2009;16(6-7):617-622.

Panossian A, Wikman G, Sarris J. Rosenroot (Rhodiola rosea): traditional use, chemical composition, pharmacology and clinical efficacy. *Phytomedicine.* 2010;17(7):481-493.

Recio MC, Giner RM, Máñez S. Immunomodulatory and antiproliferative properties of Rhodiola species. *Planta Med.* 2016;82(11-12):952-60.

Rege NN, Thatte UM, Dahanukar SA. Adaptogenic properties of six rasayana herbs used in Ayurvedic medicine. *Phytother Res.* 1999;13(4):275-291.

Thu OK, Nilsen OG, Hellum B. In vitro inhibition of cytochrome P-450 activities and quantification of constituents in a selection of commercial Rhodiola rosea products. *Pharm Biol.* 2016;54(12):3249-3256.

Vasileva LV, Getova DP, Doncheva ND, et al. Beneficial effect of commercial Rhodiola extract in rats with scopolamine-induced memory impairment on active avoidance. *J Ethnopharmacol.* 2016;193:586-591.

Wagner H, Nörr H, Winterhoff H. Plant adaptogens. *Phytomedicine.* 1994;1(1):63-76.

Xu X, Li P, Zhang P, et al. Differential effects of Rhodiola rosea on regulatory T cell differentiation and interferon-γ production in vitro and in vivo. *Mol Med Rep*. 2016;14(1):529-536.

Yokoyama NN, Denmon A, Uchio EM, et al. When anti-aging studies meet cancer chemoprevention: can anti-aging agent kill two birds with one blow? *Curr Pharmacol Rep*. 2015;1(6):420-433.

Zhang B, Wang Y, Li H, et al. Neuroprotective effects of salidroside through PI3K/Akt pathway activation in Alzheimer's disease models. *Drug Des Devel Ther*. 2016;10:1335-1343.

Zhang J, Kasim V, Xie Y-D, et al. Inhibition of PHD3 by salidroside promotes neovascularization through cell-cell communications mediated by muscle-secreted angiogenic factors. *Sci Rep*. 2017;7:43935.

Zhong L, Peng L, Fu J, Zou L, Zhao G, Zhao J. Phytochemical, antibacterial and antioxidant activity evaluation of *Rhodiola crenulata*. *Molecules*. 2020;25(16):3664.

Zhuang X, Maimaitijiang A, Li Y, et al. Salidroside inhibits high-glucose induced proliferation of vascular smooth muscle cells via inhibiting mitochondrial fission and oxidative stress. *Exp Ther Med*. 2017;14(1):515-524.

Reishi

Ahmad MF. Ganoderma lucidum: a rational pharmacological approach to surmount cancer. *J Ethnopharmacol*. 2020;260:113047.

Barbieri A, Quagliariello V, Del Vecchio V, et al. Anticancer and anti-inflammatory properties of Ganoderma lucidum extract effects on melanoma and triple-negative breast cancer treatment. *Nutrients*. 2017;9(3):210.

Gill BS, Navgeet, Kumar S. Ganoderma lucidum targeting lung cancer signaling: a review. *Tumour Biol*. 2017;39(6):1010428317707437.

Sliva D. Ganoderma lucidum (Reishi) in cancer treatment. *Integr Cancer Ther*. 2003;2(4):358-364.

Sohretoglu D, Huang S. Ganoderma lucidum polysaccharides as an anti-cancer agent. *Anticancer Agents Med Chem*. 2018;18(5):667-674.

Unlu A, Nayir E, Kirca O, Ozdogan M. Ganoderma lucidum (Reishi mushroom) and cancer. *J BUON*. 2016;21(4):792-798.

Turmeric

Bengmark S, Mesa MD, Gil A. Plant-derived health: the effects of turmeric and curcuminoids. *Nutr Hosp*. 2009;24(3):273-281.

Daily JW, Yang M, Park S. Efficacy of turmeric extracts and curcumin for alleviating the symptoms of Joint arthritis: a systematic review and meta-analysis of randomized clinical trials. *J Med Food*. 2016;19(8):717-729.

Divya CS, Pillai MR. Antitumor action of curcumin in human papillomavirus associated cells involves downregulation of viral oncogenes, prevention of NFkB and AP-1 translocation, and modulation of apoptosis. *Mol Carcinog*. 2006;45(5):320-332.

Gorabi AM, Hajighasemi S, Kiaie N, et al. Anti-fibrotic effects of curcumin and some of its analogues in the heart. *Heart Fail Rev*. 2020;25(5):731-743.

Gupta H, Gupta M, Bhargava S. Potential use of turmeric in COVID-19. *Clin Exp Dermatol*. 2020;45(7):902-903.

Gupta SC, Patchva S, Aggarwal BB. Therapeutic roles of curcumin: lessons learned from clinical trials. *AAPS J*. 2013;15(1):195-218.

He Y, Yue Y, Zheng X, Zhang K, Chen S, Du Z. Curcumin, inflammation, and chronic diseases: how are they linked? *Molecules*. 2015;20(5):9183-9213.

Hutchins-Wolfbrandt A, Mistry AM. Dietary turmeric potentially reduces the risk of cancer. *Asian Pac J Cancer Prev*. 2011;12(12):3169-3173.

Jurenka JS. Anti-inflammatory properties of curcumin, a major constituent of Curcuma longa: a review of preclinical and clinical research. *Altern Med Rev*. 2009;14(2):141-153. [published correction appears in *Altern Med Rev*. 2009;14(3):277.]

Kim Y, Clifton P. Curcumin, cardiometabolic health and dementia. *Int J Environ Res Public Health*. 2018;15(10):2093.

Kocaadam B, Şanlier N. Curcumin, an active component of turmeric (Curcuma longa), and its effects on health. *Crit Rev Food Sci Nutr*. 2017;57(13):2889-2895.

Kulczyński B, Gramza-Michałowska A. The importance of selected spices in cardiovascular diseases. *Postepy Hig Med Dosw (Online)*. 2016;70(0):1131-1141.

Kunnumakkara AB, Bordoloi D, Padmavathi G, et al. Curcumin, the golden nutraceutical: multitargeting for multiple chronic diseases. *Br J Pharmacol*. 2017;174(11):1325-1348.

Lee W-H, Loo C-Y, Bebawy M, et al. Curcumin and its derivatives: their application in neuropharmacology and neuroscience in the 21st Century. *Curr Neuropharmacol*. 2013;11(4):338-378.

Li H, Sureda A, Devkota HP, et al. Curcumin, the golden spice in treating cardiovascular diseases. *Biotechnol Adv*. 2020;38:107343.

Moghadamtousi SZ, Kadir HA, Hassandarvish P, Tajik H, Abubakar S, Zandi K. A review on antibacterial, antiviral, and antifungal activity of curcumin. *Biomed Res Int*. 2014;2014:186864.

Ng T-P, Chiam P-C, Lee T, et al. Curry consumption and cognitive function in the elderly. *Am J Epidemiol.* 2006;164(9):898-906.

Pivari F, Mingione A, Brasacchio C, Soldati L. Curcumin and type 2 diabetes mellitus: prevention and treatment. *Nutrients.* 2019;11(8):1837.

Prusty BK, Das BC. Constitutive activation of transcription factor AP-1 in cervical cancer and suppression of human papillomavirus (HPV) transcription and AP-1 activity in HeLa cells by curcumin. *Int J Cancer.* 2005;113(6):951-960.

Qin S, Huang L, Gong J, et al. Efficacy and safety of turmeric and curcumin in lowering blood lipid levels in patients with cardiovascular risk factors: a meta-analysis of randomized controlled trials. *Nutr J.* 2017;16(1):68.

Soleimani V, Sahebkar A, Hosseinzadeh H. Turmeric (Curcuma longa) and its major constituent (curcumin) as nontoxic and safe substances: review. *Phytother Res.* 2018;32(6):985-995.

Vaughn AR, Branum A, Sivamani RK. Effects of turmeric (Curcuma longa) on skin health: a systematic review of the clinical evidence. *Phytother Res.* 2016;30(8):1243-1264.

Gotu Kola

Bylka W, Znajdek-Awiżeń P, Studzińska-Sroka E, Brzezińska M. Centella asiatica in cosmetology. *Postepy Dermatol Alergol.* 2013;30(1):46-49.

Bylka W, Znajdek-Awiżeń P, Studzińska-Sroka E, Dańczak-Pazdrowska A, Brzezińska M. Centella asiatica in dermatology: an overview. *Phytother Res.* 2014;28(8):1117-1124.

Ceremuga TE, Valdivieso D, Kenner C, et al. Evaluation of the anxiolytic and antidepressant effects of asiatic acid, a compound from Gotu kola or Centella asiatica, in the male Sprague Dawley rat. *AANA J.* 2015;83(2):91-98.

Gohil KJ, Patel JA, Gajjar AK. Pharmacological review on Centella asiatica: a potential herbal cure-all. *Indian J Pharm Sci.* 2010;72(5):546-556.

Jana U, Sur TK, Maity LN, Debnath PK, Bhattacharyya D. A clinical study on the management of generalized anxiety disorder with Centella asiatica. *Nepal Med Coll J.* 2010;12(1):8-11.

Kabir AU, Samad MB, D'Costa NM, Akhter F, Ahmed A, Hannan JM. Anti-hyperglycemic activity of Centella asiatica is partly mediated by carbohydrase inhibition and glucose-fiber binding. *BMC Complement Altern Med.* 2014;14:31.

Lokanathan Y, Omar N, Ahmad Puzi NN, Saim A, Hj Idrus R. Recent updates in neuroprotective and neuroregenerative potential of Centella asiatica. *Malays J Med Sci.* 2016;23(1):4-14.

Orhan IE. Centella asiatica (L.) urban: from traditional medicine to modern medicine with neuroprotective potential. *Evid Based Complement Alternat Med.* 2012;2012:946259.

Milk Thistle

Abenavoli L, Izzo AA, Milić N, Cicala C, Santini A, Capasso R. Milk thistle (Silybum marianum): a concise overview on its chemistry, pharmacological, and nutraceutical uses in liver diseases. *Phytother Res.* 2018;32(11):2202-2213.

Aller R, Izaola O, Gómez S, et al. Effect of silymarin plus vitamin E in patients with non-alcoholic fatty liver disease. A randomized clinical pilot study. *Eur Rev Med Pharmacol Sci.* 2015;19(16):3118-3124.

Borah A, Paul R, Choudhury S, et al. Neuroprotective potential of silymarin against CNS disorders: insight into the pathways and molecular mechanisms of action. *CNS Neurosci Ther.* 2013;19(11):847-853.

Casas-Grajales S, Muriel P. Antioxidants in liver health. *World J Gastrointest Pharmacol Ther.* 2015;6(3):59-72.

Gillessen A, Schmidt HH. Silymarin as supportive treatment in liver diseases: a narrative review. *Adv Ther.* 2020;37(4):1279-1301.

Kalantari H, Shahshahan Z, Hejazi SM, Ghafghazi T, Sebghatolahi V. Effects of silybum marianum on patients with chronic hepatitis C. *J Res Med Sci.* 2011;16(3):287-290.

Mastron JK, Siveen KS, Sethi G, Bishayee A. Silymarin and hepatocellular carcinoma: a systematic, comprehensive, and critical review. *Anticancer Drugs.* 2015;26(5):475-486.

Milić N, Milosević N, Suvajdzić L, Zarkov M, Abenavoli L. New therapeutic potentials of milk thistle (Silybum marianum). *Nat Prod Commun.* 2013;8(12):1801-1810.

Ramasamy K, Agarwal R. Multitargeted therapy of cancer by silymarin. *Cancer Lett.* 2008;269(2):352-362.

Rastegarpanah M, Malekzadeh R, Vahedi H, et al. A randomized, double blinded, placebo-controlled clinical trial of silymarin in ulcerative colitis. *Chin J Integr Med.* 2015;21(12):902-906.

Saller R, Meier R, Brignoli R. The use of silymarin in the treatment of liver diseases. *Drugs.* 2001;61(14):2035-2063.

Surai PF. Silymarin as a natural antioxidant: an overview of the current evidence and perspectives. *Antioxidants (Basel).* 2015;4(1):204-247.

Vargas-Mendoza N, Madrigal-Santillán E, Morales-González A, et al. Hepatoprotective effect of silymarin. *World J Hepatol.* 2014;6(3):144-149.

Wang X, Zhang Z, Wu SC. Health benefits of *Silybum marianum*: phytochemistry, pharmacology, and applications. *J Agric Food Chem.* 2020;68(42):11644-11664.

Wei F, Liu SK, Liu XY, et al. Meta-analysis: silymarin and its combination therapy for the treatment of chronic hepatitis B. *Eur J Clin Microbiol Infect Dis*. 2013;32(5):657-669.

Xiao J, Fai So K, Liong EC, Tipoe GL. Recent advances in the herbal treatment of non-alcoholic fatty liver disease. *J Tradit Complement Med*. 2013;3(2):88-94.

Shilajit

Biswas TK, Pandit S, Mondal S, et al. Clinical evaluation of spermatogenic activity of processed Shilajit in oligospermia. *Andrologia*. 2010;42(1):48-56.

Cagno V, Donalisio M, Civra A, Cagliero C, Rubiolo P, Lembo D. In vitro evaluation of the antiviral properties of Shilajit and investigation of its mechanisms of action. *J Ethnopharmacol*. 2015;166:129-134.

Carrasco-Gallardo C, Guzmán L, Maccioni RB. Shilajit: a natural phytocomplex with potential procognitive activity. *Int J Alzheimers Dis*. 2012;2012:674142.

Das A, Datta S, Rhea B, et al. The human skeletal muscle transcriptome in response to oral shilajit supplementation. *J Med Food*. 2016;19(7):701-709.

Wilson E, Rajamanickam GV, Dubey GP, et al. Review on shilajit used in traditional Indian medicine. *J Ethnopharmacol*. 2011;136(1):1-9.

Goel RK, Banerjee RS, Acharya SB. Antiulcerogenic and antiinflammatory studies with shilajit. *J Ethnopharmacol*. 1990;29(1):95-103.

Keller JL, Housh TJ, Hill EC, Smith CM, Schmidt RJ, Johnson GO. The effects of Shilajit supplementation on fatigue-induced decreases in muscular strength and serum hydroxyproline levels. *J Int Soc Sports Nutr*. 2019;16(1):3.

Meena H, Pandey HK, Arya MC, Ahmed Z. Shilajit: a panacea for high-altitude problems. *Int J Ayurveda Res*. 2010;1(1):37-40.

Pandit S, Biswas S, Jana U, De RK, Mukhopadhyay SC, Biswas TK. Clinical evaluation of purified Shilajit on testosterone levels in healthy volunteers. *Andrologia*. 2016;48(5):570-575.

Schepetkin IA, Khlebnikov AI, Ah SY, et al. Characterization and biological activities of humic substances from mumie. *J Agric Food Chem*. 2003;51(18):5245-5254.

Surapaneni DK, Adapa SR, Preeti K, Teja GR, Veeraragavan M, Krishnamurthy S. Shilajit attenuates behavioral symptoms of chronic fatigue syndrome by modulating the hypothalamic-pituitary-adrenal axis and mitochondrial bioenergetics in rats. *J Ethnopharmacol*. 2012;143(1):91-99.

Vucskits AV, Hullár I, Bersényi A, Andrásofszky E, Kulcsár M, Szabó J. Effect of fulvic and humic acids on performance, immune response and thyroid function in rats. *J Anim Physiol Anim Nutr (Berl)*. 2010;94(6):721-728.

Wilson E, Rajamanickam GV, Dubey GP, et al. Review on shilajit used in traditional Indian medicine. *J Ethnopharmacol.* 2011;136(1):1-9.

Winkler J, Ghosh S. Therapeutic potential of fulvic acid in chronic inflammatory diseases and diabetes. *J Diabetes Res.* 2018;2018:5391014.

Chapter 10: Antimicrobial Herbs

Antibiotics and Antibiotic Resistance

Arshad N, Mehreen A, Liaqat I, Arshad M, Afrasiab H. In vivo screening and evaluation of four herbs against MRSA infections. *BMC Complement Altern Med.* 2017;17(1):498.

Buyck JM, Lemaire S, Seral C, et al. In vitro models for the study of the intracellular activity of antibiotics. *Methods Mol Biol.* 2016;1333:147-157.

Davies J, Davies D. Origins and evolution of antibiotic resistance. *Microbiol Mol Biol Rev.* 2010;74(3):417-433.

Durack J, Lynch SV. The gut microbiome: relationships with disease and opportunities for therapy. *J Exp Med.* 2019;216(1):20-40.

Gaynes R. The discovery of penicillin—new insights after more than 75 years of clinical use. *Emerg Infect Dis.* 2017;23(5):849-853.

Gupta PD, Birdi TJ. Development of botanicals to combat antibiotic resistance. *J Ayurveda Integr Med.* 2017;8(4):266-275.

Kuok CF, Hoi SO, Hoi CF, et al. Synergistic antibacterial effects of herbal extracts and antibiotics on methicillin-resistant Staphylococcus aureus: a computational and experimental study. *Exp Biol Med (Maywood).* 2017;242(7):731-743.

Lobanovska M, Pilla G. Penicillin's discovery and antibiotic resistance: lessons for the future? *Yale J Biol Med.* 2017;90(1):135-145.

Mehta RS, Lochhead P, Wang Y, et al. Association of midlife antibiotic use with subsequent cognitive function in women. *PLoS One.* 2022;17(3):e0264649.

Su T, Qiu Y, Hua X, et al. Novel opportunity to reverse antibiotic resistance: to explore traditional Chinese medicine with potential activity against antibiotics-resistance bacteria. *Front Microbiol.* 2020;11:610070.

Wencewicz TA. Crossroads of antibiotic resistance and biosynthesis. *J Mol Biol.* 2019;431(18):3370-3399.

Vanrompay D, Nguyen TLA, Cutler SJ, Butaye P. Antimicrobial resistance in *Chlamydiales, Rickettsia, Coxiella*, and other intracellular pathogens. *Microbiol Spectr.* 2018;6(2):10.1128/microbiolspec.ARBA-0003-2017.

Antimicrobial Herbs

Abreu AC, McBain AJ, Simões M. Plants as sources of new antimicrobials and resistance-modifying agents. *Nat Prod Rep.* 2012;29(9):1007-1021.

Adnan M, Ali S, Sheikh K, Amber R. Review on antibacterial activity of Himalayan medicinal plants traditionally used to treat pneumonia and tuberculosis. *J Pharm Pharmacol.* 2019;71(11):1599-1625.

Ahmad I, Aqil F. In vitro efficacy of bioactive extracts of 15 medicinal plants against ESbetaL-producing multidrug-resistant enteric bacteria. *Microbiol Res.* 2007;162(3):264-275.

An X, Bao Q, Di S, et al. The interaction between the gut microbiota and herbal medicines. *Biomed Pharmacother.* 2019;118:109252.

An X, Zhang Y, Duan L, et al. The direct evidence and mechanism of traditional Chinese medicine treatment of COVID-19. *Biomed Pharmacother.* 2021;137:111267.

Aqil F, Ahmad I. Antibacterial properties of traditionally used Indian medicinal plants. *Methods Find Exp Clin Pharmacol.* 2007;29(2):79-92.

Bibi R, Tariq A, Mussarat S, et al. Review: ethnomedicinal, phytochemical and antibacterial activities of medicinal flora of Pakistan used against Pseudomonas aeruginosa-a review. *Pak J Pharm Sci.* 2017;30(6):2285-2300.

Borges A, Saavedra MJ, Simões M. Insights on antimicrobial resistance, biofilms and the use of phytochemicals as new antimicrobial agents. *Curr Med Chem.* 2015;22(21):2590-2614.

Cock IE, Van Vuuren SF. The traditional use of southern African medicinal plants for the treatment of bacterial respiratory diseases: a review of the ethnobotany and scientific evaluations. *J Ethnopharmacol.* 2020;263:113204.

Cowan MM. Plant products as antimicrobial agents. *Clin Microbiol Rev.* 1999;12(4):564-582.

Das S. Natural therapeutics for urinary tract infections-a review. *Futur J Pharm Sci.* 2020;6(1):64.

Feng J, Leone J, Schweig S, Zhang Y. Evaluation of natural and botanical medicines for activity against growing and non-growing forms of *B. burgdorferi. Front Med (Lausanne).* 2020;7:6.

Hossan MS, Jindal H, Maisha S, et al. Antibacterial effects of 18 medicinal plants used by the Khyang tribe in Bangladesh. *Pharm Biol.* 2018;56(1):201-208.

Ma X, Leone J, Schweig S, Zhang Y. Botanical medicines with activity against stationary phase *Bartonella henselae. Cold Spring Harbor Laboratory.* Aug 28, 2020.

Madureira AM, Ramalhete C, Mulhovo S, Duarte A, Ferreira MJ. Antibacterial activity of some African medicinal plants used traditionally against infectious diseases. *Pharm Biol.* 2012;50(4):481-489.

Ríos JL, Recio MC. Medicinal plants and antimicrobial activity. *J Ethnopharmacol.* 2005;100(1-2):80-84.

Romulo A, Zuhud EAM, Rondevaldova J, Kokoska L. Screening of in vitro antimicrobial activity of plants used in traditional Indonesian medicine. *Pharm Biol.* 2018;56(1):287-293.

Silveira D, Prieto-Garcia JM, Boylan F, et al. COVID-19: is there evidence for the use of herbal medicines as adjuvant symptomatic therapy? *Front Pharmacol.* 2020;11:581840.

Vestergaard M, Ingmer H. Antibacterial and antifungal properties of resveratrol. *Int J Antimicrob Agents.* 2019;53(6):716-723.

Walusansa A, Asiimwe S, Nakavuma JL, et al. Antibiotic-resistance in medically important bacteria isolated from commercial herbal medicines in Africa from 2000 to 2021: a systematic review and meta-analysis. *Antimicrob Resist Infect Control.* 2022;11(1):11.

Zhang Y, Alvarez-Manzo H, Leone J, Schweig S, Zhang Y. Botanical medicines Cryptolepis sanguinolenta, Artemisia annua, Scutellaria baicalensis, Polygonum cuspidatum, and Alchornea cordifolia demonstrate inhibitory activity against Babesia duncani. *Front Cell Infect Microbiol.* 2021;11:624745.

Japanese Knotweed

Aluyen JK, Ton QN, Tran T, Yang AE, Gottlieb HB, Bellanger RA. Resveratrol: potential as anticancer agent. *J Diet Suppl.* 2012;9(1):45-56.

Cheng L, Jin Z, Zhao R, Ren K, Deng C, Yu S. Resveratrol attenuates inflammation and oxidative stress induced by myocardial ischemia-reperfusion injury: role of Nrf2/ARE pathway. *Int J Clin Exp Med.* 2015;8(7):10420-10428.

Cong X, Li Y, Lu N, et al. Resveratrol attenuates the inflammatory reaction induced by ischemia/reperfusion in the rat heart. *Mol Med Rep.* 2014;9(6):2528-2532.

Dolinsky VW, Dyck JR. Experimental studies of the molecular pathways regulated by exercise and resveratrol in heart, skeletal muscle and the vasculature. *Molecules.* 2014;19(9):14919-14947.

Ghanim H, Sia CL, Abuaysheh S, et al. An antiinflammatory and reactive oxygen species suppressive effects of an extract of Polygonum cuspidatum containing resveratrol. *J Clin Endocrinol Metab.* 2010;95(9):E1-E8.

Han JH, Koh W, Lee HJ, et al. Analgesic and anti-inflammatory effects of ethyl acetate fraction of Polygonum cuspidatum in experimental animals. *Immunopharmacol Immunotoxicol.* 2012;34(2):191-195.

Joshi MS, Williams D, Horlock D, et al. Role of mitochondrial dysfunction in hyperglycaemia-induced coronary microvascular dysfunction: protective role of resveratrol. *Diab Vasc Dis Res*. 2015;12(3):208-216.

Kakoti BB, Hernandez-Ontiveros DG, Kataki MS, Shah K, Pathak Y, Panguluri SK. Resveratrol and omega-3 fatty acid: its implications in cardiovascular diseases. *Front Cardiovasc Med*. 2015;2:38.

Kirino A, Takasuka Y, Nishi A, et al. Analysis and functionality of major polyphenolic components of Polygonum cuspidatum (itadori). *J Nutr Sci Vitaminol (Tokyo)*. 2012;58(4):278-286.

Kurita S, Kashiwagi T, Ebisu T, Shimamura T, Ukeda H. Content of resveratrol and glycoside and its contribution to the antioxidative capacity of Polygonum cuspidatum (Itadori) harvested in Kochi. *Biosci Biotechnol Biochem*. 2014;78(3):499-502.

Lin CJ, Lin HJ, Chen TH, et al. Polygonum cuspidatum and its active components inhibit replication of the influenza virus through toll-like receptor 9-induced interferon beta expression *PLoS One*. 2015;10(2):e0117602. [published correction appears in *PLoS One*. 2015;10(4):e0125288].

Lin SP, Chu PM, Tsai SY, Wu MH, Hou YC. Pharmacokinetics and tissue distribution of resveratrol, emodin and their metabolites after intake of Polygonum cuspidatum in rats. *J Ethnopharmacol*. 2012;144(3):671-676.

Liu Y, Ma W, Zhang P, He S, Huang D. Effect of resveratrol on blood pressure: a meta-analysis of randomized controlled trials. *Clin Nutr*. 2015;34(1):27-34.

Liu Z, Wei F, Chen LJ, et al. In vitro and in vivo studies of the inhibitory effects of emodin isolated from Polygonum cuspidatum on Coxsakievirus B_4. *Molecules*. 2013;18(10):11842-11858.

Meng C, Liu JL, Du AL. Cardioprotective effect of resveratrol on atherogenic diet-fed rats. *Int J Clin Exp Pathol*. 2014;7(11):7899-7906.

Mokni M, Hamlaoui S, Karkouch I, et al. Resveratrol provides cardioprotection after ischemia/reperfusion injury via modulation of antioxidant enzyme activities. *Iran J Pharm Res*. 2013;12(4):867-875.

Su PW, Yang CH, Yang JF, Su PY, Chuang LY. Antibacterial activities and antibacterial mechanism of Polygonum cuspidatum extracts against nosocomial drug-resistant Pathogens. *Molecules*. 2015;20(6):11119-11130.

Pasinetti GM, Wang J, Ho L, Zhao W, Dubner L. Roles of resveratrol and other grape-derived polyphenols in Alzheimer's disease prevention and treatment. *Biochim Biophys Acta*. 2015;1852(6):1202-1208.

Peng W, Qin R, Li X, Zhou H. Botany, phytochemistry, pharmacology, and potential application of Polygonum cuspidatum Sieb.et Zucc.: a review. *J Ethnopharmacol*. 2013;148(3):729-745.

Piotrowska H, Kucinska M, Murias M. Biological activity of piceatannol: leaving the shadow of resveratrol. *Mutat Res*. 2012;750(1):60-82.

Rabassa M, Zamora-Ros R, Urpi-Sarda M, Andres-Lacueva C. Resveratrol metabolite profiling in clinical nutrition research--from diet to uncovering disease risk biomarkers: epidemiological evidence. *Ann N Y Acad Sci*. 2015;1348(1):107-115.

Raj P, Zieroth S, Netticadan T. An overview of the efficacy of resveratrol in the management of ischemic heart disease. *Ann N Y Acad Sci*. 2015;1348(1):55-67.

Schwager J, Richard N, Widmer F, Raederstorff D. Resveratrol distinctively modulates the inflammatory profiles of immune and endothelial cells. *BMC Complement Altern Med*. 2017;17(1):309.

Song JH, Kim SK, Chang KW, Han SK, Yi HK, Jeon JG. In vitro inhibitory effects of Polygonum cuspidatum on bacterial viability and virulence factors of Streptococcus mutans and Streptococcus sobrinus. *Arch Oral Biol*. 2006;51(12):1131-1140.

Su PW, Yang CH, Yang JF, Su PY, Chuang LY. Antibacterial activities and antibacterial mechanism of Polygonum cuspidatum extracts against nosocomial drug-resistant pathogens. *Molecules*. 2015;20(6):11119-11130.

Wang HL, Gao JP, Han YL, et al. Comparative studies of polydatin and resveratrol on mutual transformation and antioxidative effect in vivo. *Phytomedicine*. 2015;22(5):553-559.

Xie HC, Han HP, Chen Z, He JP. A study on the effect of resveratrol on lipid metabolism in hyperlipidemic mice. *Afr J Tradit Complement Altern Med*. 2013;11(1):209-212.

Yang X, Li X, Ren J. From French paradox to cancer treatment: anti-cancer activities and mechanisms of resveratrol. *Anticancer Agents Med Chem*. 2014;14(6):806-825.

Yiu CY, Chen SY, Yang TH, et al. Inhibition of Epstein-Barr virus lytic cycle by an ethyl acetate subfraction separated from Polygonum cuspidatum root and its major component, emodin. *Molecules*. 2014;19(1):1258-1272.

Zheng H, Guo H, Hong Y, Zheng F, Wang J. The effects of age and resveratrol on the hypoxic preconditioning protection against hypoxia-reperfusion injury: studies in rat hearts and human cardiomyocytes. *Eur J Cardiothorac Surg*. 2015;48(3):375-381.

Chinese Skullcap

Butenko IG, Gladtchenko SV, Galushko SV. Anti-inflammatory properties and inhibition of leukotriene C4 biosynthesis in vitro by flavonoid baicalein from Scutellaria baicalensis georgy roots. *Agents Actions*. 1993;39 Spec No:C49-C51.

Chien CF, Wu YT, Tsai TH. Biological analysis of herbal medicines used for the treatment of liver diseases. *Biomed Chromatogr*. 2011;25(1-2):21-38.

Gasiorowski K, Lamer-Zarawska E, Leszek J, et al. Flavones from root of Scutellaria baicalensis Georgi: drugs of the future in neurodegeneration?. *CNS Neurol Disord Drug Targets*. 2011;10(2):184-191.

Huang Y, Tsang SY, Yao X, Chen ZY. Biological properties of baicalein in cardiovascular system. *Curr Drug Targets Cardiovasc Haematol Disord.* 2005;5(2):177-184.

Jung HS, Kim MH, Gwak NG, et al. Antiallergic effects of Scutellaria baicalensis on inflammation in vivo and in vitro. *J Ethnopharmacol.* 2012;141(1):345-349.

Konoshima T, Kokumai M, Kozuka M, et al. Studies on inhibitors of skin tumor promotion. XI. Inhibitory effects of flavonoids from Scutellaria baicalensis on Epstein-Barr virus activation and their anti-tumor-promoting activities. *Chem Pharm Bull (Tokyo).* 1992;40(2):531-533.

Li K, Liang Y, Cheng A, et al. Antiviral properties of Baicalin: a concise review. *Rev Bras Farmacogn.* 2021;31(4):408-419.

Li-Weber M. New therapeutic aspects of flavones: the anticancer properties of Scutellaria and its main active constituents Wogonin, Baicalein and Baicalin. *Cancer Treat Rev.* 2009;35(1):57-68.

Muluye RA, Bian Y, Alemu PN. Anti-inflammatory and antimicrobial effects of heat-clearing Chinese herbs: a current review. *J Tradit Complement Med.* 2014;4(2):93-98.

Piao HZ, Jin SA, Chun HS, Lee JC, Kim WK. Neuroprotective effect of wogonin: potential roles of inflammatory cytokines. *Arch Pharm Res.* 2004;27(9):930-936.

Shang X, He X, He X, et al. The genus Scutellaria an ethnopharmacological and phytochemical review. *J Ethnopharmacol.* 2010;128(2):279-313.

Shi H, Ren K, Lv B, et al. Baicalin from Scutellaria baicalensis blocks respiratory syncytial virus (RSV) infection and reduces inflammatory cell infiltration and lung injury in mice. *Sci Rep.* 2016;6:35851.

Yune TY, Lee JY, Cui CM, Kim HC, Oh TH. Neuroprotective effect of Scutellaria baicalensis on spinal cord injury in rats. *J Neurochem.* 2009;110(4):1276-1287.

Zhao Q, Chen XY, Martin C. *Scutellaria baicalensis*, the golden herb from the garden of Chinese medicinal plants. *Sci Bull (Beijing).* 2016;61(18):1391-1398.

Andrographis

Bertoglio JC, Baumgartner M, Palma R, et al. Andrographis paniculata decreases fatigue in patients with relapsing-remitting multiple sclerosis: a 12-month double-blind placebo-controlled pilot study. *BMC Neurol.* 2016;16:77.

Burgos RA, Hancke JL, Bertoglio JC, et al. Efficacy of an Andrographis paniculata composition for the relief of rheumatoid arthritis symptoms: a prospective randomized placebo-controlled trial. *Clin Rheumatol.* 2009;28(8):931-946.

Choudhary P, Bhowmik A, Chakdar H, et al. Understanding the biological role of PqqB in *Pseudomonas stutzeri* using molecular dynamics simulation approach. *J Biomol Struct Dyn.* 2020;1-13.

Chua LS. Review on liver inflammation and antiinflammatory activity of Andrographis paniculata for hepatoprotection. *Phytother Res.* 2014;28(11):1589-1598.

Hossain S, Urbi Z, Karuniawati H, et al. *Andrographis paniculata* (Burm. f.) Wall. ex Nees: an updated review of phytochemistry, antimicrobial pharmacology, and clinical safety and efficacy. *Life (Basel).* 2021;11(4):348.

Islam MT, Ali ES, Uddin SJ, et al. Andrographolide, a diterpene lactone from Andrographis paniculata and its therapeutic promises in cancer. *Cancer Lett.* 2018;420:129-145.

Jayakumar T, Hsieh C-Y, Lee, J-J, Sheu J-R. Experimental and clinical pharmacology of Andrographis paniculata and its major bioactive phytoconstituent andrographolide. *Evid Based Complement Alternat Med.* 2013;2013:846740.

Kishore V, Bishayee A, Putta S, et al. Multi-targeting andrographolide and its natural analogs as potential therapeutic agents. *Curr Top Med Chem.* 2017;17(8):845-857.

Koh PH, Mokhtar RA, Iqbal M. Andrographis paniculata ameliorates carbon tetrachloride (CCl(4))-dependent hepatic damage and toxicity: diminution of oxidative stress. *Redox Rep.* 2011;16(3):134-143.

Li GF, Qin YH, Du PQ. Andrographolide inhibits the migration, invasion and matrix metalloproteinase expression of rheumatoid arthritis fibroblast-like synoviocytes via inhibition of HIF-1α signaling. *Life Sci.* 2015;136:67-72.

Li ZZ, Tan JP, Wang LL, Li QH. Andrographolide benefits rheumatoid arthritis via inhibiting MAPK pathways. *Inflammation.* 2017;40(5):1599-1605.

Lim JC, Chan TK, Ng DSW, et al. Andrographolide and its analogues: versatile bioactive molecules for combating inflammation and cancer. *Clin Exp Pharmacol Physiol.* 2012;39(3):300-310.

Lu J, Ma Y, Wu J, et al. A review for the neuroprotective effects of andrographolide in the central nervous system. *Biomed Pharmacother.* 2019;117:109078.

Mishra SK, Tripathi S, Shukla A, Oh SH, Kim HM. Andrographolide and analogues in cancer prevention. *Front Biosci (Elite Ed).* 2015;7:255-266.

Mishra US, Mishra A, Kumari R, Murthy PN, Naik BS. Antibacterial activity of ethanol extract of Andrographis paniculata. *Indian J Pharm Sci.* 2009;71(4):436-438.

Murugan NA, Pandian CJ, Jeyakanthan J. Computational investigation on *Andrographis paniculata* phytochemicals to evaluate their potency against SARS-CoV-2 in comparison to known antiviral compounds in drug trials. *J Biomol Struct Dyn.* 2020;1-12.

Nugroho AE, Andrie M, Warditiani NK, et al. Antidiabetic and antihiperlipidemic effect of Andrographis paniculata (Burm. f.) Nees and andrographolide in high-fructose-fat-fed rats. *Indian J Pharmacol.* 2012; 44(3):377-381.

Rana AC, Avadhoot Y. Hepatoprotective effects of Andrographis paniculata against carbon tetrachloride-induced liver damage. *Arch Pharm Res*. 1991;14(1):93-95.

Sa-Ngiamsuntorn K, Suksatu A, Pewkliang Y, et al. Anti-SARS-CoV-2 activity of *Andrographis paniculata* extract and its major component andrographolide in human lung epithelial cells and cytotoxicity evaluation in major organ cell representatives. *J Nat Prod*. 2021;84(4):1261-1270.

Sandborn WJ, Targan SR, Byers VS, et al. Andrographis paniculata extract (HMPL-004) for active ulcerative colitis. *Am J Gastroenterol*. 2013;108(1):90-98.

Singha PK, Roy S, Dey S. Antimicrobial activity of Andrographis paniculata. *Fitoterapia*. 2003;74(7-8):692-694.

Tang T, Targan SR, Li ZS, Xu C, Byers VS, Sandborn WJ. Randomised clinical trial: herbal extract HMPL-004 in active ulcerative colitis - a double-blind comparison with sustained release mesalazine. *Aliment Pharmacol Ther*. 2011;33(2):194-202.

Thakur AK, Chatterjee SS, Kumar V. Adaptogenic potential of andrographolide: an active principle of the king of bitters (Andrographis paniculata). *J Tradit Complement Med*. 2014;5(1):42-50.

Widjajakusuma EC, Jonosewojo A, Hendriati L, et al. Phytochemical screening and preliminary clinical trials of the aqueous extract mixture of Andrographis paniculata (Burm. f.) Wall. ex Nees and Syzygium polyanthum (Wight.) Walp leaves in metformin treated patients with type 2 diabetes. *Phytomedicine*. 2019;55:137-147.

Yan J, Chen Y, He C, Yang ZZ, Lü C, Chen XS. Andrographolide induces cell cycle arrest and apoptosis in human rheumatoid arthritis fibroblast-like synoviocytes. *Cell Biol Toxicol*. 2012;28(1):47-56.

Zeng M, Jiang W, Tian Y, et al. Andrographolide inhibits arrhythmias and is cardioprotective in rabbits. *Oncotarget*. 2017;8(37):61226-61238.

Zhai ZJ, Li HW, Liu GW, et al. Andrographolide suppresses RANKL-induced osteoclastogenesis in vitro and prevents inflammatory bone loss in vivo. *Br J Pharmacol*. 2014;171(3):663-675.

Cat's Claw

Ahmed S, Anuntiyo J, Malemud CJ, Haqqi TM. Biological basis for the use of botanicals in osteoarthritis and rheumatoid arthritis: a review. *Evid Based Complement Alternat Med*. 2005;2(3):301-308.

Allen-Hall L, Arnason JT, Cano P, Lafrenie RM. Uncaria tomentosa acts as a potent TNF-alpha inhibitor through NF-kappaB. *J Ethnopharmacol*. 2010;127(3):685-693.

Araujo LCC, Feitosa KB, Murata GM, et al. Uncaria tomentosa improves insulin sensitivity and inflammation in experimental NAFLD. *Sci Rep*. 2018;8(1):11013.

Ccahuana-Vasquez RA, Santos SS, Koga-Ito CY, Jorge AO. Antimicrobial activity of Uncaria tomentosa against oral human pathogens. *Braz Oral Res*. 2007;21(1):46-50.

Ciani F, Tafuri S, Troiano A, et al. Anti-proliferative and pro-apoptotic effects of Uncaria tomentosa aqueous extract in squamous carcinoma cells. *J Ethnopharmacol*. 2018;211:285-294.

de Paula LC, Fonseca F, Perazzo F, et al. Uncaria tomentosa (cat's claw) improves quality of life in patients with advanced solid tumors. *J Altern Complement Med*. 2015;21(1):22-30.

Della Valle V. Uncaria tomentosa. *G Ital Dermatol Venereol*. 2017;152(6):651-657.

Domingues A, Sartori A, Valente LM, Golim MA, Siani AC, Viero RM. Uncaria tomentosa aqueous-ethanol extract triggers an immunomodulation toward a Th2 cytokine profile. *Phytother Res*. 2011;25(8):1229-1235.

Gonçalves C, Dinis T, Batista MT. Antioxidant properties of proanthocyanidins of Uncaria tomentosa bark decoction: a mechanism for anti-inflammatory activity. *Phytochemistry*. 2005;66(1):89-98.

Kośmider A, Czepielewska E, Kuraś M, et al. Uncaria tomentosa leaves decoction modulates differently ROS production in cancer and normal cells, and effects cisplatin cytotoxicity. *Molecules*. 2017;22(4):620.

Mammone T, Akesson C, Gan D, Giampapa V, Pero RW. A water soluble extract from Uncaria tomentosa (Cat's Claw) is a potent enhancer of DNA repair in primary organ cultures of human skin. *Phytother Res*. 2006;20(3):178-183.

Navarro-Hoyos M, Lebrón-Aguilar R, Quintanilla-López JE, et al. Proanthocyanidin characterization and bioactivity of extracts from different parts of Uncaria tomentosa L. (cat's claw). *Antioxidants (Basel)*. 2017;6(1):12.

Piscoya J, Rodriguez Z, Bustamante SA, Okuhama NN, Miller MJ, Sandoval M. Efficacy and safety of freeze-dried cat's claw in osteoarthritis of the knee: mechanisms of action of the species Uncaria guianensis. *Inflamm Res*. 2001;50(9):442-448.

Reis SR, Valente LM, Sampaio AL, et al. Immunomodulating and antiviral activities of Uncaria tomentosa on human monocytes infected with Dengue Virus-2. *Int Immunopharmacol*. 2008;8(3):468-476.

Rojas-Duran R, González-Aspajo G, Ruiz-Martel C, et al. Anti-inflammatory activity of mitraphylline isolated from Uncaria tomentosa bark. *J Ethnopharmacol*. 2012;143(3):801-804.

Sandoval M, Okuhama NN, Zhang XJ, et al. Anti-inflammatory and antioxidant activities of cat's claw (Uncaria tomentosa and Uncaria guianensis) are independent of their alkaloid content. *Phytomedicine*. 2002;9(4):325-337.

Sandoval-Chacón M, Thompson JH, Zhang XJ, et al. Antiinflammatory actions of cat's claw: the role of NF-kappaB. *Aliment Pharmacol Ther*. 1998;12(12):1279-1289.

Snow AD, Castillo GM, Nguyen BP, et al. The Amazon rain forest plant Uncaria tomentosa (cat's claw) and its specific proanthocyanidin constituents are potent inhibitors and reducers of both brain plaques and tangles. *Sci Rep*. 2019;9(1):561.

Williams JE. Review of antiviral and immunomodulating properties of plants of the Peruvian rainforest with a particular emphasis on Una de Gato and Sangre de Grado. *Altern Med Rev*. 2001;6(6):567-579.

Garlic/Allicin

Ankri S, Mirelman D. Antimicrobial properties of allicin from garlic. *Microbes Infect*. 1999;1(2):125-129.

Ban JO, Oh JH, Kim TM, et al. Anti-inflammatory and arthritic effects of thiacremonone, a novel sulfur compound isolated from garlic via inhibition of NF-kappaB. *Arthritis Res Ther*. 2009;11(5):R145.

Borlinghaus J, Albrecht F, Gruhlke MC, Nwachukwu ID, Slusarenko AJ. Allicin: chemistry and biological properties. *Molecules*. 2014;19(8):12591-12618.

Chan JY-Y, Yuen AC-Y, Chan RY-K, Chan S-W. A review of the cardiovascular benefits and antioxidant properties of allicin. *Phytother Res*. 2013;27(5):637-646.

Chen K, Xie K, Liu Z, et al. Preventive effects and mechanisms of garlic on dyslipidemia and gut microbiome dysbiosis. *Nutrients*. 2019;11(6):1225.

Coppi A, Cabinian M, Mirelman D, Sinnis P. Antimalarial activity of allicin, a biologically active compound from garlic cloves. *Antimicrob Agents Chemother*. 2006;50(5):1731-1737.

Corral MJ, Benito-Peña E, Jiménez-Antón MD, Cuevas L, Moreno-Bondi MC, Alunda JM. Allicin induces calcium and mitochondrial dysregulation causing necrotic death in leishmania. *PLoS Negl Trop Dis*. 2016;10(3):e0004525.

Feng Y, Zhu X, Wang Q, et al. Allicin enhances host pro-inflammatory immune responses and protects against acute murine malaria infection. *Malar J*. 2012;11:268.

Fratianni F, Riccardi R, Spigno P, et al. Biochemical characterization and antimicrobial and antifungal activity of two endemic varieties of garlic (Allium sativum L.) of the Campania region, Southern Italy. *J Med Food*. 2016;19(7):686-691.

Gonen A, Harats D, Rabinkov A, et al. The antiatherogenic effect of allicin: possible mode of action. *Pathobiology*. 2005;72(6):325-334.

Gu X, Wu H, Fu P. Allicin attenuates inflammation and suppresses HLA-B27 protein expression in ankylosing spondylitis mice. *Biomed Res Int*. 2013;2013:171573.

Guo N, Wu X, Yu L, et al. In vitro and in vivo interactions between fluconazole and allicin against clinical isolates of fluconazole-resistant Candida albicans determined by alternative methods. *FEMS Immunol Med Microbiol.* 2010;58(2):193-201.

Harris JC, Cottrell SL, Plummer S, Lloyd D. Antimicrobial properties of Allium sativum (garlic). *Appl Microbiol Biotechnol.* 2001;57(3):282-286.

Hsing AW, Chokkalingam AP, Gao YT et al. Allium vegetables and risk of prostate cancer: a population-based study. *J Natl Cancer Inst.* 2002;94(21):1648-1651.

Jiang XW, Zhang Y, Song GD, et al. Clinical evaluation of allicin oral adhesive tablets in the treatment of recurrent aphthous ulceration. *Oral Surg Oral Med Oral Pathol Oral Radiol.* 2012;113(4):500-504.

Kyung KH. Antimicrobial properties of allium species. *Curr Opin Biotechnol.* 2012;23(2):142-147.

Lawson LD, Gardner CD. Composition, stability, and bioavailability of garlic products used in a clinical trial. *J Agric Food Chem.* 2005;53(16):6254-6261.

Li XH, Li CY, Lu JM, Tian RB, Wei J. Allicin ameliorates cognitive deficits ageing-induced learning and memory deficits through enhancing of Nrf2 antioxidant signaling pathways. *Neurosci Lett.* 2012;514(1):46-50.

Lissiman E, Bhasale AL, Cohen M. Garlic for the common cold. *Cochrane Database Syst Rev.* 2014;2014(11):CD006206.

Liu C, Cao F, Tang QZ, et al. Allicin protects against cardiac hypertrophy and fibrosis via attenuating reactive oxygen species-dependent signaling pathways. *J Nutr Biochem.* 2010;21(12):1238-1250.

Louis XL, Murphy R, Thandapilly SJ, Yu L, Netticadan T. Garlic extracts prevent oxidative stress, hypertrophy and apoptosis in cardiomyocytes: a role for nitric oxide and hydrogen sulfide. *BMC Complement Altern Med.* 2012;12:140.

Majewski M. Allium sativum: facts and myths regarding human health. *Rocz Panstw Zakl Hig.* 2014;65(1):1-8.

McMahon FG, Vargas R. Can garlic lower blood pressure? A pilot study. *Pharmacotherapy.* 1993;13(4):406-407.

Nicastro HL, Ross SA, Milner JA. Garlic and onions: their cancer prevention properties. *Cancer Prev Res (Phila).* 2015;8(3):181-189.

O'Gara EA, Hill DJ, Maslin DJ. Activities of garlic oil, garlic powder, and their diallyl constituents against Helicobacter pylori. *Appl Environ Microbiol.* 2000;66(5):2269-2273.

Panyod S, Wu WK, Chen PC, et al. Atherosclerosis amelioration by allicin in raw garlic through gut microbiota and trimethylamine-N-oxide modulation. *NPJ Biofilms Microbiomes.* 2022;8(1):4.

Rana SV, Pal R, Vaiphei K, Sharma SK, Ola RP. Garlic in health and disease. *Nutr Res Rev.* 2011;24(1):60-71.

Ranjbar-Omid M, Arzanlou M, Amani M, Shokri Al-Hashem SK, Amir Mozafari N, Peeri Doghaheh H. Allicin from garlic inhibits the biofilm formation and urease activity of Proteus mirabilis in vitro. *FEMS Microbiol Lett.* 2015;362(9):fnv049.

Ribeiro M, Alvarenga L, Cardozo LFMF, et al. From the distinctive smell to therapeutic effects: garlic for cardiovascular, hepatic, gut, diabetes and chronic kidney disease. *Clin Nutr.* 2021;40(7):4807-4819.

Salama AA, AbouLaila M, Terkawi MA, et al. Inhibitory effect of allicin on the growth of Babesia and Theileria equi parasites. *Parasitol Res.* 2014;113(1):275-283.

Si XB, Zhang XM, Wang S, Lan Y, Zhang S, Huo LY. Allicin as add-on therapy for *Helicobacter pylori* infection: a systematic review and meta-analysis. *World J Gastroenterol.* 2019;25(39):6025-6040.

Shang A, Cao SY, Xu XY, et al. Bioactive compounds and biological functions of garlic (*Allium sativum* L.). *Foods.* 2019;8(7):246.

Shouk R, Abdou A, Shetty K, Sarkar D, Eid AH. Mechanisms underlying the antihypertensive effects of garlic bioactives. *Nutr Res.* 2014;34(2):106-115.

Tsubura A, Lai YC, Kuwata M, Uehara N, Yoshizawa K. Anticancer effects of garlic and garlic-derived compounds for breast cancer control. *Anticancer Agents Med Chem.* 2011;11(3):249-253.

Viswanathan V, Phadatare AG, Mukne A. Antimycobacterial and antibacterial activity of Allium sativum bulbs. *Indian J Pharm Sci.* 2014;76(3):256-261.

Wallock-Richards D, Doherty CJ, Doherty L, et al. Garlic revisited: antimicrobial activity of allicin-containing garlic extracts against Burkholderia cepacia complex. *PLoS One.* 2014;9(12):e112726.

Wu X, Santos RR, Fink-Gremmels J. Analyzing the antibacterial effects of food ingredients: model experiments with allicin and garlic extracts on biofilm formation and viability of Staphylococcus epidermidis. *Food Sci Nutr.* 2015;3(2):158-168.

Yang LJ, Fan L, Liu ZQ, et al. Effects of allicin on CYP2C19 and CYP3A4 activity in healthy volunteers with different CYP2C19 genotypes. *Eur J Clin Pharmacol.* 2009;65(6):601-608.

Yoshida S, Kasuga S, Hayashi N, Ushiroguchi T, Matsuura H, Nakagawa S. Antifungal activity of ajoene derived from garlic. *Appl Environ Microbiol.* 1987;53(3):615-617.

Zardast M, Namakin K, Kaho JE, Hashemi SS. Assessment of antibacterial effect of garlic in patients infected with *Helicobacter pylori* using urease breath test. *Avicenna J Phytomed.* 2016;6(5):495-501.

COVID-19

Ahmad A, Rehman MU, Alkharfy KM. An alternative approach to minimize the risk of coronavirus (Covid-19) and similar infections. *Eur Rev Med Pharmacol Sci.* 2020;24(7):4030-4034.

Alschuler L, Weil A, Horwitz R, et al. Integrative considerations during the COVID-19 pandemic. *Explore (NY).* 2020;16(6):354-356.

An X, Zhang Y, Duan L, et al. The direct evidence and mechanism of traditional Chinese medicine treatment of COVID-19. *Biomed Pharmacother.* 2021;137:111267.

Ang L, Lee HW, Kim A, Lee JA, Zhang J, Lee MS. Herbal medicine for treatment of children diagnosed with COVID-19: a review of guidelines. *Complement Ther Clin Pract.* 2020;39:101174.

Ben-Shabat S, Yarmolinsky L, Porat D, Dahan A. Antiviral effect of phytochemicals from medicinal plants: applications and drug delivery strategies. *Drug Deliv Transl Res.* 2020;10(2):354-367.

Hensel A, Bauer R, Heinrich M, et al. Challenges at the time of COVID-19: opportunities and innovations in antivirals from nature. *Planta Med.* 2020;86(10):659-664.

Huang YF, Bai C, He F, Xie Y, Zhou H. Review on the potential action mechanisms of Chinese medicines in treating Coronavirus Disease 2019 (COVID-19). *Pharmacol Res.* 2020;158;104939.

Levy E, Delvin E, Marcil V, Spahis S. Can phytotherapy with polyphenols serve as a powerful approach for the prevention and therapy tool of novel coronavirus disease 2019 (COVID-19)? *Am J Physiol Endocrinol Metab.* 2020;319(4):E689-E708.

Ng JY. Global research trends at the intersection of coronavirus disease 2019 (COVID-19) and traditional, integrative, and complementary and alternative medicine: a bibliometric analysis. *BMC Complement Med Ther.* 2020;20(1):353.

Ngwa W, Kumar R, Thompson D, et al. Potential of flavonoid-Inspired phytomedicines against COVID-19. *Molecules.* 2020;25(11):2707.

Owoyele BV, Bakare AO, Ologe MO. Bromelain: a review on its potential as a therapy for the management of Covid-19. *Niger J Physiol Sci.* 2020;35(1):10-19.

Portella CFS, Ghelman R, Abdala CVM, Schveitzer MC. Evidence map on the contributions of traditional, complementary and integrative medicines for health care in times of COVID-19. *Integr Med Res.* 2020;9(3):100473.

Shahzad F, Anderson D, Najafzadeh M. The antiviral, anti-inflammatory effects of natural medicinal herbs and mushrooms and SARS-CoV-2 infection. *Nutrients.* 2020;12(9):2573.

Silveira D, Prieto-Garcia JM, Boylan F, et al. COVID-19: is there evidence for the use of herbal medicines as adjuvant symptomatic therapy? *Front Pharmacol.* 2020;11:581840.

Yang Y, Islam MS, Wang J, Li Y, Chen X. Traditional Chinese medicine in the treatment of patients infected with 2019-New Coronavirus (SARS-CoV-2): a review and perspective. *Int J Biol Sci*. 2020;16(10):1708-1717.

Zahedipour F, Hosseini SA, Sathyapalan T, et al. Potential effects of curcumin in the treatment of COVID-19 infection. *Phytother Res*. 2020;34(11):2911-2920.

Zhang DH, Zhang X, Peng B, et al. Network pharmacology suggests biochemical rationale for treating COVID-19 symptoms with a traditional Chinese medicine. *Commun Biol*. 2020;3(1):466.

Zhang HT, Huang MX, Liu X, et al. Evaluation of the adjuvant efficacy of natural herbal medicine on COVID-19: a retrospective matched case-control study. *Am J Chin Med*. 2020;48(4):779-792.

Zhang Y, Li Y, Wang X, et al. Herbal plants coordinate COVID-19 in multiple dimensions - an insight analysis for clinically applied remedies. *Int J Med Sci*. 2020;17(18):3125-3145.

Chapter 11: Nourish

Abdel-Aal el-SM, Akhtar H, Zaheer K, Ali R. Dietary sources of lutein and zeaxanthin carotenoids and their role in eye health. *Nutrients*. 2013;5(4):1169-1185.

Abdul QA, Yu BP, Chung HY, Jung HA, Choi JS. Epigenetic modifications of gene expression by lifestyle and environment. *Arch Pharm Res*. 2017;40(11):1219-1237.

Aldret RL, Bellar D. A double-blind, cross-over study to examine the effects of maritime pine extract on exercise performance and postexercise inflammation, oxidative stress, muscle soreness, and damage. *J Diet Suppl*. 2020;17(3):309-320.

Allen BG, Bhatia SK, Anderson CM, et al. Ketogenic diets as an adjuvant cancer therapy: history and potential mechanism. *Redox Biol*. 2014;2:963-70.

Dean L. Methylenetetrahydrofolate reductase deficiency. In: Pratt V, McLeod H, Dean L, et al., eds. *Medical Genetics Summaries* [Internet]. National Center for Biotechnology Information; 2012 [updated Oct 27, 2016]. https://www.ncbi.nlm.nih.gov/books/NBK66131/

Gardener H, Moon YP, Rundek T, Elkind MSV, Sacco RL. Diet soda and sugar-sweetened soda consumption in relation to incident diabetes in the northern Manhattan study. *Curr Dev Nutr*. 2018;2(5):nzy008.

Glenn AJ, Lo K, Jenkins DJA, et al. Relationship between a plant-based dietary portfolio and risk of cardiovascular disease: findings from the Women's Health Initiative Prospective Cohort Study. *J Am Heart Assoc*. 2021;10(16):e021515.

Halton TL, Willett WC, Liu S, et al. Low-carbohydrate-diet score and the risk of coronary heart disease in women. *N Engl J Med*. 2006;355(19):1991-2002.

Huang Z, Huang Q, Ji L, et al. Epigenetic regulation of active Chinese herbal components for cancer prevention and treatment: a follow-up review. *Pharmacol Res.* 2016;114:1-12.

Jenkins DJ, Wong JM, Kendall CW, et al. The effect of a plant-based low-carbohydrate ("Eco-Atkins") diet on body weight and blood lipid concentrations in hyperlipidemic subjects. *Arch Intern Med.* 2009;169(11):1046-1054. [published correction appears in *Arch Intern Med.* 2009;169(16):1490.]

Kapelner A, Vorsanger M. Starvation of cancer via induced ketogenesis and severe hypoglycemia. *Med Hypotheses.* 2015;84(3):162-168.

Lagiou P, Sandin S, Lof M, Trichopoulos D, Adami HO, Weiderpass E. Low carbohydrate-high protein diet and incidence of cardiovascular diseases in Swedish women: prospective cohort study. *BMJ.* 2012;344:e4026.

Landrigan PJ, Straif K. Aspartame and cancer - new evidence for causation. *Environ Health.* 2021;20(1):42.

Legaki E, Gazouli M. Influence of environmental factors in the development of inflammatory bowel diseases. *World J Gastrointest Pharmacol Ther.* 2016;7(1):112-125.

Lobo V, Patil A, Phatak A, Chandra N. Free radicals, antioxidants and functional foods: impact on human health. *Pharmacogn Rev.* 2010;4(8):118-126.

Mangin M, Sinha R, Fincher K. Inflammation and vitamin D: the infection connection. *Inflamm Res.* 2014;63(10):803-819.

Masino SA, Ruskin DN. Ketogenic diets and pain. *J Child Neurol.* 2013;28(8):993-1001.

Minich DM, Brown BI. A review of dietary (phyto)nutrients for glutathione support. *Nutrients.* 2019;11(9):2073.

Ruskin DN, Masino SA. The nervous system and metabolic dysregulation: emerging evidence converges on ketogenic diet therapy. *Front Neurosci.* 2012;6:33.

Sadowska-Bartosz I, Bartosz G. Prevention of protein glycation by natural compounds. *Molecules.* 2015;20(2):3309-3334.

Schwalfenberg GK. The alkaline diet: is there evidence that an alkaline pH diet benefits health? *J Environ Public Health.* 2012;2012:727630.

Stephens L, Whitehouse J, Polley M. Western herbal medicine, epigenetics, and endometriosis. *J Altern Complement Med.* 2013 Nov;19(11):853-859.

Thakur VS, Deb G, Babcook MA, Gupta S. Plant phytochemicals as epigenetic modulators: role in cancer chemoprevention. *AAPS J.* 2014;16(1):151-163.

Vidali S, Aminzadeh S, Lambert B, et al. Mitochondria: the ketogenic diet--a metabolism-based therapy. *J Biochem Cell Biol.* 2015;63:55-59.

Wahls TL, Chenard CA, Snetselaar LG. Review of two popular eating plans within the multiple sclerosis community: low saturated fat and modified paleolithic. *Nutrients*. 2019;11(2):352.

Winter G, Hart RA, Charlesworth RPG, Sharpley CF. Gut microbiome and depression: what we know and what we need to know. *Rev Neurosci*. 2018;29(6):629-643.

Omega-3 Fatty Acids

Berge K, Musa-Veloso K, Harwood M, Hoem N, Burri L. Krill oil supplementation lowers serum triglycerides without increasing low-density lipoprotein cholesterol in adults with borderline high or high triglyceride levels. *Nutr Res*. 2014;34(2):126-133.

Bunea R, El Farrah K, Deutsch L. Evaluation of the effects of Neptune Krill Oil on the clinical course of hyperlipidemia. *Altern Med Rev*. 2004;9(4):420-428.

Deutsch L. Evaluation of the effect of Neptune Krill Oil on chronic inflammation and arthritic symptoms. *J Am Coll Nutr*. 2007;26(1):39-48.

Elagizi A, Lavie CJ, O'Keefe E, Marshall K, O'Keefe JH, Milani RV. An update on omega-3 polyunsaturated fatty acids and cardiovascular health. *Nutrients*. 2021;13(1):204.

Kidd PM. Omega-3 DHA and EPA for cognition, behavior, and mood: clinical findings and structural-functional synergies with cell membrane phospholipids. *Altern Med Rev*. 2007;12(3):207-227.

Maki KC, Reeves MS, Farmer M, et al. Krill oil supplementation increases plasma concentrations of eicosapentaenoic and docosahexaenoic acids in overweight and obese men and women. *Nutr Res*. 2009;29(9):609-615.

Nobili V, Alisi A, Musso G, Scorletti E, Calder PC, Byrne CD. Omega-3 fatty acids: mechanisms of benefit and therapeutic effects in pediatric and adult NAFLD. *Crit Rev Clin Lab Sci*. 2016;53(2):106-120.

Ramprasath VR, Eyal I, Zchut S, Jones PJ. Enhanced increase of omega-3 index in healthy individuals with response to 4-week n-3 fatty acid supplementation from krill oil versus fish oil. *Lipids Health Dis*. 2013;12:178.

Rupp H, Wagner D, Rupp T, Schulte LM, Maisch B. Risk stratification by the "EPA+DHA level" and the "EPA/AA ratio" focus on anti-inflammatory and antiarrhythmogenic effects of long-chain omega-3 fatty acids. *Herz*. 2004;29(7):673-685. [published correction appears in *Herz*. 2004;29(8):805.]

Schuchardt JP, Schneider I, Meyer H, Neubronner J, von Schacky C, Hahn A. Incorporation of EPA and DHA into plasma phospholipids in response to different omega-3 fatty acid formulations--a comparative bioavailability study of fish oil vs. krill oil. *Lipids Health Dis*. 2011;10:145.

Suganuma K, Nakajima H, Ohtsuki M, Imokawa G. Astaxanthin attenuates the UVA-induced up-regulation of matrix-metalloproteinase-1 and skin fibroblast elastase in human dermal fibroblasts. *J Dermatol Sci.* 2010;58(2):136-142.

Tou JC, Jaczynski J, Chen YC. Krill for human consumption: nutritional value and potential health benefits. *Nutr Rev.* 2007;65(2):63-77.

Ulven SM, Kirkhus B, Lamglait A, et al. Metabolic effects of krill oil are essentially similar to those of fish oil but at lower dose of EPA and DHA, in healthy volunteers. *Lipids.* 2011;46(1):37-46.

Yoon HS, Cho HH, Cho S, Lee SR, Shin MH, Chung JH. Supplementing with dietary astaxanthin combined with collagen hydrolysate improves facial elasticity and decreases matrix metalloproteinase-1 and -12 expression: a comparative study with placebo. *J Med Food.* 2014;17(7):810-816.

Yoshihisa Y, Rehman MU, Shimizu T. Astaxanthin, a xanthophyll carotenoid, inhibits ultraviolet-induced apoptosis in keratinocytes. *Exp Dermatol.* 2014;23(3):178-183.

Lutein/Zeaxanthin

Bernstein PS, Li B, Vachali PP, et al. Lutein, zeaxanthin, and meso-zeaxanthin: the basic and clinical science underlying carotenoid-based nutritional interventions against ocular disease. *Prog Retin Eye Res.* 2016;50:34-66.

Hobbs RP, Bernstein PS. Nutrient supplementation for age-related macular degeneration, cataract, and dry eye. *J Ophthalmic Vis Res.* 2014;9(4):487-493.

McCusker MM, Durrani K, Payette MJ, Suchecki J. An eye on nutrition: the role of vitamins, essential fatty acids, and antioxidants in age-related macular degeneration, dry eye syndrome, and cataract. *Clin Dermatol.* 2016;34(2):276-285.

Meinke MC, Friedrich A, Tscherch K, et al. Influence of dietary carotenoids on radical scavenging capacity of the skin and skin lipids. *Eur J Pharm Biopharm.* 2013;84(2):365-373.

Roberts JE, Dennison J. The photobiology of lutein and zeaxanthin in the eye. *J Ophthalmol.* 2015;2015:687173.

Roberts RL, Green J, Lewis B. Lutein and zeaxanthin in eye and skin health. *Clin Dermatol.* 2009;27(2):195-201.

Scripsema NK, Hu DN, Rosen RB. Lutein, zeaxanthin, and meso-zeaxanthin in the clinical management of eye disease. *J Ophthalmol.* 2015;2015:865179.

French Maritime Pine Bark

Bianchi S, Kroslakova I, Janzon R, Mayer I, Saake B, Pichelin F. Characterization of condensed tannins and carbohydrates in hot water bark extracts of European softwood species. *Phytochemistry.* 2015;120:53-61.

Furumura M, Sato N, Kusaba N, Takagaki K, Nakayama J. Oral administration of French maritime pine bark extract (Flavangenol(®)) improves clinical symptoms in photoaged facial skin. *Clin Interv Aging*. 2012;7:275-286.

McGrath KC, Li XH, McRobb LS, Heather AK, Gangoda SVS. Inhibitory effect of a French maritime pine bark extract-based nutritional supplement on TNF-α-induced inflammation and oxidative stress in human coronary artery endothelial cells. *Evid Based Complement Alternat Med*. 2015;2015:260530. [published correction appears in *Evid Based Complement Alternat Med*. 2018;2018:5642129.]

Nakayama S, Kishimoto Y, Saita E, et al. Pine bark extract prevents low-density lipoprotein oxidation and regulates monocytic expression of antioxidant enzymes. *Nutr Res*. 2015;35(1):56-64.

Tagashira H, Miyamoto A, Kitamura S, et al. UVB stimulates the expression of endothelin B receptor in human melanocytes via a sequential activation of the p38/MSK1/CREB/MITF pathway which can be interrupted by a French maritime pine bark extract through a direct inactivation of MSK1. *PLoS One*. 2015;10(6):e0128678.

Multivitamin

Chen F, Du M, Blumberg JB, et al. Association between dietary supplement use, nutrient intake, and mortality among US adults: a cohort study. *Ann Intern Med*. 2019;170(9):604-613.

Jenkins, DJA, Spence JD, Giovannucci EL, et al. Supplemental vitamins and minerals for CVD prevention and treatment. *J Am Coll Cardiol*. 2018;71(22):2570-2584.

Chapter 12: Purify

Franco LS, Shanahan DF, Fuller RA. A review of the benefits of nature experiences: more than meets the eye. *Int J Environ Res Public Health*. 2017;14(8):864.

Kim JH, Lee JK, Kim HG, Kim KB, Kim HR. Possible effects of radiofrequency electromagnetic field exposure on central nerve system. *Biomol Ther (Seoul)*. 2019;27(3):265-275.

Kıvrak EG, Yurt KK, Kaplan AA, Alkan I, Altun G. Effects of electromagnetic fields exposure on the antioxidant defense system. *J Microsc Ultrastruct*. 2017;5(4):167-176.

Li Q, Kobayashi M, Inagaki H, et al. A day trip to a forest park increases human natural killer activity and the expression of anti-cancer proteins in male subjects. *J Biol Regul Homeost Agents*. 2010;24(2):157-165.

Li Q, Morimoto K, Kobayashi M, et al. A forest bathing trip increases human natural killer activity and expression of anti-cancer proteins in female subjects. *J Biol Regul Homeost Agents*. 2008;22(1):45-55.

Li Q, Morimoto K, Kobayashi M, et al. Visiting a forest, but not a city, increases human natural killer activity and expression of anti-cancer proteins. *Int J Immunopathol Pharmacol.* 2008;21(1):117-127.

Li Q, Kobayashi M, Wakayama Y, et al. Effect of phytoncide from trees on human natural killer cell function. *Int J Immunopathol Pharmacol.* 2009;22(4):951-959.

Park SH, Kim D, Kim J, Moon Y. Effects of mycotoxins on mucosal microbial infection and related pathogenesis. *Toxins (Basel).* 2015;7(11):4484-4502.

Perez V, Alexander D, Bailey W. Air ions and mood outcomes: a review and meta-analysis. *BMC Psychiatry.* 2013;13:29.

Siņicina N, Skromulis A, Martinovs A. Amount of air ions depending on indoor plant activity. *Environment Technology Resources, Proceedings of the 10th International Scientific and Practical Conference.* 2015; Volume II: 267-273.

Chlorella

Kwak JH, Baek SH, Woo Y, et al. Beneficial immunostimulatory effect of short-term Chlorella supplementation: enhancement of natural killer cell activity and early inflammatory response (randomized, double-blinded, placebo-controlled trial). *Nutr J.* 2012;11:53.

Morita K, Ogata M, Hasegawa T. Chlorophyll derived from Chlorella inhibits dioxin absorption from the gastrointestinal tract and accelerates dioxin excretion in rats. *Environ Health Perspect.* 2001;109(3):289-294.

Panahi Y, Darvishi B, Jowzi N, Beiraghdar F, Sahebkar A. Chlorella vulgaris: a multifunctional dietary supplement with diverse medicinal properties. *Curr Pharm Des.* 2016;22(2):164-173.

Ryu NH, Lim Y, Park JE, et al. Impact of daily Chlorella consumption on serum lipid and carotenoid profiles in mildly hypercholesterolemic adults: a double-blinded, randomized, placebo-controlled study. *Nutr J.* 2014;13:57.

Takekoshi H, Suzuki G, Chubachi H, Nakano M. Effect of Chlorella pyrenoidosa on fecal excretion and liver accumulation of polychlorinated dibenzo-p-dioxin in mice. *Chemosphere.* 2005;59(2):297-304.

Glutathione/NAC

Bavarsad Shahripour R, Harrigan MR, Alexandrov AV. N-acetylcysteine (NAC) in neurological disorders: mechanisms of action and therapeutic opportunities. *Brain Behav.* 2014;4(2):108-122.

Calverley P, Rogliani P, Papi A. Safety of N-acetylcysteine at high doses in chronic respiratory diseases: a review. *Drug Saf.* 2021;44(3):273-290.

Hagen TM, Bai C, Jones DP. Stimulation of glutathione absorption in rat small intestine by alpha-adrenergic agonists. *FASEB J.* 1991;5(12):2721-2727.

Hunjan MK, Evered DF. Absorption of glutathione from the gastro-intestinal tract. *Biochim Biophys Acta.* 1985;815(2):184-188.

Kumar P, Liu C, Hsu JW, et al. Glycine and N-acetylcysteine (GlyNAC) supplementation in older adults improves glutathione deficiency, oxidative stress, mitochondrial dysfunction, inflammation, insulin resistance, endothelial dysfunction, genotoxicity, muscle strength, and cognition: Results of a pilot clinical trial. *Clin Transl Med.* 2021;11(3):e372.

McKinley-Barnard S, Andre T, Morita M, Willoughby DS. Combined L-citrulline and glutathione supplementation increases the concentration of markers indicative of nitric oxide synthesis. *J Int Soc Sports Nutr.* 2015;12:27.

Minich DM, Brown BI. A review of dietary (phyto)nutrients for glutathione support. *Nutrients.* 2019;11(9):2073.

Richie JP Jr, Nichenametla S, Neidig W, et al. Randomized controlled trial of oral glutathione supplementation on body stores of glutathione. *Eur J Nutr.* 2015;54(2):251-263.

Schwalfenberg GK. N-acetylcysteine: a review of clinical usefulness (an old drug with new tricks). *J Nutr Metab.* 2021;2021:9949453.

Shi Z, Puyo CA. N-acetylcysteine to combat COVID-19: an evidence review. *Ther Clin Risk Manag.* 2020;16:1047-1055.

Wong KK, Lee SWH, Kua KP. N-acetylcysteine as adjuvant therapy for COVID-19 - a perspective on the current state of the evidence. *J Inflamm Res.* 2021;14:2993-3013.

See Chapter 9 references for milk thistle.

Chapter 13: Calm

Bostock S, Crosswell AD, Prather AA, Steptoe A. Mindfulness on-the-go: effects of a mindfulness meditation app on work stress and well-being. *J Occup Health Psychol.* 2019;24(1):127-138.

Hilton L, Hempel S, Ewing BA, et al. Mindfulness meditation for chronic pain: systematic review and meta-analysis. *Ann Behav Med.* 2017;51(2):199-213.

Househam AM, Peterson CT, Mills PJ, Chopra D. The effects of stress and meditation on the immune system, human microbiota, and epigenetics. *Adv Mind Body Med.* 2017;31(4):10-25.

Jahnke R, Larkey L, Rogers C, Etnier J, Lin F. A comprehensive review of health benefits of qigong and tai chi. *Am J Health Promot.* 2010;24(6):e1-e25.

Rusch HL, Rosario M, Levison LM, et al. The effect of mindfulness meditation on sleep quality: a systematic review and meta-analysis of randomized controlled trials. *Ann N Y Acad Sci.* 2019;1445(1):5-16.

Saeed SA, Cunningham K, Bloch RM. Depression and anxiety disorders: benefits of exercise, yoga, and meditation. *Am Fam Physician*. 2019;99(10):620-627.

Wielgosz J, Goldberg SB, Kral TRA, Dunne JD, Davidson RJ. Mindfulness meditation and psychopathology. *Annu Rev Clin Psychol*. 2019;15:285-316.

Yeung A, Chan JSM, Cheung JC, Zou L. Qigong and tai-chi for mood regulation. *Focus (Am Psychiatr Publ)*. 2018;16(1):40-47.

L-theanine

Hidese S, Ogawa S, Ota M, et al. Effects of L-theanine administration on stress-related symptoms and cognitive functions in healthy adults: a randomized controlled trial. *Nutrients*. 2019;11(10):2362.

Hidese S, Ota M, Wakabayashi C, et al. Effects of chronic L-theanine administration in patients with major depressive disorder: an open-label study. *Acta Neuropsychiatr*. 2017;29(2):72-79.

Juszkiewicz A, Glapa A, Basta P, et al. The effect of L-theanine supplementation on the immune system of athletes exposed to strenuous physical exercise. *J Int Soc Sports Nutr*. 2019;16(1):7.

Kelly SP, Gomez-Ramirez M, Montesi JL, Foxe JJ. L-theanine and caffeine in combination affect human cognition as evidenced by oscillatory alpha-band activity and attention task performance. *J Nutr*. 2008;138(8):1572S-1577S.

Kim S, Jo K, Hong KB, Han SH, Suh HJ. GABA and L-theanine mixture decreases sleep latency and improves NREM sleep. *Pharm Biol*. 2019;57(1):65-73.

Kim TI, Lee YK, Park SG, et al. L-theanine, an amino acid in green tea, attenuates beta-amyloid-induced cognitive dysfunction and neurotoxicity: reduction in oxidative damage and inactivation of ERK/p38 kinase and NF-kappaB pathways. *Free Radic Biol Med*. 2009;47(11):1601-1610.

Kimura K, Ozeki M, Juneja LR, Ohira H. L-theanine reduces psychological and physiological stress responses. *Biol Psychol*. 2007;74(1):39-45.

Li C, Tong H, Yan Q, et al. L-theanine improves immunity by altering TH2/TH1 cytokine balance, brain neurotransmitters, and expression of phospholipase C in rat hearts. *Med Sci Monit*. 2016;22:662-669.

Nathan PJ, Lu K, Gray M, Oliver C. The neuropharmacology of L-theanine(N-ethyl-L-glutamine): a possible neuroprotective and cognitive enhancing agent. *J Herb Pharmacother*. 2006;6(2):21-30.

Nobre AC, Rao A, Owen GN. L-theanine, a natural constituent in tea, and its effect on mental state. *Asia Pac J Clin Nutr*. 2008;(17 Suppl 1):167-168.

Williams JL, Everett JM, D'Cunha NM, et al. The effects of green tea amino acid L-theanine consumption on the ability to manage stress and anxiety levels: a systematic review. *Plant Foods Hum Nutr*. 2020;75(1):12-23.

Yoto A, Motoki M, Murao S, Yokogoshi H. Effects of L-theanine or caffeine intake on changes in blood pressure under physical and psychological stresses. *J Physiol Anthropol.* 2012;31(1):28.

Passionflower

Akhondzadeh S, Kashani L, Mobaseri M, Hosseini SH, Nikzad S, Khani M. Passionflower in the treatment of opiates withdrawal: a double-blind randomized controlled trial. *J Clin Pharm Ther.* 2001;26(5):369-373.

Akhondzadeh S, Naghavi HR, Vazirian M, Shayeganpour A, Rashidi H, Khani M. Passionflower in the treatment of generalized anxiety: a pilot double-blind randomized controlled trial with oxazepam. *J Clin Pharm Ther.* 2001;26(5):363-367.

Anheyer D, Lauche R, Schumann D, Dobos G, Cramer H. Herbal medicines in children with attention deficit hyperactivity disorder (ADHD): a systematic review. *Complement Ther Med.* 2017;30:14-23.

Elsas SM, Rossi DJ, Raber J, et al. Passiflora incarnata L. (Passionflower) extracts elicit GABA currents in hippocampal neurons in vitro, and show anxiogenic and anticonvulsant effects in vivo, varying with extraction method. *Phytomedicine.* 2010;17(12):940-949.

Grundmann O, Wang J, McGregor GP, Butterweck V. Anxiolytic activity of a phytochemically characterized Passiflora incarnata extract is mediated via the GABAergic system. *Planta Med.* 2008;74(15):1769-1773.

Movafegh A, Alizadeh R, Hajimohamadi F, Esfehani F, Nejatfar M. Preoperative oral Passiflora incarnata reduces anxiety in ambulatory surgery patients: a double-blind, placebo-controlled study. *Anesth Analg.* 2008;106(6):1728-1732.

Ngan A, Conduit R. A double-blind, placebo-controlled investigation of the effects of Passiflora incarnata (passionflower) herbal tea on subjective sleep quality. *Phytother Res.* 2011;25(8):1153-1159.

Otify A, George C, Elsayed A, Farag MA. Mechanistic evidence of Passiflora edulis (Passifloraceae) anxiolytic activity in relation to its metabolite fingerprint as revealed via LC-MS and chemometrics. *Food Funct.* 2015;6(12):3807-3817.

Villet S, Vacher V, Colas A, et al. Open-label observational study of the homeopathic medicine Passiflora Compose for anxiety and sleep disorders. *Homeopathy.* 2016;105(1):84-91.

Wohlmuth H, Penman KG, Pearson T, Lehmann RP. Pharmacognosy and chemotypes of passionflower (Passiflora incarnata L.). *Biol Pharm Bull.* 2010;33(6):1015-1018.

Lemon Balm

Alijaniha F, Naseri M, Afsharypuor S, et al. Heart palpitation relief with Melissa officinalis leaf extract: double blind, randomized, placebo controlled trial of efficacy and safety. *J Ethnopharmacol.* 2015;164:378-384.

Haybar H, Javid AZ, Haghighizadeh MH, et al. The effects of Melissa officinalis supplementation on depression, anxiety, stress, and sleep disorder in patients with chronic stable angina. *Clin Nutr ESPEN*. 2018;26:47-52.

Ibarra A, Feuillere N, Roller M, Lesburgere E, Beracochea D. Effects of chronic administration of Melissa officinalis L. extract on anxiety-like reactivity and on circadian and exploratory activities in mice. *Phytomedicine Int J Phytother Phytopharm*. 2010;17(6):397-403.

Kennedy DO, Wake G, Savelev S, et al. Modulation of mood and cognitive performance following acute administration of single doses of Melissa officinalis (lemon balm) with human CNS nicotinic and muscarinic receptor-binding properties. *Neuropsychopharmacology*. 2003;28(10):1871-1881.

Mirabi P, Namdari M, Alamolhoda S, Mojab F. The effect of Melissa officinalis extract on the severity of primary dysmenorrhea. *Iran J Pharm Res IJPR*. 2017;16(Suppl):171-177.

Miraj S, Rafieian-Kopaei, Kiani S. Melissa officinalis L: a review study with an antioxidant prospective. *J Evid-Based Complement Altern Med*. 2017;22(3):385-394.

Ozarowski M, Mikolajczak PL, Piasecka A, et al. Influence of the Melissa officinalis leaf extract on long-term memory in scopolamine animal model with assessment of mechanism of action. *Evid Based Complement Alternat Med*. 2016;2016:e9729818.

Ranjbar M, Firoozabadi A, Salehi A, et al. Effects of herbal combination (Melissa officinalis L. and Nepeta menthoides Boiss. & Buhse) on insomnia severity, anxiety and depression in insomniacs: Randomized placebo controlled trial. *Integr Med Res*. 2018;7(4):328-332.

Schnitzler P, Schuhmacher A, Astani A, Reichling J. Melissa officinalis oil affects infectivity of enveloped herpesviruses. *Phytomedicine Int J Phytother Phytopharm*. 2008;15(9):734-740.

Soodi M, Naghdi N, Hajimehdipoor H, Choopani S, Sahraei E. Memory-improving activity of Melissa officinalis extract in naïve and scopolamine-treated rats. *Res Pharm Sci*. 2014;9(2):107.

See Chapter 5 references for ashwagandha.

Chapter 14: Move

Carmack CL, Boudreaux E, Amaral-Melendez M, Brantley PJ, de Moor C. Aerobic fitness and leisure physical activity as moderators of the stress-illness relation. *Ann Behav Med*. 1999;21(3):251-257.

Denham J. Exercise and epigenetic inheritance of disease risk. *Acta Physiol (Oxf)*. 2018;222(1):10.1111/apha.12881.

Fernandes J, Arida RM, Gomez-Pinilla F. Physical exercise as an epigenetic modulator of brain plasticity and cognition. *Neurosci Biobehav Rev*. 2017;80:443-456.

Rea IM. Towards ageing well: Use it or lose it: Exercise, epigenetics and cognition. *Biogerontology*. 2017;18(4):679-691.

Santos L, Elliott-Sale KJ, Sale C. Exercise and bone health across the lifespan. *Biogerontology*. 2017;18(6):931-946.

Tudor-Locke C, Craig CL, Thyfault JP, Spence JC. A step-defined sedentary lifestyle index: <5000 steps/day. *Appl Physiol Nutr Metab*. 2013;38(2):100-114.

Wallace RG, Twomey LC, Custaud M-A, et al. The role of epigenetics in cardiovascular health and ageing: a focus on physical activity and nutrition. *Mech Ageing Dev*. 2018;174:76-85.

CBD oil

Bergamaschi MM, Queiroz RH, Zuardi AW, Crippa JA. Safety and side effects of cannabidiol, a Cannabis sativa constituent. *Curr Drug Saf*. 2011;6(4):237-249.

Bitencourt RM, Takahashi RN. Cannabidiol as a therapeutic alternative for post-traumatic stress disorder: from bench research to confirmation in human trials. *Front Neurosci*. 2018;12:502.

Blessing EM, Steenkamp MM, Manzanares J, Marmar CR. Cannabidiol as a potential treatment for anxiety disorders. *Neurotherapeutics*. 2015;12(4):825-836.

Bruni N, Pepa CD, Oliaro-Bosso S, et al. Cannabinoid delivery systems for pain and inflammation treatment. *Molecules*. 2018;23(10):E2478.

Burstein S. Cannabidiol (CBD) and its analogs: a review of their effects on inflammation. *Bioorg Med Chem*. 2015;23(7):1377-1385.

Burstein SH, Zurier RB. Cannabinoids, endocannabinoids, and related analogs in inflammation. *AAPS J*. 2009;11(1):109-119.

Crippa JA, Guimaraes FS, Campos AC, Zuardi AW. Translational investigation of the therapeutic potential of cannabidiol (CBD): toward a new age. *Front Immunol*. 2018;9:2009.

De Gregorio D, McLaughlin RJ, Posa L, et al. Cannabidiol modulates serotonergic transmission and reverses both allodynia and anxiety-like behavior in a model of neuropathic pain. *Pain*. 2019;160(1):136-150.

Devinsky O, Marsh E, Friedman D, et al. Cannabidiol in patients with treatment-resistant epilepsy: an open-label interventional trial. *Lancet Neurol*. 2016;15(3):270-278.

Devinsky O, Cilio MR, Cross H, et al. Cannabidiol: pharmacology and potential therapeutic role in epilepsy and other neuropsychiatric disorders. *Epilepsia*. 2014;55(6):791-802.

Grotenhermen F, Russo E, Zuardi AW. Even high doses of oral cannabidiol do not cause THC-like effects in humans: comment on Merrick et al. *Cannabis and Cannabinoid Research*. 2016;1(1):102-112. *Cannabis Cannabinoid Res*. 2017;2(1):1-4.

Hasenoehrl C, Storr M, Schicho R. Cannabinoids for treating inflammatory bowel diseases: where are we and where do we go? *Expert Rev Gastroenterol Hepatol.* 2017;11(4):329-337.

Hazekamp A. The trouble with CBD oil. *Med Cannabis Cannabinoids.* 2018;1:65-72.

Hilderbrand RL. Hemp & cannabidiol: what is a medicine? *Mo Med.* 2018;115(4):306-309.

Hurd YL, Yoon M, Manini AF, et al. Early phase in the development of cannabidiol as a treatment for addiction: opioid relapse takes initial center stage. *Neurotherapeutics.* 2015;12(4):807-815.

Iffland K, Grotenhermen F. An update on safety and side effects of cannabidiol: a review of clinical data and relevant animal studies. *Cannabis Cannabinoid Res.* 2017;2(1):139-154.

Katsuyama S, Mizoguchi H, Kuwahata H, et al. Involvement of peripheral cannabinoid and opioid receptors in β-caryophyllene-induced antinociception. *Eur J Pain.* 2013;17(5):664-675.

Laprairie RB, Bagher AM, Kelly MEM, Denovan-Wright EM. Cannabidiol is a negative allosteric modulator of the cannabinoid CB1 receptor. *Br J Pharmacol.* 2015;172(20):4790-4805.

Lee JLC, Bertoglio LJ, Guimaraes FS, Stevenson CW. Cannabidiol regulation of emotion and emotional memory processing: relevance for treating anxiety-related and substance abuse disorders. *Br J Pharmacol.* 2017;174(19):3242-3256.

Leweke FM, Piomelli D, Pahlisch F, et al. Cannabidiol enhances anandamide signaling and alleviates psychotic symptoms of schizophrenia. *Transl Psychiatry.* 2012;2(3):e94.

Massi P, Solinas M, Cinquina V, Parolaro D. Cannabidiol as potential anticancer drug. *Br J Clin Pharmacol.* 2013;75(2):303-312.

Peres FF, Lima AC, Hallak JEC, et al. Cannabidiol as a promising strategy to treat and prevent movement disorders? *Front Pharmacol.* 2018;9:482.

Pickrell WO, Robertson NP. Cannabidiol as a treatment for epilepsy. *J Neurol.* 2017;264(12):2506-2508.

Prud'homme M, Cata R, Jutras-Aswad D. Cannabidiol as an intervention for addictive behaviors: a systematic review of the evidence. *Subst Abuse.* 2015;9:33-38.

Rudroff T, Sosnoff J. Cannabidiol to improve mobility in people with multiple sclerosis. *Front Neurol.* 2018;9:183.

Russo EB, Marcu J. Cannabis pharmacology: the usual suspects and a few promising leads. *Adv Pharmacol.* 2017;80:67-134.

Russo EB. Cannabidiol claims and misconceptions. *Trends Pharmacol Sci.* 2017;38(3):198-201.

Schoedel KA, Szeto I, Setnik B, et al. Abuse potential assessment of cannabidiol (CBD) in recreational polydrug users: a randomized, double-blind, controlled trial. *Epilepsy Behav.* 2018;88:162-171.

Solowij N, Broyd SJ, Beale C, et al. Therapeutic effects of prolonged cannabidiol treatment on psychological symptoms and cognitive function in regular cannabis users: a pragmatic open-label clinical trial. *Cannabis Cannabinoid Res*. 2018;3(1):21-34.

Viudez-Martínez A, García-Gutiérrez MS, Manzanares J. Cannabidiol regulates the expression of hypothalamus-pituitary-adrenal axis-related genes in response to acute restraint stress. *J Psychopharmacol*. 2018;32(12):1379-1384.

Wu H-Y, Huang C-H, Lin Y-H, et al. Cannabidiol induced apoptosis in human monocytes through mitochondrial permeability transition pore-mediated ROS production. *Free Radic Biol Med*. 2018;124:311-318.

Collagen

Bello AE, Oesser S. Collagen hydrolysate for the treatment of osteoarthritis and other joint disorders: a review of the literature. *Curr Med Res Opin*. 2006;22(11):2221-2232.

Bolke L, Schlippe G, Gerß J, Voss W. A collagen supplement improves skin hydration, elasticity, roughness, and density: results of a randomized, placebo-controlled, blind study. *Nutrients*. 2019;11(10):2494.

Borumand M, Sibilla S. Daily consumption of the collagen supplement Pure Gold Collagen® reduces visible signs of aging. *Clin Interv Aging*. 2014;9:1747-1758. [published correction appears in *Clin Interv Aging*. 2020;15:131.]

Czajka A, Kania EM, Genovese L, et al. Daily oral supplementation with collagen peptides combined with vitamins and other bioactive compounds improves skin elasticity and has a beneficial effect on joint and general wellbeing. *Nutr Res*. 2018;57:97-108.

García-Coronado JM, Martínez-Olvera L, Elizondo-Omaña RE, et al. Effect of collagen supplementation on osteoarthritis symptoms: a meta-analysis of randomized placebo-controlled trials. *Int Orthop*. 2019;43(3):531-538.

Lugo JP, Saiyed ZM, Lane NE. Efficacy and tolerability of an undenatured type II collagen supplement in modulating knee osteoarthritis symptoms: a multicenter randomized, double-blind, placebo-controlled study. *Nutr J*. 2016;15:14.

Sangsuwan W, Asawanonda P. Four-weeks daily intake of oral collagen hydrolysate results in improved skin elasticity, especially in sun-exposed areas: a randomized, double-blind, placebo-controlled trial. *J Dermatolog Treat*. 2021;32(8):991-996.

Chapter 15: Defend

See Chapter 10 references for antimicrobial herbs.

Chapter 16: Andropause

Campion S, Catlin N, Heger N, et al. Male reprotoxicity and endocrine disruption. *Exp Suppl.* 2012;101:315-360.

Ricci E, Vigano P, Cipriani S, et al. Coffee and caffeine intake and male infertility: a systematic review. *Nutr J.* 2017;16:37.

Grossmann M, Thomas MC, Panagiotopoulos S, et al. Low testosterone levels are common and associated with insulin resistance in men with diabetes. *J Clin Endocrinol Metab.* 2008;93(5):1834-1840.

Hwang K, Miner M. Controversies in testosterone replacement therapy: testosterone and cardiovascular disease. *Asian J Androl.* 2015;17(2):187-191.

Kloner RA, Carson C 3rd, Dobs A, Kopecky S, Mohler ER 3rd. Testosterone and cardiovascular disease. *J Am Coll Cardiol.* 2016;67(5):545-557.

Kurniawan LB, Adnan E; Windarwati, Mulyono B. Insulin resistance and testosterone level in Indonesian young adult males. *Rom J Intern Med.* 2020;58(2):93-98.

Levine H, Jørgensen N, Martino-Andrade A, et al. Temporal trends in sperm count: a systematic review and meta-regression analysis. *Hum Reprod Update.* 2017;23(6):646-659.

Etminan M, Skeldon SC, Goldenberg SL, Carleton B, Brophy JM. Testosterone therapy and risk of myocardial infarction: a pharmacoepidemiologic study. *Pharmacotherapy.* 2015;35(1):72-78.

Rao PM, Kelly DM, Jones TH. Testosterone and insulin resistance in the metabolic syndrome and T2DM in men. *Nat Rev Endocrinol.* 2013;9(8):479-493.

Salas-Huetos A, Bulló M, Salas-Salvadó J. Dietary patterns, foods and nutrients in male fertility parameters and fecundability: a systematic review of observational studies. *Hum Reprod Update.* 2017;23(4):371-389.

Travison TG, Araujo AB, O'Donnell AB, et al. A population-level decline in serum testosterone levels in American men. *J Clin Endocrinol Metab.* 2007;92(1):196-202.

Eurycoma

Abd Jalil MA, Shuid AN, Muhammad N. Role of medicinal plants and natural products on osteoporotic fracture healing. *Evid Based Complement Alternat Med.* 2012;2012:714512.

Bhat R, Karim AA. Tongkat Ali (Eurycoma longifolia Jack): a review on its ethnobotany and pharmacological importance. *Fitoterapia.* 2010;81(7):669-679.

George A, Suzuki N, Abas AB, et al. Immunomodulation in middle-aged humans via the ingestion of Physta® standardized root water extract of Eurycoma longifolia Jack--a randomized, double-blind, placebo-controlled, parallel study. *Phytother Res.* 2016;30(4):627-635.

George A, Henkel R. Phytoandrogenic properties of Eurycoma longifolia as natural alternative to testosterone replacement therapy. *Andrologia.* 2014;46(7):708-721.

Girish S, Kumar S, Aminudin N. Tongkat Ali (Eurycoma longifolia): a possible therapeutic candidate against Blastocystis sp. *Parasit Vectors.* 2015;8:332.

Hajjouli S, Chateauvieux S, Tieten M-H, et al. Eurycomanone and eurycomanol from Eurycoma longifolia Jack as regulators of signaling pathways involved in proliferation, cell death and inflammation. *Molecules.* 2014;19(9):14649-14666.

Han YM, Woo S-U, Choi MS, et al. Antiinflammatory and analgesic effects of Eurycoma longifolia extracts. *Arch Pharm Res.* 2016;39(3):421-428.

Han YM, Kim IS, Rehman SU, et al. In vitro evaluation of the effects of Eurycoma longifolia extract on CYP-mediated drug metabolism. *Evid Based Complement Alternat Med.* 2015; 2015:631329.

Henkel R, Wang R, Bassett SH, et al. Tongkat Ali as a potential herbal supplement for physically active male and female seniors — a pilot study. *Phytother Res.* 2014;28(4):544-550.

Husen R, Pihie AH, Nallappan M. Screening for antihyperglycaemic activity in several local herbs of Malaysia. *J Ethnopharmacol.* 2004;95(2-3):205-208.

Ismail SB, Mohammad WMZW, George A, et al. Randomized clinical trial on the use of PHYSTA freeze-dried water extract of Eurycoma longifolia for the improvement of quality of life and sexual well-being in men. *Evid Based Complement Alternat Med.* 2012;2012:429268.

Khanijo T, Jiraungkoorskul W. Review ergogenic effect of Long Jack, Eurycoma longifolia. *Pharmacogn Rev.* 2016;10(20):139-142.

Lahrita L, Kato E, Kawabata J. Uncovering potential of Indonesian medicinal plants on glucose uptake enhancement and lipid suppression in 3T3-L1 adipocytes. *J Ethnopharmacol.* 2015;168:229-236.

Leitão AE, Vieira MCS, Pelegrini A, da Silva EL, Guimarães ACA. A 6-month, double-blind, placebo-controlled, randomized trial to evaluate the effect of Eurycoma longifolia (Tongkat Ali) and concurrent training on erectile function and testosterone levels in androgen deficiency of aging males (ADAM). *Maturitas.* 2021;145:78-85.

Low BS, Das PK, Chan KL. Standardized quassinoid-rich Eurycoma longifolia extract improved spermatogenesis and fertility in male rats via the hypothalamic-pituitary-gonadal axis. *J Ethnopharmacol.* 2013;145(3):706-714.

Meng D, Li X, Han L, Zhang L, An W, Li X. Four new quassinoids from the roots of Eurycoma longifolia Jack. *Fitoterapia.* 2014;92:105-110.

Miyake K, Tezuka Y, Awale S, Li F, Kadota S. Quassinoids from Eurycoma longifolia. *J Nat Prod.* 2009;72(12):2135-2140.

Osman A, Jordan B, Lessard PA, et al. Genetic diversity of Eurycoma longifolia inferred from single nucleotide polymorphisms. *Plant Physiol*. 2003;131(3):1294-1301.

Rehman SU, Choe K, Yoo HH. Review on a traditional herbal medicine, Eurycoma longifolia Jack (Tongkat Ali): its traditional uses, chemistry, evidence-based pharmacology and toxicology. *Molecules*. 2016;21(3):331.

Talbott SM, Talbott JA, George A, Pugh M. Effect of Tongkat Ali on stress hormones and psychological mood state in moderately stressed subjects. *J Int Soc Sports Nutr*. 2013;10(1):28.

Thu HE, Mohamed IN, Hussain Z, et al. Eurycoma longifolia as a potential adoptogen of male sexual health: a systematic review on clinical studies. *Chin J Nat Med*. 2017;15(1):71-80.

Thu HE, Mohamed IN, Hussain Z, Shuid AN. Eurycoma longifolia as a potential alternative to testosterone for the treatment of osteoporosis: exploring time-mannered proliferative, differentiative and morphogenic modulation in osteoblasts. *J Ethnopharmacol*. 2017;195:143-158.

Thu HE, Hussain Z, Mohamed IN, Shuid AN. Eurycoma longifolia, a potential phytomedicine for the treatment of cancer: evidence of p53-mediated apoptosis in cancerous cells. *Curr Drug Targets*. 2018;19(10):1109-1126.

Tong KL, Chan KL, AbuBakar S, et al. The in vitro and in vivo anti-cancer activities of a standardized quassinoids composition from Eurycoma longifolia on LNCaP human prostate cancer cells. *PLoS One*. 2015;10(3):e0121752.

Tran TV, Malainer C, Schwaiger S, et al. NF-κB inhibitors from Eurycoma longifolia. *J Nat Prod*. 2014;77(3):483-488.

Tung NH, Uto T, Hai NT, et al. Quassinoids from the root of Eurycoma longifolia and their antiproliferative activity on human cancer cell lines. *Pharmacogn Mag*. 2017;13(51):459-462.

Udani JK, George AA, Musthapa M, et al. Effects of a proprietary freeze-dried water extract of Eurycoma longifolia (physta) and polygonum minus on sexual performance and well-being in men: a randomized, double-blind, placebo-controlled study. *Evid Based Complement Alternat Med*. 2014;2014:179529.

Epimedium

Cheng H, Feng S, Shen S, et al. Extraction, antioxidant and antimicrobial activities of Epimedium acuminatum Franch. polysaccharide. *Carbohydr Polym*. 2013;96(1):101-108.

Cheng H, Feng S, Jia X, et al. Structural characterization and antioxidant activities of polysaccharides extracted from Epimedium acuminatum. *Carbohydr Polym*. 2013;92(1):63-68.

Dietz BM, Hijirahimkhan A, Dunlap TL, Bolton JL. Botanicals and their bioactive phytochemicals for women's health. *Pharmacol Rev*. 2016;68(4):1026-1073.

Fan Y, Ren M, Hou W, et al. The activation of Epimedium polysaccharide-propolis flavone liposome on Kupffer cells. *Carbohydr Polym*. 2015;133:613-623.

Guo L, Lui J, Hu Y, et al. Astragalus polysaccharide and sulfated epimedium polysaccharide synergistically resist the immunosuppression. *Carbohydr Polym*. 2012;90(2):1055-1060.

Ma H, He X, Li M, et al. The genus Epimedium: an ethnopharmacological and phytochemical review. *J Ethnopharmacol*. 2011;134(3):519-541.

Indran IR, Liang RLZ, Min TE, Yong E-L. Preclinical studies and clinical evaluation of compounds from the genus Epimedium for osteoporosis and bone health. *Pharmacol Ther*. 2016;162:188-205.

Ming LG, Chen KM, Xian CJ. Functions and action mechanisms of flavonoids genistein and icariin in regulating bone remodeling. *J Cell Physiol*. 2013;228(3):513-521.

Sze SC, Tong Y, Ng TB, et al. Herba Epimedii: anti-oxidative properties and its medical implications. *Molecules*. 2010;15(11):7861-7870.

Tan H-L, Chan K-G, Pusparajah P, et al. Anti-cancer properties of the naturally occurring aphrodisiacs: icariin and its derivatives. *Front Pharmacol*. 2016;7:191.

Wang ZY, Liu J-G, Li H, Yang H-M. Pharmacological effects of active components of Chinese herbal medicine in the treatment of Alzheimer's disease: a review. *Am J Chin Med*. 2016;44(8):1525-1541.

Wu H, Lien EJ, Lien LL. Chemical and pharmacological investigations of Epimedium species: a survey. *Prog Drug Res*. 2003;60:1-57.

Wu Y, Li Y, Liu C, et al. Structural characterization of an acidic Epimedium polysaccharide and its immune-enhancement activity. *Carbohydr Polym*. 2016;138:134-142.

Yin L-L, Lin L-L, Zhang L, Lin L. Epimedium flavonoids ameliorate experimental autoimmune encephalomyelitis in rats by modulating neuroinflammatory and neurotrophic responses. *Neuropharmacology*. 2012;63(5):851-862.

Zhai YK, Guo X, Pan Y-L, et al. A systematic review of the efficacy and pharmacological profile of Herba Epimedii in osteoporosis therapy. *Pharmazie*. 2013;68(9):713-722.

Zhang W, Li R, Wang S, Mu F, Jia P. Effect of Chinese traditional herb Epimedium grandiflorum C. Morren and its extract Icariin on osteoarthritis via suppressing NF-kappaB pathway. *Indian J Exp Biol*. 2013;51(4):313-321.

Zhou J, Ma YH, Zhou Z, et al. Intestinal absorption and metabolism of Epimedium flavonoids in osteoporosis rats. *Drug Metab Dispos*. 2015;43(10):1590-1600.

Ashwagandha

Lopresti AL, Smith SJ, Malvi H, Kodgule R. An investigation into the stress-relieving and pharmacological actions of an ashwagandha (Withania somnifera) extract: a randomized, double-blind, placebo-controlled study. *Medicine (Baltimore).* 2019;98(37):e17186.

Chapter 17: Blood Sugar Control

See Chapters 2 and 11 for additional references.

Herbs and Natural Substances for Blood Glucose Control

Arun LB, Arunachalam AM, Arunachalam KD, Annamalai SK, Kumar KA. In vivo anti-ulcer, anti-stress, anti-allergic, and functional properties of gymnemic acid isolated from Gymnema sylvestre R Br. *BMC Complement Altern Med.* 2014;14:70.

Cuong DM, Arasu MV, Jeon J, et al. Medically important carotenoids from *Momordica charantia* and their gene expressions in different organs. *Saudi J Biol Sci.* 2017;24(8):1913-1919.

Efird JT, Choi YM, Davies SW, Mehra S, Anderson EJ, Katunga LA. Potential for improved glycemic control with dietary Momordica charantia in patients with insulin resistance and pre-diabetes. *Int J Environ Res Public Health.* 2014;11(2):2328-2345.

Goyal S, Gupta N, Chatterjee S. Investigating therapeutic potential of Trigonella foenum-graecum L. as our defense mechanism against several human diseases. *J Toxicol.* 2016;2016:1250387.

Kandhari K, Paudel S, Raina K, et al. Comparative pre-clinical efficacy of Chinese and Indian cultivars of bitter melon (*Momordica charantia*) against pancreatic cancer. *J Cancer Prev.* 2021;26(4):266-276.

Khan V, Najmi AK, Akhtar M, Aqil M, Mujeeb M, Pillai KK. A pharmacological appraisal of medicinal plants with antidiabetic potential. *J Pharm Bioallied Sci.* 2012;4(1):27-42.

Kimura I. Medical benefits of using natural compounds and their derivatives having multiple pharmacological actions. *Yakugaku Zasshi.* 2006;126(3):133-143.

Ma X, Egawa T, Kimura H, et al. Berberine-induced activation of 5'-adenosine monophosphate-activated protein kinase and glucose transport in rat skeletal muscles. *Metabolism.* 2010;59(11):1619-1627.

Miura T, Takagi S, Ishida T. Management of diabetes and its complications with Banaba (Lagerstroemia speciosa L.) and corosolic acid. *Evid Based Complement Alternat Med.* 2012;2012:871495.

Nahas R, Moher M. Complementary and alternative medicine for the treatment of type 2 diabetes. *Can Fam Physician.* 2009;55(6):591-596.

Pérez-Rubio KG, Gonzalez-Ortiz M, Martinez-Abundis E, et al. Effect of berberine administration on metabolic syndrome, insulin sensitivity, and insulin secretion. *Metab Syndr Relat Disord.* 2013;11(5):366-369.

Rao CV. Immunomodulatory effects of *Momordica charantia* extract in the prevention of oral cancer. *Cancer Prev Res (Phila).* 2018;11(4):185-186.

Wang Y, Zidichouski JA. Update on the benefits and mechanisms of action of the bioactive vegetal alkaloid berberine on lipid metabolism and homeostasis. *Cholesterol.* 2018;2018:7173920.

Yin J, Xing H, Ye J. Efficacy of berberine in patients with type 2 diabetes mellitus. *Metabolism.* 2008;57(5):712-717.

Zare R, Nadjarzadeh A, Zarshenas MM, Shams M, Heydari M. Efficacy of cinnamon in patients with type II diabetes mellitus: a randomized controlled clinical trial. *Clin Nutr.* 2019;38(2):549-556.

Zhang Y, Li X, Zou D, et al. Treatment of type 2 diabetes and dyslipidemia with the natural plant alkaloid berberine. *J Clin Endocrinol Metab.* 2008;93(7):2559-2565.

Zuñiga LY, González-Ortiz M, Martínez-Abundis E. Effect of Gymnema sylvestre administration on metabolic syndrome, insulin sensitivity, and insulin secretion. *J Med Food.* 2017;20(8):750-754.

Metformin

Nir Barzilai, Crandall JP, Kritchevsky SB, Espeland MA. Metformin as a tool to target aging. *Cell Metab.* 2016;23(6):1060-1065.

Podhorecka M, Ibanez B, Dmoszyńska A. Metformin - its potential anti-cancer and anti-aging effects. *Postepy Hig Med Dosw (Online).* 2017;71(0):170-175.

Chapter 18: Bone Health

Chen W, Melamed ML, Abramowitz MK. Serum bicarbonate and bone mineral density in US adults. *Am J Kidney Dis.* 2015;65(2):240-248.

Dawson-Hughes B, Harris SS, Palermo NJ, Castaneda-Sceppa C, Rasmussen HM, Dallal GE. Treatment with potassium bicarbonate lowers calcium excretion and bone resorption in older men and women. *J Clin Endocrinol Metab.* 2009;94(1):96-102.

Demontiero O, Vidal C, Duque G. Aging and bone loss: new insights for the clinician. *Ther Adv Musculoskelet Dis.* 2012;4(2):61-76.

Fardellone P, Séjourné A, Blain H, Cortet B, Thomas T; GRIO Scientific Committee. Osteoporosis: is milk a kindness or a curse? *Joint Bone Spine.* 2017;84(3):275-281.

Hwang YC, Jeong IK, Ahn KJ, Chung HY. The effects of Acanthopanax senticosus extract on bone turnover and bone mineral density in Korean postmenopausal women. *J Bone Miner Metab.* 2009;27(5):584-590.

International Osteoporosis Foundation. www.iofbonehealth.org

Reyes-Garcia R, Mendoza N, Palacios S, et al. Effects of daily intake of calcium and vitamin D-enriched milk in healthy postmenopausal women: a randomized, controlled, double-blind nutritional study. *J Womens Health (Larchmt).* 2018;27(5):561-568.

Rovenský J, Stancíková M, Masaryk P, Svík K, Istok R. Eggshell calcium in the prevention and treatment of osteoporosis. *Int J Clin Pharmacol Res.* 2003;23(2-3):83-92.

Santos L, Elliott-Sale KJ, Sale C. Exercise and bone health across the lifespan. *Biogerontology.* 2017;18(6):931-946.

Vitamin D

Aranow C. Vitamin D and the immune system. *J Investig Med.* 2011;59(6):881-886.

Ascherio A, Munger KL, White R, et al. Vitamin D as an early predictor of multiple sclerosis activity and progression. *JAMA Neurol.* 2014;71(3):306-314.

Garland CF, Kim JJ, Mohr SB, et al. Meta-analysis of all-cause mortality according to serum 25-hydroxyvitamin D. *Am J Public Health.* 2014;104(8):e43-e50.

Ginde AA, Mansbach JM, Camargo CA Jr. Association between serum 25-hydroxyvitamin D level and upper respiratory tract infection in the Third National Health and Nutrition Examination Survey. *Arch Intern Med.* 2009;169(4):384-390.

Jorde R, Sneve M, Figenschau Y, Svartberg J, Waterloo K. Effects of vitamin D supplementation on symptoms of depression in overweight and obese subjects: randomized double blind trial. *J Intern Med.* 2008;264(6):599-609.

Lee J, van Hecke O, Roberts N. Vitamin D: a rapid review of the evidence for treatment or prevention in COVID-19. The Centre for Evidence-Based Medicine. May 1, 2020. https://www.cebm.net/covid-19/vitamin-d-a-rapid-review-of-the-evidence-for-treatment-or-prevention-in-covid-19/

Lips P, Eekhoff M, van Schoor N, et al. Vitamin D and type 2 diabetes. *J Steroid Biochem Mol Biol.* 2017;173:280-285.

Liu X, Baylin A, Levy PD. Vitamin D deficiency and insufficiency among US adults: prevalence, predictors and clinical implications. *Br J Nutr.* 2018;119(8):928-936.

National Institutes of Health. Vitamin D: fact sheet for health professionals. https://ods.od.nih.gov/factsheets/VitaminD-HealthProfessional/

Northwestern University. One size doesn't fit all for vitamin D and men: African-American men in northern regions especially need high doses of supplements. *ScienceDaily*. September 20, 2011. www.sciencedaily.com/releases/2011/09/110920100100.htm

Raharusun P, Priambada S, Budiarti C, Agung E, Budi C. Patterns of COVID-19 mortality and Vitamin D: an Indonesian study. April 26, 2020. https://www.readcube.com/articles/10.2139%2Fssrn.3585561

Rhodes LE, Webb AR, Fraser HI, et al. Recommended summer sunlight exposure levels can produce sufficient (> or =20 ng ml(-1)) but not the proposed optimal (> or =32 ng ml(-1)) 25(OH)D levels at UK latitudes. *J Invest Dermatol*. 2010;130(5):1411-1418.

T.H. Chan School of Public Health, Harvard University. The nutrition source. Vitamin D. March 2020. https://www.hsph.harvard.edu/nutritionsource/vitamin-d/

Chapter 19: Brain Health

Bartol TM, Bromer C, Kinney J, et al. Nanoconnectomic upper bound on the variability of synaptic plasticity. *Elife*. 2015;4:e10778.

Cardoso SM, Empadinhas N. The microbiome-mitochondria dance in prodromal Parkinson's disease. *Front Physiol*. 2018;9:471.

De Chiara G, Marcocci ME, Sgarbanti R, et al. Infectious agents and neurodegeneration. *Mol Neurobiol*. 2012;46(3):614-638.

Fumagalli M, Lombardi M, Gressens P, Verderio C. How to reprogram microglia toward beneficial functions. *Glia*. 2018;66(12):2531-2549.

Goldman SA, Kuypers NJ. How to make an oligodendrocyte. *Development*. 2015;142(23):3983-3995.

Hickman S, Izzy S, Sen P, Morsett L, El Khoury J. Microglia in neurodegeneration. *Nat Neurosci*. 2018;21(10):1359-1369.

Hirschberg S, Gisevius B, Duscha A, Haghikia A. Implications of diet and the gut microbiome in neuroinflammatory and neurodegenerative diseases. *Int J Mol Sci*. 2019;20(12):3109.

Jiang C, Li G, Huang P, Liu Z, Zhao B. The gut microbiota and Alzheimer's disease. *J Alzheimers Dis*. 2017;58(1):1-15.

Khakh BS, Sofroniew MV. Diversity of astrocyte functions and phenotypes in neural circuits. *Nat Neurosci*. 2015;18(7):942-952.

Kuhn S, Gritti L, Crooks D, Dombrowski Y. Oligodendrocytes in development, myelin generation and beyond. *Cells*. 2019;8(11):1424.

Maass W, Papadimitriou CH, Vempala S, Legenstein R. Brain computation: a computer science perspective. In: Steffen B, Woeginger G, eds. *Computing and Software Science. Lecture Notes in Computer Science*, vol 10000. Springer; 2019:184-199.

MacDonald AB. Spirochetal cyst forms in neurodegenerative disorders...hiding in plain sight. *Med Hypotheses.* 2006;67(4):819-832.

Nasrabady SE, Rizvi B, Goldman JE, Brickman AM. White matter changes in Alzheimer's disease: a focus on myelin and oligodendrocytes. *Acta Neuropathol Commun.* 2018;6(1):22.

Nayak D, Roth TL, McGavern DB. Microglia development and function. *Annu Rev Immunol.* 2014;32:367-402.

Paoli A, Bianco A, Damiani E, Bosco G. Ketogenic diet in neuromuscular and neurodegenerative diseases. *Biomed Res Int.* 2014;2014:474296.

Plog BA, Nedergaard M. The glymphatic system in central nervous system health and disease: past, present, and future. *Annu Rev Pathol.* 2018;13:379-394.

Sohrab SS, Suhail M, Ali A, et al. Role of viruses, prions and miRNA in neurodegenerative disorders and dementia. *Virusdisease.* 2018;29(4):419-433.

Soung A, Klein RS. Viral Encephalitis and neurologic diseases: focus on astrocytes. *Trends Mol Med.* 2018;24(11):950-962.

Wang HX, Wang YP. Gut microbiota-brain axis. *Chin Med J (Engl).* 2016;129(19):2373-2380.

Zhou L, Miranda-Saksena M, Saksena NK. Viruses and neurodegeneration. *Virol J.* 2013;10:172.

Alzheimer's

Allen HB. Alzheimer's disease: assessing the role of spirochetes, biofilms, the immune system, and amyloid-β with regard to potential treatment and prevention. *J Alzheimers Dis.* 2016;53(4):1271-1276.

Alonso R, Pisa D, Fernández-Fernández AM, Carrasco L. Infection of fungi and bacteria in brain tissue from elderly persons and patients With Alzheimer's disease. *Front Aging Neurosci.* 2018;10:159.

Angelucci F, Cechova K, Amlerova J, Hort J. Antibiotics, gut microbiota, and Alzheimer's disease. *J Neuroinflammation.* 2019;16(1):108.

Azam S, Haque ME, Kim IS, Choi DK. Microglial turnover in ageing-related neurodegeneration: therapeutic avenue to intervene in disease progression. *Cells.* 2021;10(1):150.

Blanc F, Philippi N, Cretin B, et al. Lyme neuroborreliosis and dementia. *J Alzheimers Dis.* 2014;41(4):1087-1093.

Emery DC, Shoemark DK, Batstone TE, et al. 16S rRNA next generation sequencing analysis shows bacteria in Alzheimer's post-mortem brain. *Front Aging Neurosci.* 2017;9:195.

Franceschi F, Ojetti V, Candelli M, et al. Microbes and Alzheimer' disease: lessons from H. pylori and GUT microbiota. *Eur Rev Med Pharmacol Sci*. 2019;23(1):426-430.

Frost GR, Li YM. The role of astrocytes in amyloid production and Alzheimer's disease. *Open Biol*. 2017;7(12):170228.

Hu X, Wang T, Jin F. Alzheimer's disease and gut microbiota. *Sci China Life Sci*. 2016;59(10):1006-1023.

Itzhaki RF, Lathe R, Balin BJ, et al. Microbes and Alzheimer's disease. *J Alzheimers Dis*. 2016;51(4):979-984.

La Rosa F, Clerici M, Ratto D, et al. The gut-brain axis in Alzheimer's disease and omega-3. A critical overview of clinical trials. *Nutrients*. 2018;10(9):1267.

Moir RD, Lathe R, Tanzi RE. The antimicrobial protection hypothesis of Alzheimer's disease. *Alzheimers Dement*. 2018;14(12):1602-1614.

Nayeri Chegeni T, Sarvi S, Moosazadeh M, et al. Is Toxoplasma gondii a potential risk factor for Alzheimer's disease? A systematic review and meta-analysis. *Microb Pathog*. 2019;137:103751.

Pearson HA, Peers C. Physiological roles for amyloid beta peptides. *J Physiol*. 2006;575(Pt 1):5-10.

Pisa D, Alonso R, Fernández-Fernández AM, Rábano A, Carrasco L. Polymicrobial infections In brain tissue from Alzheimer's disease patients. *Sci Rep*. 2017;7(1):5559.

Sevigny J, Chiao P, Bussière T, et al. The antibody aducanumab reduces Aβ plaques in Alzheimer's disease. *Nature*. 2016;537(7618):50-56.

Amyloid

Brothers HM, Gosztyla ML, Robinson SR. The physiological roles of amyloid-β peptide hint at new ways to treat Alzheimer's disease. *Front Aging Neurosci*. 2018;10:118.

Frost GR, Li YM. The role of astrocytes in amyloid production and Alzheimer's disease. *Open Biol*. 2017;7(12):170228.

Pearson HA, Peers C. Physiological roles for amyloid beta peptides. *J Physiol*. 2006;575(Pt 1):5-10.

Zhan X, Stamova B, Sharp FR. Lipopolysaccharide associates with amyloid plaques, neurons and oligodendrocytes in Alzheimer's disease brain: a review. *Front Aging Neurosci*. 2018;10:42.

Glymphatic System

Benveniste H, Liu X, Koundal S, Sanggaard S, Lee H, Wardlaw J. The glymphatic system and waste clearance with brain aging: a review. *Gerontology*. 2019;65(2):106-119.

Jessen NA, Munk AS, Lundgaard I, Nedergaard M. The glymphatic system: a beginner's guide. *Neurochem Res*. 2015;40(12):2583-2599.

Kim YK, Nam KI, Song J. The glymphatic system in diabetes-induced dementia. *Front Neurol.* 2018;9:867.

Nedergaard M, Goldman SA. Glymphatic failure as a final common pathway to dementia. *Science.* 2020;370(6512):50-56.

Brain Fog

Ross AJ, Medow MS, Rowe PC, Stewart JM. What is brain fog? An evaluation of the symptom in postural tachycardia syndrome. *Clin Auton Res.* 2013;23(6):305-311.

Stefano GB. Historical insight into infections and disorders associated with neurological and psychiatric sequelae similar to long COVID. *Med Sci Monit.* 2021;27:e931447.

Theoharides TC, Cholevas C, Polyzoidis K, Politis A. Long-COVID syndrome-associated brain fog and chemofog: luteolin to the rescue. *Biofactors.* 2021;47(2):232-241.

Theoharides TC, Stewart JM, Hatziagelaki E, Kolaitis G. Brain "fog," inflammation and obesity: key aspects of neuropsychiatric disorders improved by luteolin. *Front Neurosci.* 2015;9:225.

Yelland GW. Gluten-induced cognitive impairment ("brain fog") in coeliac disease. *J Gastroenterol Hepatol.* 2017;(32 Suppl 1):90-93.

Bacopa

Benson S, Downey LA, Stough C, Wetherell M, Zangara A, Scholey A. An acute, double-blind, placebo-controlled cross-over study of 320 mg and 640 mg doses of Bacopa monnieri (CDRI 08) on multitasking stress reactivity and mood. *Phytother Res.* 2014;28(4):551-559.

Calabrese C, Gregory WL, Leo M, Kraemer D, Bone K, Oken B. Effects of a standardized Bacopa monnieri extract on cognitive performance, anxiety, and depression in the elderly: a randomized, double-blind, placebo-controlled trial. *J Altern Complement Med.* 2008;14(6):707-713.

Dave UP, Dingankar SR, Saxena VS, et al. An open-label study to elucidate the effects of standardized Bacopa monnieri extract in the management of symptoms of attention-deficit hyperactivity disorder in children. *Adv Mind Body Med.* 2014;28(2):10-15.

Morgan A, Stevens J. Does Bacopa monnieri improve memory performance in older persons? Results of a randomized, placebo-controlled, double-blind trial. *J Altern Complement Med.* 2010;16(7):753-759.

Pravina K, Ravindra KR, Goudar KS, et al. Safety evaluation of BacoMind in healthy volunteers: a phase I study. *Phytomedicine.* 2007;14(5):301-308.

Saini N, Singh D, Sandhir R. Neuroprotective effects of Bacopa monnieri in experimental model of dementia. *Neurochem Res.* 2012;37(9):1928-1937.

Sarris J, McIntyre E, Camfield DA. Plant-based medicines for anxiety disorders, part 2: a review of clinical studies with supporting preclinical evidence. *CNS Drugs*. 2013;27(4):301-319. [published correction appears in *CNS Drugs*. 2013;27(8):675. Dosage error in article text.]

Shinomol GK, Muralidhara, Bharath MM. Exploring the role of "Brahmi" (Bacopa monnieri and Centella asiatica) in brain function and therapy. *Recent Pat Endocr Metab Immune Drug Discov*. 2011;5(1):33-49.

Lion's Mane

Diling C, Xin Y, Chaoqun Z, et al. Extracts from *Hericium erinaceus* relieve inflammatory bowel disease by regulating immunity and gut microbiota. *Oncotarget*. 2017;8(49):85838-85857.

Jiang S, Wang S, Sun Y, Zhang Q. Medicinal properties of Hericium erinaceus and its potential to formulate novel mushroom-based pharmaceuticals. *Appl Microbiol Biotechnol*. 2014;98(18):7661-7670.

Khan MA, Tania M, Liu R, Rahman MM. Hericium erinaceus: an edible mushroom with medicinal values. *J Complement Integr Med*. 2013;10:/j/jcim.2013.10.issue-1/jcim-2013-0001/jcim-2013-0001.xml.

Lai PL, Naidu M, Sabaratnam V, et al. Neurotrophic properties of the Lion's mane medicinal mushroom, Hericium erinaceus (higher Basidiomycetes) from Malaysia. *Int J Med Mushrooms*. 2013;15(6):539-554.

Mori K, Inatomi S, Ouchi K, Azumi Y, Tuchida T. Improving effects of the mushroom Yamabushitake (Hericium erinaceus) on mild cognitive impairment: a double-blind placebo-controlled clinical trial. *Phytother Res*. 2009;23(3):367-372.

Nagano M, Shimizu K, Kondo R, et al. Reduction of depression and anxiety by 4 weeks Hericium erinaceus intake. *Biomed Res*. 2010;31(4):231-237.

Qin M, Geng Y, Lu Z, et al. Anti-inflammatory effects of ethanol extract of lion's mane medicinal mushroom, Hericium erinaceus (agaricomycetes), in mice with ulcerative colitis. *Int J Med Mushrooms*. 2016;18(3):227-234.

Ren Z, Qin T, Qiu F, et al. Immunomodulatory effects of hydroxyethylated Hericium erinaceus polysaccharide on macrophages RAW264.7. *Int J Biol Macromol*. 2017;105(Pt 1):879-885.

Tsai-Teng T, Chin-Chu C, Li-Ya L, et al. Erinacine A-enriched Hericium erinaceus mycelium ameliorates Alzheimer's disease-related pathologies in APPswe/PS1dE9 transgenic mice. *J Biomed Sci*. 2016;23(1):49.

Wong KH, Naidu M, David RP, Bakar R, Sabaratnam V. Neuroregenerative potential of lion's mane mushroom, Hericium erinaceus (Bull.: Fr.) Pers. (higher Basidiomycetes), in the treatment of peripheral nerve injury (review). *Int J Med Mushrooms*. 2012;14(5):427-446.

Ginkgo

Gauthier S, Schlaefke S. Efficacy and tolerability of Ginkgo biloba extract EGb 761® in dementia: a systematic review and meta-analysis of randomized placebo-controlled trials. *Clin Interv Aging.* 2014;9:2065-2077.

Hashiguchi M, Ohta Y, Shimizu M, Maruyama J, Mochizuki M. Meta-analysis of the efficacy and safety of Ginkgo biloba extract for the treatment of dementia. *J Pharm Health Care Sci.* 2015;1:14.

Nabavi SM, Habtemariam S, Daglia M, et al. Neuroprotective effects of ginkgolide B against ischemic stroke: a review of current literature. *Curr Top Med Chem.* 2015;15(21):2222-2232.

Solfrizzi V, Panza F. Plant-based nutraceutical interventions against cognitive impairment and dementia: meta-analytic evidence of efficacy of a standardized Gingko biloba extract. *J Alzheimers Dis.* 2015;43(2):605-611.

Tan MS, Yu JT, Tan CC, et al. Efficacy and adverse effects of ginkgo biloba for cognitive impairment and dementia: a systematic review and meta-analysis. *J Alzheimers Dis.* 2015;43(2):589-603.

Yang G, Wang Y, Sun J, Zhang K, Liu J. Ginkgo biloba for mild cognitive impairment and Alzheimer's disease: a systematic review and meta-analysis of randomized controlled trials. *Curr Top Med Chem.* 2016;16(5):520 528.

Chapter 20: Cardiovascular Health

Adams DD. The great cholesterol myth; unfortunate consequences of Brown and Goldstein's mistake. *QJM.* 2011;104(10):867-870.

Bautch VL, Caron KM. Blood and lymphatic vessel formation. *Cold Spring Harb Perspect Biol.* 2015;7(3):a008268.

Bayram A, Erdogan MB, Eksi F, Yamak B. Demonstration of Chlamydophila pneumoniae, Mycoplasma pneumoniae, Cytomegalovirus, and Epstein-Barr virus in atherosclerotic coronary arteries, nonrheumatic calcific aortic and rheumatic stenotic mitral valves by polymerase chain reaction. *Anadolu Kardiyol Derg.* 2011;11(3):237-43.

Becker RC. The role of blood viscosity in the development and progression of coronary artery disease. *Cleve Clin J Med.* 1993;60(5):353-358.

Celik T, Balta S, Ozturk C, Iyisoy A. Whole blood viscosity and cardiovascular diseases: a forgotten old player of the game. *Med Princ Pract.* 2016;25(5):499-500.

de Almeida AJPO, Ribeiro TP, de Medeiros IA. Aging: molecular pathways and Implications on the cardiovascular system. *Oxid Med Cell Longev.* 2017;2017:7941563.

Ercan M, Konukoglu D, Erdem Yeşim T. Association of plasma viscosity with cardiovascular risk factors in obesity: an old marker, a new insight. *Clin Hemorheol Microcirc.* 2006;35(4):441-446.

Félix-Redondo FJ, Grau M, Fernández-Bergés D. Cholesterol and cardiovascular disease in the elderly. Facts and gaps. *Aging Dis*. 2013;4(3):154-169.

Forkosh E, Ilan Y. The heart-gut axis: new target for atherosclerosis and congestive heart failure therapy. *Open Heart*. 2019;6(1):e000993.

Galkina E, Ley K. Immune and inflammatory mechanisms of atherosclerosis (*). *Annu Rev Immunol*. 2009;27:165-197.

Koren O, Spor A, Felin J, et al. Human oral, gut, and plaque microbiota in patients with atherosclerosis. *Proc Natl Acad Sci U S A*. 2011;108(Suppl 1):4592-4598.

Lanter BB, Sauer K, Davies DG. Bacteria present in carotid arterial plaques are found as biofilm deposits which may contribute to enhanced risk of plaque rupture. *mBio*. 2014;5(3):e01206-e1214.

Lowe GD, Lee AJ, Rumley A, Price JF, Fowkes FG. Blood viscosity and risk of cardiovascular events: the Edinburgh Artery Study. *Br J Haematol*. 1997;96(1):168-173.

Marques da Silva R, Caugant DA, Eribe ER, et al. Bacterial diversity in aortic aneurysms determined by 16S ribosomal RNA gene analysis. *J Vasc Surg*. 2006;44(5):1055-1060.

Ott SJ, El Mokhtari NE, Musfeldt M, et al. Detection of diverse bacterial signatures in atherosclerotic lesions of patients with coronary heart disease. *Circulation*. 2006;113(7):929-937.

Parthasarathy S, Raghavamenon A, Garelnabi MO, Santanam N. Oxidized low-density lipoprotein. *Methods Mol Biol*. 2010;610:403-417.

Tang WH, Kitai T, Hazen SL. Gut microbiota in cardiovascular health and disease. *Circ Res*. 2017;120(7):1183-1196.

Wang Z, Zhao Y. Gut microbiota derived metabolites in cardiovascular health and disease. *Protein Cell*. 2018;9(5):416-431.

Microbes/Carditis

Blauwet LA, Cooper LT. Myocarditis. *Prog Cardiovasc Dis*. 2010;52(4):274-288.

Bracamonte-Baran W, Čiháková D. Cardiac autoimmunity: myocarditis. *Adv Exp Med Biol*. 2017;1003:187-221.

Bush LM, Vazquez-Pertejo MT. Tick borne illness-Lyme disease. *Dis Mon*. 2018;64(5):195-212.

Cooper LT Jr. Myocarditis. *N Engl J Med*. 2009;360(15):1526-1538.

Guzik TJ, Mohiddin SA, Dimarco A, et al. COVID-19 and the cardiovascular system: implications for risk assessment, diagnosis, and treatment options. *Cardiovasc Res*. 2020;116(10):1666-1687.

Herath HMLY, Jayasundara JMHD, Senadhira SDN, Kularatne SAM, Kularatne WKS. Spotted fever rickettsioses causing myocarditis and ARDS: a case from Sri Lanka. *BMC Infect Dis*. 2018;18(1):705.

Holland TL, Baddour LM, Bayer AS, Hoen B, Miro JM, Fowler VG Jr. Infective endocarditis. *Nat Rev Dis Primers*. 2016;2:16059.

Ki YJ, Kim DM, Yoon NR, Kim SS, Kim CM. A case report of scrub typhus complicated with myocarditis and rhabdomyolysis. *BMC Infect Dis*. 2018;18(1):551.

Kitai T, Tang WHW. Gut microbiota in cardiovascular disease and heart failure. *Clin Sci (Lond)*. 2018;132(1):85-91.

Kostić T, Momčilović S, Perišić ZD, et al. Manifestations of Lyme carditis. *Int J Cardiol*. 2017;232:24-32.

Kushawaha A, Brown M, Martin I, Evenhuis W. Hitch-hiker taken for a ride: an unusual cause of myocarditis, septic shock and adult respiratory distress syndrome. *BMJ Case Rep*. 2013;2013:bcr2012007155.

Lasrado N, Yalaka B, Reddy J. Triggers of inflammatory heart disease. *Front Cell Dev Biol*. 2020;8:192.

Leone O, Pieroni M, Rapezzi C, Olivotto I. The spectrum of myocarditis: from pathology to the clinics. *Virchows Arch*. 2019;475(3):279-301.

Myers F, Mishra PE, Cortez D, Schleiss MR. Chest palpitations in a teenager as an unusual presentation of Lyme disease: case report. *BMC Infect Dis*. 2020;20(1):730.

Okaro U, Addisu A, Casanas B, Anderson B. Bartonella species, an emerging cause of blood-culture-negative endocarditis. *Clin Microbiol Rev*. 2017;30(3):709-746.

Oktay AA, Dibs SR, Friedman H. Sinus pause in association with Lyme carditis. *Tex Heart Inst J*. 2015;42(3):248-250.

Ørbæk M, Lebech AM, Helleberg M. The clinical spectrum of tularemia–two cases. *IDCases*. 2020;21:e00890.

Revilla-Martí P, Cecilio-Irazola Á, Gayán-Ordás J, Sanjoaquín-Conde I, Linares-Vicente JA, Oteo JA. Acute myopericarditis associated with tickborne *Rickettsia sibirica mongolitimonae*. *Emerg Infect Dis*. 2017;23(12):2091-2093.

Rivera OJ, Nookala V. Lyme carditis. In: *StatPearls*. StatPearls Publishing; February 15, 2022.

Rose NR. Viral myocarditis. *Curr Opin Rheumatol*. 2016;28(4):383-389.

Shah SS, McGowan JP. Rickettsial, ehrlichial and Bartonella infections of the myocardium and pericardium. *Front Biosci*. 2003;8:e197-e201.

Trøseid M, Andersen GØ, Broch K, Hov JR. The gut microbiome in coronary artery disease and heart failure: current knowledge and future directions. *EBioMedicine*. 2020;52:102649.

Yeung C, Baranchuk A. Diagnosis and treatment of Lyme carditis: JACC review topic of the week. *J Am Coll Cardiol*. 2019;73(6):717-726. [published correction appears in *J Am Coll Cardiol*. 2019;74(21):2709-2711.]

Herbs for Cardiovascular

Al Disi SS, Anwar MA, Eid AH. Anti-hypertensive herbs and their mechanisms of action: part I. *Front Pharmacol*. 2016;6:323.

Anwar MA, Al Disi SS, Eid AH. Anti-hypertensive herbs and their mechanisms of action: part II. *Front Pharmacol*. 2016;7:50.

Bayan L, Koulivand PH, Gorji A. Garlic: a review of potential therapeutic effects. *Avicenna J Phytomed*. 2014;4(1):1-14.

Pereira CPM, Souza ACR, Vasconcelos AR, Prado PS, Name JJ. Antioxidant and anti-inflammatory mechanisms of action of astaxanthin in cardiovascular diseases (Review). *Int J Mol Med*. 2021;47(1):37-48.

See Chapter 5 for references on hawthorn.

See Chapter 9 for references on milk thistle and garlic.

See Chapter 11 for references on maritime pine bark.

Chapter 21: Gastrointestinal Health

Bassotti G, de Roberto G, Castellani D, Sediari L, Morelli A. Normal aspects of colorectal motility and abnormalities in slow transit constipation. *World J Gastroenterol*. 2005;11(18):2691-2696.

Bharucha AE, Lacy BE. Mechanisms, evaluation, and management of chronic constipation. *Gastroenterology*. 2020;158(5):1232-1249.e3.

Bures J, Cyrany J, Kohoutova D, et al. Small intestinal bacterial overgrowth syndrome. *World J Gastroenterol*. 2010;16(24):2978-2990.

Concon J, Newburg D, Eades S. Lectins in wheat gluten proteins. *J Agric Food Chem*. 1983;31:939-941.

Freed DL. Do dietary lectins cause disease? *BMJ*. 1999;318(7190):1023-1024.

Hamid R, Masood A. Dietary lectins as disease causing toxicants. *Pakistan J Nutr*. 2009;8(3):293-303.

Iebba V, Totino V, Gagliardi A, et al. Eubiosis and dysbiosis: the two sides of the microbiota. *New Microbiol*. 2016;39(1):1-12.

Israelyan N, Del Colle A, Li Z, et al. Effects of serotonin and slow-release 5-hydroxytryptophan on gastrointestinal motility in a mouse model of depression. *Gastroenterology*. 2019;157(2):507-521.e4.

Jones MP, Bratten JR. Small intestinal motility. *Curr Opin Gastroenterol.* 2008;24(2):164-172.

Losurdo G, Salvatore D'Abramo F, Indellicati G, Lillo C, Ierardi E, Di Leo A. The influence of small intestinal bacterial overgrowth in digestive and extra-intestinal disorders. *Int J Mol Sci.* 2020;21(10):3531.

Majee SB, Biswas GR, Exploring plant lectins in diagnosis, prophylaxis, and therapy. *J Med Plant Res.* 2013;7(47):3444-3451.

Martinez KB, Leone V, Chang EB. Western diets, gut dysbiosis, and metabolic diseases: are they linked? *Gut Microbes.* 2017;8(2):130-142.

Nachbar M, Oppenheim JD. Lectins in the United States diet, a survey of lectins in commonly consumed foods and a review of the literature. *Am J Clin Nutr.* 1980;88(11):2338-2345.

Rao SSC, Bhagatwala J. Small intestinal bacterial overgrowth: clinical features and therapeutic management. *Clin Transl Gastroenterol.* 2019;10(10):e00078.

Tomasello G, Mazzola M, Leone A, et al. Nutrition, oxidative stress and intestinal dysbiosis: influence of diet on gut microbiota in inflammatory bowel diseases. *Biomed Pap Med Fac Univ Palacky Olomouc Czech Repub.* 2016;160(4):461-466.

Weiss GA, Hennet T. Mechanisms and consequences of intestinal dysbiosis. *Cell Mol Life Sci.* 2017;74(16):2959-2977.

Dandelion

González-Castejón M, Visioli F, Rodriguez-Casado A. Diverse biological activities of dandelion. *Nutr Rev.* 2012;70(9):534-47.

Kenny O, Brunton MP, Walsh D, et al. Characterisation of antimicrobial extracts from dandelion root (Taraxacum officinale) using LC-SPE-NMR. *Phytother Res.* 2015;29(4):526-532.

Martinez M, Poirrier P, Chamy R, et al. Taraxacum officinale and related species–an ethnopharmacological review and its potential as a commercial medicinal plant. *J Ethnopharmacol.* 2015;169:244-262.

Ovadje P, Ammar S, Guerrero JA, et al. Dandelion root extract affects colorectal cancer proliferation and survival through the activation of multiple death signalling pathways. *Oncotarget.* 2016;7(45).

Schütz K, Carle R, Schieber A. Taraxacum, a review on its phytochemical and pharmacological profile. *J Ethnopharmacol.* 2006;107(3):313-323.

Spelman K, Conroy RS, Spelman K. The diuretic effect in human subjects of an extract of Taraxacum officinale folium over a single day. *J Altern Complement Med.* 2009;15(8):929-934.

Choi UK, Lee O-H, Yim JH, et al. Hypolipidemic and antioxidant effects of dandelion (Taraxacum officinale) root and leaf on cholesterol-fed rabbits. *Int J Mol Sci.* 2010;11(1):67-78.

Wirngo FE, Lambert MN, Jeppesen PB. The physiological effects of dandelion (Taraxacum officinale) in type 2 diabetes. *Rev Diabet Stud.* 2016;13(2-3):113-131.

Yarnell E, Abascal K. Review article: dandelion (Taraxacum officinale and T mongolicum). *Int Med J.* 2009;8(2):35-38.

Cardamon/Fennel

Cárdenas Garza GR, Elizondo Luévano JH, Bazaldúa Rodríguez AF, et al. Benefits of cardamom (*Elettaria cardamomum* (L.) Maton) and turmeric (*Curcuma longa* L.) extracts for their applications as natural anti-inflammatory adjuvants. *Plants (Basel).* 2021;10(9):1908.

Parham S, Kharazi AZ, Bakhsheshi-Rad HR, et al. Antioxidant, antimicrobial and antiviral properties of herbal materials. *Antioxidants (Basel).* 2020;9(12):1309.

Rauf A, Akram M, Semwal P, et al. Antispasmodic potential of medicinal plants: a comprehensive review. *Oxid Med Cell Longev.* 2021;2021:4889719.

Bitters

Chou WL. Therapeutic potential of targeting intestinal bitter taste receptors in diabetes associated with dyslipidemia. *Pharmacol Res.* 2021;170:105693.

Depoortere I. Taste receptors of the gut: emerging roles in health and disease. *Gut.* 2014;63(1):179-190.

McMullen MK, Whitehouse JM, Towell A. Bitters: time for a new paradigm. *Evid Based Complement Alternat Med.* 2015;2015:670504.

Sternini C. Taste receptors in the gastrointestinal tract. IV. Functional implications of bitter taste receptors in gastrointestinal chemosensing. *Am J Physiol Gastrointest Liver Physiol.* 2007;292(2):G457-G461.

Berberine

Imenshahidi M, Hosseinzadeh H. Berberine and barberry (Berberis vulgaris): a clinical review. *Phytother Res.* 2019;33(3):504-523.

Rauf A, Abu-Izneid T, Khalil AA, et al. Berberine as a potential anticancer agent: a comprehensive review. *Molecules.* 2021;26(23):7368.

Wang Y, Zidichouski JA. Update on the benefits and mechanisms of action of the bioactive vegetal alkaloid berberine on lipid metabolism and homeostasis. *Cholesterol.* 2018;2018:7173920.

Zhang L, Wu X, Yang R, et al. Effects of berberine on the gastrointestinal microbiota. *Front Cell Infect Microbiol.* 2021;10:588517.

See Chapter 12 for references on chlorella.

Chapter 22: Joint Health

Akkiraju H, Nohe A. Role of chondrocytes in cartilage formation, progression of osteoarthritis and cartilage regeneration. *J Dev Biol.* 2015;3(4):177-192.

Birch HL, Thorpe CT, Rumian AP. Specialisation of extracellular matrix for function in tendons and ligaments. *Muscles Ligaments Tendons J.* 2013;3(1):12-22.

Caminer AC, Haberman R, Scher JU. Human microbiome, infections, and rheumatic disease. *Clin Rheumatol.* 2017;36(12):2645-2653.

Carter JD, Inman RD, Whittum-Hudson J, Hudson AP. Chlamydia and chronic arthritis. *Ann Med.* 2012;44(8):784-792.

de Molon RS, Rossa C Jr, Thurlings RM, Cirelli JA, Koenders MI. Linkage of periodontitis and rheumatoid arthritis: current evidence and potential biological interactions. *Int J Mol Sci.* 2019;20(18):4541.

Grab DJ, Kennedy R, Philipp MT. Borrelia burgdorferi possesses a collagenolytic activity. *FEMS Microbiol Lett.* 1996;144(1):39-45.

Harrington DJ. Bacterial collagenases and collagen-degrading enzymes and their potential role in human disease. *Infect Immun.* 1996;64(6):1885-1891.

Jadhav P, Jiang Y, Jarr K, Layton C, Ashouri JF, Sinha SR. Efficacy of dietary supplements in inflammatory bowel disease and related autoimmune diseases. *Nutrients.* 2020;12(7):2156.

Jansson E, Backman A, Hakkarainen K, Miettinen A, Seniusová B. Mycoplasmas and arthritis. *Z Rheumatol.* 1983;42(6):315-319.

Jeng CM, Cheng TC, Kung CH, Hsu HC. Yoga and disc degenerative disease in cervical and lumbar spine: an MR imaging-based case control study. *Eur Spine J.* 2011;20(3):408-413.

Johnson S, Sidebottom D, Brucker F, Collins D. Identification of Mycoplasma fermentans in synovial fluid samples from arthritis patients with inflammatory disease. *J Clin Microbiol.* 2000;38(1):90-93.

Johnson S, Bruckner F, Collins D. Distribution of Mycoplasma pneumoniae and Mycoplasma salivarium in the synovial fluid of arthritis patients. *J Clin Microbiol.* 2007;45(3):953-957.

Karataş E, Kul A, Tepecik E. Association between rheumatoid arthritis and apical periodontitis: a cross-sectional study. *Eur Endod J.* 2020;5(2):155-158.

Rashid T, Ebringer A. Autoimmunity in rheumatic diseases Is Induced by microbial infections via cross reactivity or molecular mimicry. *Autoimmune Dis.* 2012;2012:539282.

Scher JU. The microbiome in psoriasis and psoriatic arthritis: joints. *J Rheumatol Suppl.* 2018;94:32-35.

Scherer HU, Häupl T, Burmester GR. The etiology of rheumatoid arthritis. *J Autoimmun.* 2020;110:102400.

Schett G. How does joint remodeling work?: new insights in the molecular regulation of the architecture of joints. *Cell Adh Migr.* 2007;1(2):102-103.

Siala M, Gdoura R, Fourati H, et al. Broad-range PCR, cloning and sequencing of the full 16S rRNA gene for detection of bacterial DNA in synovial fluid samples of Tunisian patients with reactive and undifferentiated arthritis. *Arthritis Res Ther.* 2009;11(4):R102.

Tamer TM. Hyaluronan and synovial joint: function, distribution and healing. *Interdiscip Toxicol.* 2013;6(3):111-125.

Vural M, Gilbert B, Üstün I, Caglar S, Finckh A. Mini-review: human microbiome and rheumatic diseases. *Front Cell Infect Microbiol.* 2020;10:491160.

Zeidler H, Hudson AP. Coinfection of Chlamydiae and other bacteria in reactive arthritis and spondyloarthritis: need for future research. *Microorganisms.* 2016;4(3):E30.

Herbal and Natural Supplements for Joints

Bruyère O, Altman RD, Reginster JY. Efficacy and safety of glucosamine sulfate in the management of osteoarthritis: evidence from real-life setting trials and surveys. *Semin Arthritis Rheum.* 2016;45(4 Suppl):S12-S17.

Conrozier T, Mathieu P, Bonjean M, Marc JF, Renevier JL, Balblanc JC. A complex of three natural anti-inflammatory agents provides relief of osteoarthritis pain. *Altern Ther Health Med.* 2014;(20 Suppl 1):32-37.

Raynauld JP, Pelletier JP, Abram F, Dodin P, Delorme P, Martel-Pelletier J. Long-term effects of glucosamine and chondroitin sulfate on the progression of structural changes in knee osteoarthritis: six-year followup data from the osteoarthritis initiative. *Arthritis Care Res (Hoboken).* 2016;68(10):1560-1566.

Walker AF, Bundy R, Hicks SM, Middleton RW. Bromelain reduces mild acute knee pain and improves well-being in a dose-dependent fashion in an open study of otherwise healthy adults. *Phytomedicine.* 2002;9(8):681-686.

Chapter 23: Menopause

Ambler D, Bieber E, Diamond M. Sexual function in elderly women: a review of current literature. *Rev Obstet Gynecol.* 2012;5(1):16-27.

Depypere HT, Comhaire FH. Herbal preparations for the menopause: beyond isoflavones and black cohosh. *Maturitas.* 2014;77(2):191-194.

Garrison R, Chambliss WG. Effect of a proprietary Magnolia and Phellodendron extract on weight management: a pilot, double-blind, placebo-controlled clinical trial. *Altern Ther Health Med*. 2006;12(1):50-54.

Kalman DS, Feldman S, Feldman R, Schwartz HI, Krieger DR, Garrison R. Effect of a proprietary Magnolia and Phellodendron extract on stress levels in healthy women: a pilot, double-blind, placebo-controlled clinical trial. *Nutr J*. 2008;7:11.

Maltais ML, Desroches J, Dionne IJ. Changes in muscle mass and strength after menopause. *J Musculoskelet Neuronal Interact*. 2009;9(4):186-197.

Neuhouser M, Aragaki AK, Prentice RL, et al. Overweight, obesity, and postmenopausal invasive breast cancer risk: a secondary analysis of the Women's Health Initiative Randomized Clinical Trials. *JAMA Oncol*. 2015;1(5):611-621.

Rodgers K, Udesky JO, Rudel RA, Brody JG. Environmental chemicals and breast cancer: an updated review of epidemiological literature informed by biological mechanisms. *Environ Res*. 2018;160:152-182.

Talbott SM, Talbott JA, Pugh M., Effect of Magnolia officinalis and Phellodendron amurense (Relora®) on cortisol and psychological mood state in moderately stressed subjects. *J Int Soc Sports Nutr*. 2013;10(1):37.

Vitex

Arentz S, Abbott JA, Smith CA, Bensoussan A. Herbal medicine for the management of polycystic ovary syndrome (PCOS) and associated oligo/amenorrhoea and hyperandrogenism; a review of the laboratory evidence for effects with corroborative clinical findings. *BMC Complement Altern Med*. 2014;14:511.

Jang SH, Kim DI, Choi MS. Effects and treatment methods of acupuncture and herbal medicine for premenstrual syndrome/premenstrual dysphoric disorder: systematic review. *BMC Complement Altern Med*. 2014;14:11.

Mirghafourvand M, Mohammad-Alizadeh-Charandabi S, Ahmadpour P, Javadzadeh Y. Effects of Vitex agnus and Flaxseed on cyclic mastalgia: a randomized controlled trial. *Complement Ther Med*. 2016;24:90-95.

Schellenberg R, Zimmermann C, Drewe J, Hoexter G, Zahner C. Dose-dependent efficacy of the Vitex agnus castus extract Ze 440 in patients suffering from premenstrual syndrome. *Phytomedicine*. 2012;19(14):1325-1331.

van Die MD, Burger HG, Teede HJ, Bone KM. Vitex agnus-castus extracts for female reproductive disorders: a systematic review of clinical trials. *Planta Med*. 2013;79(7):562-575.

See Chapter 5 for references on ashwagandha.

See Chapter 13 for references on L-theanine.

Chapter 24: Prostate Health

Barykova YA, Logunov DY, Shmarov MM, et al. Association of Mycoplasma hominis infection with prostate cancer. *Oncotarget*. 2011;2(4):289-297.

da Silva APB, Alluri LSC, Bissada NF, Gupta S. Association between oral pathogens and prostate cancer: building the relationship. *Am J Clin Exp Urol*. 2019;7(1):1-10.

Erturhan SM, Bayrak O, Pehlivan S, et al. Can mycoplasma contribute to formation of prostate cancer? *Int Urol Nephrol*. 2013;45(1):33-38.

Fang C, Wu L, Zhu C, Xie WZ, Hu H, Zeng XT. A potential therapeutic strategy for prostatic disease by targeting the oral microbiome. *Med Res Rev*. 2021;41(3):1812-1834.

Garbas K, Zapała P, Zapała Ł, Radziszewski P. The role of microbial factors in prostate cancer development--an up-to-date review. *J Clin Med*. 2021;10(20):4772.

Irajian G, Sharifi M, Mirkalantari S, Mirnejad R, Jalali Nadoushan MR, Ghorbanpour N. Molecular detection of Ureaplasma urealyticum from prostate tissues using PCR-RFLP, Tehran, Iran. *Iran J Pathol*. 2016;11(2):138-143.

Leheste JR, Ruvolo KE, Chrostowski JE, et al. *P. acnes*-driven disease pathology: current knowledge and future directions. *Front Cell Infect Microbiol*. 2017;7:81.

Magri V, Boltri M, Cai T, et al. Multidisciplinary approach to prostatitis. *Arch Ital Urol Androl*. 2019;90(4):227-248.

Magri V, Perletti G, Stamatiou K, Montanari E, Trinchieri A. Lithogenic potential of Ureaplasma in chronic prostatitis. *Urol Int*. 2021;105(3-4):328-333.

Miyake M, Ohnishi K, Hori S, et al. *Mycoplasma genitalium* infection and chronic inflammation in human prostate cancer: detection using prostatectomy and needle biopsy specimens. *Cells*. 2019;8(3):212.

Pernar C, Ebot EM, Wilson KM, Mucci LA. The epidemiology of prostate cancer. *Cold Spring Harb Perspect Med*. 2018:a030361.

Perry A, Lambert P. Propionibacterium acnes: infection beyond the skin. *Expert Rev Anti Infect Ther*. 2011;9(12):1149-1156.

Porter CM, Shrestha E, Peiffer LB, Sfanos KS. The microbiome in prostate inflammation and prostate cancer. *Prostate Cancer Prostatic Dis*. 2018;21(3):345-354.

Puhr M, De Marzo A, Isaacs W, et al. Inflammation, microbiota, and prostate cancer. *Eur Urol Focus*. 2016;2(4):374-382.

Rogers MB. Mycoplasma and cancer: in search of the link. *Oncotarget*. 2011;2(4):271-273.

Sfanos KS, Isaacs WB, De Marzo AM. Infections and inflammation in prostate cancer. *Am J Clin Exp Urol.* 2013;1(1):3-11.

Sha S, Ni L, Stefil M, Dixon M, Mouraviev V. The human gastrointestinal microbiota and prostate cancer development and treatment. *Investig Clin Urol.* 2020;61(Suppl 1):S43-S50.

Shannon BA, Garrett KL, Cohen RJ. Links between Propionibacterium acnes and prostate cancer. *Future Oncol.* 2006;2(2):225-232.

Tantengco OAG, Aquino IMC, de Castro Silva M, Rojo RD, Abad CLR. Association of mycoplasma with prostate cancer: a systematic review and meta-analysis. *Cancer Epidemiol.* 2021;75:102021.

Yow MA, Tabrizi SN, Severi G, et al. Detection of infectious organisms in archival prostate cancer tissues. *BMC Cancer.* 2014;14:579.

Herbs and Natural Supplements for Prostate Health

Crocetto F, Boccellino M, Barone B, et al. The crosstalk between prostate cancer and microbiota inflammation: nutraceutical products are useful to balance this interplay? *Nutrients.* 2020;12(9):2648.

Komakech R, Yim NII, Shim KS, et al. Root extract of a micropropagated *Prunus africana* medicinal plant induced apoptosis in human prostate cancer cells (PC-3) via Caspase-3 activation. *Evid Based Complement Alternat Med.* 2022;2022:8232851.

Komakech R, Kang Y, Lee JH, Omujal F. A review of the potential of phytochemicals from *Prunus africana* (Hook f.) Kalkman stem bark for chemoprevention and chemotherapy of prostate cancer. *Evid Based Complement Alternat Med.* 2017;2017:3014019.

Kwon Y. Use of saw palmetto (*Serenoa repens*) extract for benign prostatic hyperplasia. *Food Sci Biotechnol.* 2019;28(6):1599-1606.

Chapter 25: Skin Health

Jhawar N, Wang JV, Saedi N. Oral collagen supplementation for skin aging: A fad or the future? *J Cosmet Dermatol.* 2020;19(4):910-912.

Rinnerhaler M, Bischof J, Streubel MK, Trost A, Richter K. Oxidative stress in aging human skin. *Biomolecules.* 2015;5(2):545-589.

Wong QYA, Chew FT. Defining skin aging and its risk factors: a systematic review and meta-analysis. *Sci Rep.* 2021;11(1):22075.

Zhang S, Duan E. Fighting against skin aging: the way from bench to bedside. *Cell Transplant.* 2018;27(5):729-738.

See Chapter 11 for supplements to benefit skin.

Chapter 26: Sleep

Donga E, Romijn JA. Sleep characteristics and insulin sensitivity in humans. *Handb Clin Neurol*. 2014;124:107-14.

Egan BM. Insulin resistance and the sympathetic nervous system. *Curr Hypertens Rep*. 2003;5(3):247-254.

Grandner MA, Seixas A, Shetty S, Shenoy S. Sleep duration and diabetes risk: population trends and potential mechanisms. *Curr Diab Rep*. 2016;16(11):106.

Hayaishi O. Sleep-wake regulation by prostaglandins D2 and E2. *J Biol Chem*. 1988;263(29):14593-14596.

Huang ZL, Urade Y, Hayaishi O. The role of adenosine in the regulation of sleep. *Curr Top Med Chem*. 2011;11(8):1047-1057.

Huang ZL, Zhang Z, Qu WM. Roles of adenosine and its receptors in sleep-wake regulation. *Int Rev Neurobiol*. 2014;119:349-371.

Krystal AD, Benca RM, Kilduff TS. Understanding the sleep-wake cycle: sleep, insomnia, and the orexin system. *J Clin Psychiatry*. 2013;(74 Suppl 1):3-20.

Kumar S, Rai S, Hsieh KC, McGinty D, Alam MN, Szymusiak R. Adenosine A(2A) receptors regulate the activity of sleep regulatory GABAergic neurons in the preoptic hypothalamus. *Am J Physiol Regul Integr Comp Physiol*. 2013;305(1):R31-R41.

Lazarus M, Shen HY, Cherasse Y, et al. Arousal effect of caffeine depends on adenosine A2A receptors in the shell of the nucleus accumbens. *J Neurosci*. 2011;31(27):10067-10075.

Liu A, Kushida CA, Reaven GM. Habitual shortened sleep and insulin resistance: an independent relationship in obese individuals. *Metabolism*. 2013;62(11):1553-1556.

Liu JT, Lee I-H, Wang C-H, et al. Cigarette smoking might impair memory and sleep quality. *J Formos Med Assoc*. 2013;112(5):287-290.

Siegel JM. The neurotransmitters of sleep. *J Clin Psychiatry*. 2004;65(Suppl 16):4-7.

Herbs/Natural Substances

Kim S, Jo K, Hong K-B, Han SH, Soo HJ. GABA and L-theanine mixture decreases sleep latency and improves NREM sleep. *Pharm Biol*. 2019;57(1):65.

Oketch-Rabah HA, Madden EF, Roe AL, Betz JM. United States Pharmacopeia (USP) safety review of gamma-aminobutyric acid (GABA). *Nutrients*. 2021;13(8):2742.

Shin YY, Byun J-I, Chung S-E, et al. Effect of low and high-dose GABA from unpolished rice-germ on timing and quality of sleep: a randomized double-blind placebo-controlled trial. *J Sleep Med*. 2016;13(2):60-66.

See Chapter 13 for additional references for calming supplements.

Index

Page numbers in **bold** indicate figures, charts, or diagrams.

gastrointestinal issues, 173, 365–369, 427. *See also* digestion

gastrointestinal side effects, 157, 251, 343, 396

gelatin, 279

generally recognized as safe (GRAS), 178, 268, 314

genetic risk of chronic illness, 43

genetic risk of heart disease, 354

ginger (*Zingiber officinale*), 411, 459
  tea, 291, 293, 377

Ginkgo biloba, 343–344, 459

ginseng, Asian (*Panax ginseng*), 139, 455

ginseng, Siberian (*Eleutherococcus senticosus*), 139, 458

Gladstar, Rosemary, 160

Glucophage (metformin), 175, 317

glucosamine, 386, 418

glucose, 45, 272, 308. *See also* blood glucose, sugar

glutathione, 92, 179, 252

gluten, 214, 218

glycation, 45, 278, 308, 312–313, 335, 382

glycine, 436

Glycyrrhiza spp. (licorice), 134, 461

glymphatic drainage system, 334, 335

gotu kola (*Centella asiatica*), 170, 174–175, 459

gout, 382

Graedon, Joe and Terry, 160

grains, 111–112, 214–215, 218, 325, 367

granulocytes, 201

GRAS. *See* generally recognized as safe

guinea hen weed (*Petiveria alliacea*), 150, 407–408

gut. *See* gastrointestinal issues, intestines

gut-brain connection, 369

Gymnema sylvestre, 316, 460

gynecologists, 394

H

habits, health and, 43

habituation, 134, 135

Hadza tribe, 109

hair loss, 396

handwashing, 286

hawthorn (*Crataegus* spp.), 100–102, 140, 356–357, 460

HDL. *See* cholesterol

headaches, 64, 343, 405

healing, 38–40, 424, 425

health care, routine
  blood chemistries, 444
  checkups, 355, 359, 394
  follow-up exams, 448
  testing, 444–445
  well visits, 447

healthcare providers
  types of, 447, 448, 450–452
  when to see, 294, 359, 394, 405, 437–438

healthcare system, 359–362, 443, 447–448
  limits of 5, 6–7, 8, 10, 18, 19, 20, 35

health coaches, 452

hearing loss, 343

heart. *See* cardiovascular disease, cardiovascular health

Notes

Notes

Notes

Notes

Notes

Notes

Notes

Notes